Handbook of Food and Nutrition

Handbook of Food and Nutrition

Edited by Margo Field

SYRAWOOD
PUBLISHING HOUSE
New York

Published by Syrawood Publishing House,
750 Third Avenue, 9th Floor,
New York, NY 10017, USA
www.syrawoodpublishinghouse.com

Handbook of Food and Nutrition
Edited by Margo Field

International Standard Book Number: 978-1-68286-621-4 (Hardback)

Cataloging-in-Publication Data

Handbook of food and nutrition / edited by Margo Field.
p. cm.
Includes bibliographical references and index.
ISBN 978-1-68286-621-4
1. Food. 2. Nutrition. I. Field, Margo.
RA601 .H36 2018
363.192--dc23

Printed in China.

TABLE OF CONTENTS

PREFACE

This book unravels the recent studies in the field of food science and nutrition. Food science is the study of food, its deterioration, processing, and its production and consumption pattern. It uses the methods of engineering to analyze food. Similarly, nutrition science deals with the study of nutrients present in the food. Nutrients are divided into macro nutrients and micro nutrients. This book presents researches and studies performed by experts across the globe. The various advancements in food and nutrition science are glanced at and their applications as well as ramifications are looked at in detail. Students, researchers, experts and all associated with the field will benefit alike from this book.

This book is a comprehensive compilation of works of different researchers from varied parts of the world. It includes valuable experiences of the researchers with the sole objective of providing the readers (learners) with a proper knowledge of the concerned field. This book will be beneficial in evoking inspiration and enhancing the knowledge of the interested readers.

In the end, I would like to extend my heartiest thanks to the authors who worked with great determination on their chapters. I also appreciate the publisher's support in the course of the book. I would also like to deeply acknowledge my family who stood by me as a source of inspiration during the project.

Editor

1

Allergens of *Arachis hypogaea* and the effect of processing on their detection by ELISA

Amjad Iqbal[1,2], Farooq Shah[2], Muhammad Hamayun[3], Ayaz Ahmad[4], Anwar Hussain[3], Muhammad Waqas[5], Sang-Mo Kang[5] and In-Jung Lee[5]*

[1]Department of Food Safety and Food Quality, University of Gent, Gent, Belgium; [2]Department of Agriculture, Abdul Wali Khan University Mardan, Mardan, Pakistan; [3]Department of Botany, Abdul Wali Khan University Mardan, Mardan, Pakistan; [4]Department of Biotechnology, Abdul Wali Khan University Mardan, Mardan, Pakistan; [5]School of Applied Biosciences, College of Agriculture and Life Science, Kyungpook National University, Daegu, South Korea

Abstract

Food allergies are an emerging public health problem in industrialized areas of the world. They represent a considerable health problem in these areas because of the relatively high number of reported cases. Usually, food allergens are proteins or glycoproteins with a molecular mass ranging from 10 to 70 kDa. Among the food allergies, peanut is accounted to be responsible for more than 50% of the food allergy fatalities. Threshold doses for peanut allergenic reactions have been found to range from as low as 100 µg to 1 g of peanut protein, which equal to 400 µg to 4 g peanut meal. Allergens from peanut are mainly seed storage proteins that are composed of conglutin, vicilin, and glycinin families. Several peanut proteins have been identified to induce allergic reactions, particularly Ara h 1–11. This review is mainly focused on different classes of peanut allergens, the effect of thermal and chemical treatment of peanut allergens on the IgY binding and detectability of these allergens by enzyme linked immunosorbent assay (ELISA) to provide knowledge for food industry.

Keywords: *peanut proteins*; *anaphylaxis*; *conglutin*; *vicilin*; *glycinin*; *allergens processing*

Food allergies are becoming a main public health concern in well-established areas, which represents a significant threat to human health in recent years (1, 2). The occurrence of food allergies has amplified over the years, which has confronted both allergologists and food scientists with serious challenges. The term 'food allergy' has been defined by the European Academy of Allergology and Clinical Immunology (EAACI) as '... a hypersensitivity reaction initiated by immunological mechanisms'. Food allergens are actually the constituents in foods that aggravate immunological reactions. The adverse/hypersensitive reactions to foods might be poisonous or non-poisonous reactions; the latter might be immune-mediated or non-immune-mediated opposing reactions. The food's adverse effect that involves the immune system reaction is an absolutely IgE-mediated allergy (3). Generally, the most common allergenic food worldwide includes peanut, tree nuts, milk, soybean, crustacean, egg, fish, and wheat. Among the offending food, peanuts are the main culprits that cause severe allergies and even life-threatening anaphylactic shocks (4).

The cultivation of peanut or groundnut (*Arachis hypogaea* L.), began in Bolivia, South America, but today it is grown throughout various ecological zones of the world. The crop was initially grown by the natives during European expansion in the sixteenth century and was thereafter grown in Europe, Africa, Asia, and the Pacific Islands. Peanut belongs to the family Fabaceae or legumes and is the world's third important oil and food crop, following soybean and cotton. Asian countries, including India and China, and the United States have been the leading producers for more than 25 years and provide 70% of the world's peanuts. Peanuts are grown mainly for human consumption in the form of whole seed or processed to produce butter, cooking oil, and various other products.

Beside all these benefits, peanuts have some proteins known as peanut allergens. These allergens are of particular interest because of the reported life-threatening consequences of anaphylactic shock. Peanut allergy causes significant health-care problems globally and currently affects 0.6–1.5% of the children in developed countries (5). The prevalence is, however, different in different parts of the world and is increasing in developed nations (6). There is less peanut allergy in China than in the United States, despite similar levels of peanut consumption (7), possibly because of differences in food preparation. For example, dry roasted peanuts are more allergic than boiled or fried peanuts. Nevertheless, it remains unclear why the peanut allergy prevalence is lower in China than in Europe and America (8–12).

Presently, peanut allergy diagnostic includes double-blind, placebo-controlled food challenge (DBPCFC), the specific skin prick test (SPT), the basophil activation test, and the measurement of specific IgE (13, 14). The major reason in the failure of these tests is the existence of the 'peanut-sensitized' individuals. Those individuals, despite of having peanut-specific IgE antibodies, consume peanuts without any symptoms. Among a group of 8-year-old children, only 10% had peanut-specific IgE antibodies, but only approximately 2% were truly allergic (15).

Nowadays, the ELISA technique is the most commonly used immunoassay in the laboratories of the food industry to detect and quantify hidden allergens in food. ELISA has been successfully used over the years as a preferred method to detect allergens in meat and meat products, fish and fish products, milk and milk products, soyabean, nuts and nut-based products, and fruit juices and ingredients (16, 17). The method has the advantages of high sensitivity, low cost, fast application, ease of use, reliability, and speed. With ELISA tests, allergens or specific marker proteins can be detected by colorimetric reaction after the binding of the antigen with a specific enzyme-labeled antibody.

Composition of peanut proteins

The presence of the various proteins in the tested peanut samples from different parts of the world was found same, but the amounts were different. Beside this, the IgE-binding properties of different peanut varieties were also the same as Koppelman et al. (18). Highly processed oil (acid extracted, heat distilled), on the other hand, does not contain peanut protein and can safely be consumed by allergic patients. However, the cold-pressed or cold-extruded peanut oils, with processing at lower temperatures, may contain traces of peanut protein and may induce allergic reactions in allergic subjects (19).

Allergens in peanut

The seeds of peanut contain over 32 different proteins (20) but only 18 have been reported to have an allergen property and 11 have been identified (21). Among the various isolated allergens from peanut (Ara h 1–11), Ara h 2 and Ara h 6 are the most important with regard to food allergy (22). Indeed, peanut allergens, in particular, are more important than other food allergens because they have shown to be extremely resistant to digestion, denaturation from heat, acidity, alkali, and proteolytic activities (23, 24). Allergens that have been isolated include cupin (vicilin-type, 7S globulin), conglutin (2S albumin), cupin (legumin-type, 11S globulin, glycinin), cupin (legumin-type, 11S, glycinin), profilin, pathogenesis-related protein, PR-10, nonspecific lipid-transfer protein 1, 14 kDa oleosin, and 16 kDa oleosin (20). Lipid-transfer proteins (LTPs) are heat stable and resistant to proteolytic digestion (25) and can cross-react with a broad range of food allergens (26). Due to the extreme resistance of LTPs to pepsin digestion, LTPs in particular are potentially severe food allergens (27).

Properties of peanut allergens

Ara h 1

Ara h 1 or conarachin belongs to the vicilin family, a seed storage proteins (globulins). The molecular weight of this glycoprotein is about 65,000. This protein is similar to the conglycinin from soy proteins with the major IgE epitopes within this extension region. Ara h 1 is a protein with high thermal stability but showed minor structural changes in 5M urea. It has also been observed that few of the IgE-binding epitopes of Ara h1 are resistant to pepsin degradation (28).

Ara h 2

Ara h 2 is a glycoprotein of 17.5 kDa and was initially identified from crude peanut extracts. Ara h 2, a glycoprotein with an isoelectric point (pI) of 5.2 that resembles to a protein from 2S albumin family, that is, delta conglutin. Ara h 2 is known to be a storage protein that can act as a trypsin inhibitor (25). The Ara h 2 is an aciduric protein that can withstand degradation by digestive enzymes, which might be why it is recognized by serum IgE from most peanut-allergic patients (29).

Ara h 3

Peanut is one of the well-known sources of allergens, and among those allergens, Ara h 3 is the major and complex one (30). Ara h 3 is a single-chain polypeptide of 60 kDa and belongs to 11S storage protein from the glycinin family with a less stable response to the enzymatic (pepsin) action than the Ara h 2 and Ara h 6 (31). The extensively proteolytically processed protein is bound by disulphide bridges and is found in trimeric and hexameric structures. This oligomeric structure limits the determination of allerginisity of the Ara h 3, as there is no specific IgE available but the polyclonal antibody raised against the oligomers will solve this problem (32).

Ara h 4

Ara h 4 has 35.9 kDa acidic subunit with a pI of 5.5, and the amino acid sequences of both Ara h 3 and Ara h 4 are 91% identical and considered isoallergens (33).

Ara h 5

Profilinin or Ara h 5 is a 12 to 15 kDa monomeric actin-binding protein present in all eukaryotic cells. It was reported to be a minor allergen in birch pollen but is now considered a ubiquitous panallergen found in peanuts, hazelnuts, pear, tomato, and so on. Profiling has been involved in the birch-mugwort-celery-spice syndrome, and several studies concluded that this protein can also play role in patients allergic to hazelnut, celery, carrot, peanuts, peach, pear, apple, potato, tomato, and pumpkin seed. However, recent studies suggested that profilin sensitization has little or no clinical relevance (34).

Ara h 6

Ara h 6, a 15 kDa allergen, has been isolated, and is recognized by 20 out of 29 peanut-allergic patients on IgE-immunoblot. The potent biological functionality of Ara h 6 is demonstrated by the degranulation of basophils, even at concentrations below 10 pg/mL, and by positive skin prick reactions. Ara h 6 has homology to Ara h 2, especially in the middle part and at the C-terminal part of the protein. This demonstrates that at least part of the epitopes of Ara h 6 is cross-reactive with epitopes on Ara h 2. The potent biological functionality of Ara h 6 is demonstrated by the release of histamine from basophils; even at concentrations below 10 μg/ml (35).

Ara h 7

Another storage protein from conglutin family is an Ara h 7 with 15.8 kDa *Mw* and pI of 5.6. The amino acid sequence of Ara h 7 is 53% similar to Ara h 6, while 35% similar to Ara h 2 (33), but are less stable than both due to conservation of only two disulphide bonding. Schmidt et al., (36) enriched and separated peanut proteins of molecular weight less than 20 kDa on 2D gel electrophoresis. After mass spectroscopic analysis, two isoallergens were found, one of which had an additional pro-peptide cleavage point. Furthermore, the putative cleavage point demonstrates the biological function of conglutins as an amylase/trypsin inhibitor.

Ara h 8

Unlike Ara h 1–6, which are seed storage proteins, Ara h 8 belongs to pathogenesis-related protein family PR–10. Ara h 8 is also heat labile and prone to proteolytic digestion. This allergen is homologous with birch pollen allergen and because of its cross-reactivity, it is very important for birch pollen allergic patients (33, 37, 38).

Ara h 9

Ara h 9 is a nonspecific lipid-transfer protein 1, which was indentified clearly in 2009 (39). There two isoforms of Ara h 9 have been established, and the amino acid sequences of both isoforms are 90% identical. Beside similar IgE reactivity, both also have 60–70% identical amino acid sequence with LTPs from other food (e.g. hazelnut, chestnut, almond, peach, pear, plum, cherry, strawberry, lentils, lupin, sunflower, beans, pea) (40, 41).

Ara h 10 and Ara h 11

Both types of peanut allergens belong to the oleosin family. Ara h 10 is approximately 16 kDa, while Ara h 11 is 14 kD. Both can be obtained from oil bodies of peanut and need to be studied in depth (20).

Sensitization to peanut proteins

Peanut allergy usually presents after a period of sensitization to peanut. However, some children have severe reactions as a result of their apparent first exposure to some allergens through breast milk (42). Several studies have documented an epidemiologic relationship between the increased consumption of peanut by pregnant and breast-feeding mothers and the likelihood of the allergic sensitization of their children. These studies suggest a transfer of maternal dietary peanut protein to breast milk may predispose at-risk children to occult sensitization. Since sensitization requires prior exposure to generate allergen-specific IgE, the sensitizing exposure must be occult, in many cases. According to Vadas et al., (43), peanut proteins appeared with 1 to 3 h following oral ingestion. Both low- and high-molecular weight proteins with mobilities corresponding to Ara h 1 and Ara h 2 were secreted intact into breast milk with no evidence of degradation (18). The mechanism of action of sensitization was given by Poulsen (44) (Fig. 1).

Effect of processing on the detection of allergens

For many foods, thermal processing is necessary and unavoidable and may include drying, baking, frying, microwave treatment, roasting, frying, or boiling. It is often thought that thermal processing may affect the structure of the protein, which in turn influences the

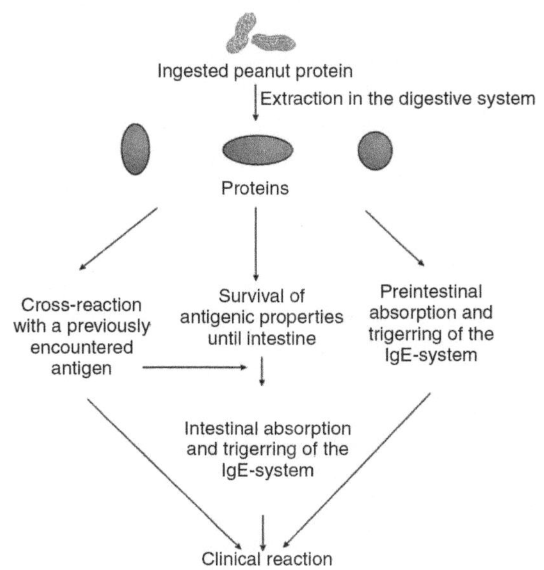

Fig. 1. Sequence leading to sensitization and elicitation of a food allergic reaction to a food.

detection of the proteins or allergens. The extent of the physicochemical impact on protein structure and functionality depends largely on the intrinsic characteristics of protein, the temperature applied, the duration of heat treatment, and the pH. The loss of tertiary structure can create new epitopes, e.g. by unfolding and exposing the formerly hidden sites, as well as destroying the existing sites (29, 45). Typically, the loss of secondary structure occurs at a temperature between 55°C and 70°C, the cleavage of disulfide bonds occurs at 70°C – 80°C, the formation of new intra/intermolecular interactions and rearrangements of the disulfide bonds at 80°C – 90°C, and the formation of aggregates at 90°C – 100°C. Besides those physical transformations, the chemical modification of protein may also occur at high temperatures, such as 100°C – 125°C. One of the most important reactions is that of protein amino groups with sugars, leading to an impressive cocktail of advance glycation end products, such as Millard reaction products. Thermal processing will also reduce the solubility of target protein, which can reduce the extractability of soluble proteins, the basis for the detectability of allergenic food constituents in food products. Roasted peanuts, for instance, are widely used for food businesses to enhance the flavor of the raw ingredient, yet the allergenic protein is less soluble in the aqueous solutions required for detection (8). In addition, antigen recognition by immunological detection is adversely affected by processing because it can denature, alter, or remove proteins so that they are no longer detectable by the antibodies used in the assays. Millard reaction products have been shown to have an inhibitory effect on IgE binding of proteins (46).

Effect of heat treatment of peanut proteins on IgY binding

Iqbal and Ateeq (24) observed the effect of heat treatment on the detectability of peanut proteins by Chicken IgYs (Fig. 2). The concentration of peanut proteins in PBS before heat treatment shows a good sensitivity, but after heat treatment there was a low detection of peanut concentration, which could be correlated to the loss of IgY binding due to conformational changes of peanut proteins. After certain period of time, the protein concentration became constant because of heat stable fractions, which is an indication that certain fractions of epitopes were not affected by heat and hence retained their IgY binding capacity (24, 47).

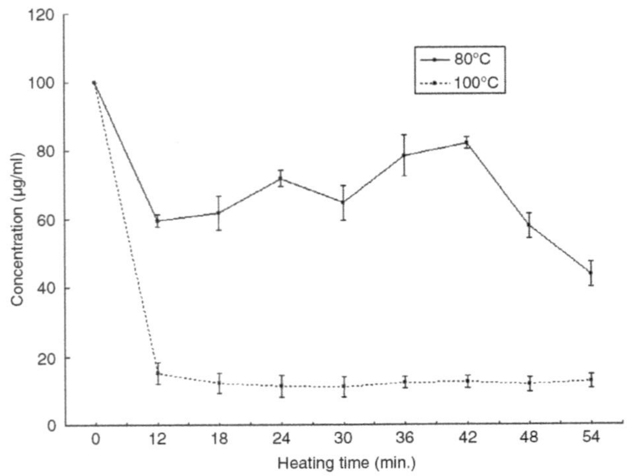

Fig. 2. Detectability of peanut proteins after heat treatment at 80°C and 100°C in PBS (24).

Effect of pH on the detectability of peanut proteins

Heating peanut antigens at 100°C in normal, acidic, and alkali conditions has an effect on the IgY binding. This might be due to the conformational changes of the protein molecules because both antibodies and antigens are proteins and can be affected by the changes in pH. The alkaline and acidic conditions have almost the same negative effect on the binding of IgY, but the severity in alkaline conditions can be high (Fig. 3). The denaturation of proteins in alkaline conditions might be marginally faster because of the hydrolysis of proteins that occurs faster in alkaline conditions than in acidic conditions (24).

Effect of reducing sugar of peanut proteins on IgY binding

The effect of heating in 20 mM glucose at 100°C can results in a Maillard reaction between an amino acid (peanut proteins) and a reducing sugar (glucose). The Maillard products may interfere with the IgY binding by altering the protein resulting in the antibody not being able to recognize the antigen protein anymore (Fig. 4) (24).

Conclusion

Many foods require thermal processing from an aromatic and microbial point of view, which includes drying,

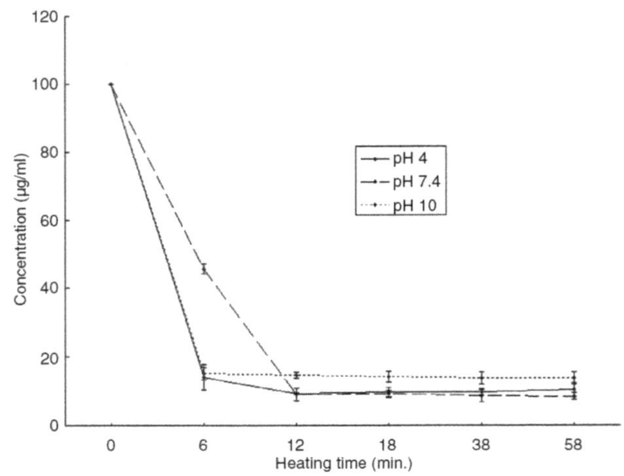

Fig. 3. Detectability of peanut protein after heat treatment at 100°C in PBS buffer at pH 4, pH 7.4 and pH 10 (24).

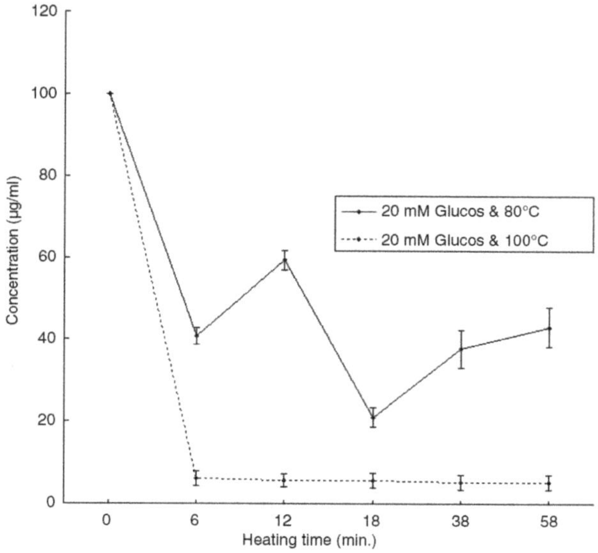

Fig. 4. Detectability of peanut protein after heat treatment at 80°C in 20 mM glucose solution and 100°C in 20 mM glucose solution (24).

baking, frying, microwave treatment, roasting, frying, or boiling. It is possible that such processing may affect the structure of the protein, which in turn influences the detection of these proteins or allergens. The extent of physicochemical impact on protein structure and functionality depends largely on the intrinsic characteristics of proteins, the temperature applied, the duration of heat treatment, and the pH. Thermal processing may reduce the solubility of the target protein, which is the basis for the detectability of allergenic food constituents in food products. Certainly peanuts are the most common of the allergens and are a good source of allergenic proteins. Roasting these proteins (allergens) might change the confirmation of the native protein to a protein with high allergenicity and low detection. Therefore, a cheap, robust, and reliable biochemical method is needed to protect the consumer from life-threatening allergens. Enzyme linked immunosorbent assay is one of the best options to overcome these hurdles. The method is not as sensitive as polymerase chain reaction, but is still cheap, offers high throughput, and is reliable enough to detect altered allergenic protein fractions. Also, different processing conditions can completely change the protein's immunochemical characteristics; the risk of masking the antigen is high. This is much more likely to happen when using monoclonal antibodies, which are specific for a particular protein, but using polyclonal antibodies, reduces this risk.

Acknowledgements

This study was supported by the Agenda Program (Project No. PJ01099002), Rural Development Administration, Republic of Korea.

Conflict of interest and funding

The authors have not received any funding or benefits from industry or elsewhere to conduct this study.

References

1. Burks A, Tang M, Sicherer S, Muraro A, Eigenmann PA, Ebisawa M, et al. ICON: food allergy. J Allergy Clin Immunol 2012; 129(4): 906–20.
2. Sicherer SH, Sampson HA. Food allergy. J Allergy Clin Immunol 2010; 125(2): S116–25.
3. Katz Y, Rajuan N, Goldberg MR, Eisenberg E, Heyman E, Cohen A, et al. Early exposure to cow's milk protein is protective against IgE-mediated cow's milk protein allergy. J Allergy Clin Immunol 2010; 126(1): 77–82. e1.
4. Finkelman FD. Peanut allergy and anaphylaxis. Curr Opin Immunol 2010; 22(6): 783–8.
5. Venter C, Hasan Arshad S, Grundy J, Pereira B, Bernie Clayton C, Voigt K, et al. Time trends in the prevalence of peanut allergy: three cohorts of children from the same geographical location in the UK. Allergy 2010; 65(1): 103–8.
6. Du Toit G, Katz Y, Sasieni P, Mesher D, Maleki SJ, Fisher HR, et al. Early consumption of peanuts in infancy is associated with a low prevalence of peanut allergy. J Allergy Clin Immunol 2008; 122(5): 984–91.
7. Sampson HA. Update on food allergy. J Allergy Clin Immunol 2004; 113(5): 805–19.
8. Poms RE, Anklam E. Effects of chemical, physical, and technological processes on the nature of food allergens. J AOAC Int 2004; 87(6): 1466–74.
9. Cong Y-J, Lou F, Xue W-T, Li L-F, Wang J, Zhang H. The effect of cooking methods on the allergenicity of peanut. Food Agric Immunol 2007; 18(1): 53–65.
10. Chung S-Y, Butts CL, Maleki SJ, Champagne ET. Linking peanut allergenicity to the processes of maturation, curing, and roasting. J Agric Food Chem 2003; 51(15): 4273–7.
11. Piersma SR, Gaspari M, Hefle SL, Koppelman SJ. Proteolytic processing of the peanut allergen Ara h 3. Mol Nutr Food Res 2005; 49(8): 744–55.
12. Kopper RA, Odum NJ, Sen M, Helm RM, Stanley JS, Burks AW. Peanut protein allergens: the effect of roasting on solubility and allergenicity. Int Arch Allergy Immunol 2005; 136(1): 16–22.
13. Lieberman JA, Sicherer SH. Diagnosis of food allergy: epicutaneous skin tests, in vitro tests, and oral food challenge. Curr Allergy Asthma Rep 2011; 11(1): 58–64.
14. Hamilton RG, MacGlashan DW Jr., Saini SS. IgE antibody-specific activity in human allergic disease. Immunol Res 2010; 47(1–3): 273–84.
15. Nicolaou N, Murray C, Belgrave D, Poorafshar M, Simpson A, Custovic A. Quantification of specific IgE to whole peanut extract and peanut components in prediction of peanut allergy. J Allergy Clin Immunol 2011; 127(3): 684–5.
16. Asensio L, González I, García T, Martín R. Determination of food authenticity by enzyme-linked immunosorbent assay (ELISA). Food Control 2008; 19(1): 1–8.
17. You J, Li D, Qiao S, Wang Z, He P, Ou D, et al. Development of a monoclonal antibody-based competitive ELISA for detection of β-conglycinin, an allergen from soybean. Food Chem 2008; 106(1): 352–60.
18. Koppelman SJ, Vlooswijk RAA, Knippels LMJ, Hessing M, Knol EF, Van Reijsen FC, et al. Quantification of major peanut allergens Ara h 1 and Ara h 2 in the peanut varieties Runner, Spanish, Virginia, and Valencia, bred in different parts of the world. Allergy 2001; 56(2): 132–7.

19. du Plessis K, Steinman H. Practical aspects of adverse reactions to peanut. Curr Allergy Clin Immunol 2004; 17: 10–14.
20. Pele M. Peanut allergens. Romanian Biotechnol Lett 2010; 15(2): 5205.
21. Krause S, Latendorf T, Schmidt H, Darcan-Nicolaisen Y, Reese G, Petersen A, et al. Peanut varieties with reduced Ara h 1 content indicating no reduced allergenicity. Mol Nutr Food Res 2010; 54(3): 381–7.
22. Porterfield HS, Murray KS, Schlichting DG, Chen X, Hansen KC, Duncan MW, et al. Effector activity of peanut allergens: a critical role for Ara h 2, Ara h 6, and their variants. Clin Exp Allergy 2009; 39(7): 1099–108.
23. Koppelman SJ, Hefle SL, Taylor SL, de Jong GAH. Digestion of peanut allergens Ara h 1, Ara h 2, Ara h 3, and Ara h 6: A comparative in vitro study and partial characterization of digestion-resistant peptides. Mol Nutr Food Res 2010; 54(12): 1711–21.
24. Iqbal A, Ateeq N. Effect of processing on the detectability of peanut protein by ELISA. Food Chem 2013; 141: 1651–4.
25. Maleki SJ, Viquez O, Jacks T, Dodo H, Champagne ET, Chung S-Y, et al. The major peanut allergen, Ara h 2, functions as a trypsin inhibitor, and roasting enhances this function. J Allergy Clin Immunol 2003; 112(1): 190–5.
26. Asero R, Mistrello G, Roncarolo D, Amato S, Caldironi G, Barocci F, et al. Immunological cross-reactivity between lipid transfer proteins from botanically unrelated plant-derived foods: a clinical study. Allergy 2002; 57(10): 900–6.
27. Asero R, Mistrello G, Roncarolo D, de Vries SC, Gautier MF, Ciurana CLF, et al. Lipid transfer protein: a pan-allergen in plant-derived foods that is highly resistant to pepsin digestion. Int Arch Allergy Immunol 2000; 122(1): 20–32.
28. Maleki SJ, Chung S-Y, Champagne ET, Raufman J-P. The effects of roasting on the allergenic properties of peanut proteins. J Allergy Clin Immunol 2000; 106(4): 763–8.
29. Sen M, Kopper R, Pons L, Abraham EC, Burks AW, Bannon GA. Protein structure plays a critical role in peanut allergen stability and may determine immunodominant IgE-binding epitopes. J Immunol 2002; 169(2): 882–7.
30. Jin T, Guo F, Chen Y-W, Howard A, Zhang Y-Z. Crystal structure of Ara h 3, a major allergen in peanut. Mol Immunol 2009; 46(8): 1796–804.
31. Koppelman SJ, Hefle SL, Taylor SL, de Jong GA. Digestion of peanut allergens Ara h 1, Ara h 2, Ara h 3, and Ara h 6: a comparative in vitro study and partial characterization of digestionp-resistant peptides. Mol Nutr Food Res 2010; 54(12): 1711–21.
32. Yusnawan E, Marquis CP, Lee NA. Purification and characterization of Ara h1 and Ara h3 from four peanut market types revealed higher order oligomeric structures. J Agric Food Chem 2012; 60(41): 10352–8.
33. Wen HW, Borejsza-Wysocki W, DeCory TR, Durst RA. Peanut allergy, peanut allergens, and methods for the detection of peanut contamination in food products. Compr Rev Food Sci Food Saf 2007; 6(2): 47–58.
34. Asero R, Mistrello G, Roncarolo D, Amato S, Zanoni D, Barocci F, et al. Detection of clinical markers of sensitization to profilin in patients allergic to plant-derived foods. J Allergy Clin Immunol 2003; 112(2): 427–32.
35. Koppelman SJ, De Jong GAH, Laaper-Ertmann M, Peeters K, Knulst AC, Hefle SL, et al. Purification and immunoglobulin E-binding properties of peanut allergen Ara h 6: evidence for cross-reactivity with Ara h 2. Clin Exp Allergy 2005; 35(4): 490–7.
36. Schmidt H, Krause S, Gelhaus C, Petersen A, Janssen O, Becker W-M. Detection and structural characterization of natural Ara h 7, the third peanut allergen of the 2S albumin family. J Proteome Res 2010; 9(7): 3701–9.
37. Mittag D, Akkerdaas J, Ballmer-Weber BK, Vogel L, Wensing M, Becker W-M, et al. Ara h 8, a Bet v 1-homologous allergen from peanut, is a major allergen in patients with combined birch pollen and peanut allergy. J Allergy Clin Immunol 2004; 114(6): 1410–17.
38. Riecken S, Lindner B, Petersen A, Jappe U, Becker W-M. Purification and characterization of natural Ara h 8, the Bet v 1 homologous allergen from peanut, provides a novel isoform. Biol Chem 2008; 389(4): 415–23.
39. Krause S, Reese G, Randow S, Zennaro D, Quaratino D, Palazzo P, et al. Lipid transfer protein (Ara h 9) as a new peanut allergen relevant for a Mediterranean allergic population. J Allergy Clin Immunol 2009; 124(4): 771–8. e5.
40. Mari A, Riecken S, Quaratino D, Zennaro D, Reese G, Petersen A, et al. Identification of a lipid transfer protein (LTP) in peanut extract and cloning of two LTP isoallergens. J Allergy Clin Immunol 2008; 121(2): S212.
41. Lauer I, Dueringer N, Pokoj S, Rehm S, Zoccatelli G, Reese G, et al. The non-specific lipid transfer protein, Ara h 9, is an important allergen in peanut. Clin Exp Allergy 2009; 39(9): 1427–37.
42. Taylor SL, Hefle SL. Will genetically modified foods be allergenic? Journal Allergy Clin Immunol 2001; 107(5): 765.
43. Vadas P, Wai Y, Burks W, Perelman B. Detection of peanut allergens in breast milk of lactating women. JAMA 2001; 285(13): 1746–8.
44. Poulsen LK. In search of a new paradigm: mechanisms of sensitization and elicitation of food allergy*. Allergy 2005; 60(5): 549–58.
45. Davis PJ, Smales CM, James DC. How can thermal processing modify the antigenicity of proteins? Allergy 2001; 56(Suppl 67): 56–60.
46. Chung S-Y, Champagne ET. Allergenicity of Maillard reaction products from peanut proteins. J Agric Food Chem 1999; 47(12): 5227–31.
47. Kiio J, De Meulenaer B. Immunochemical detection of peanut (Arachis hypogaea L.) proteins using chicken antibodies. Food Agric Immunol 2012; 23(3): 217–26.

***In-Jung Lee**
School of Applied Bioscience
College of Agriculture and Life Science
Kyungpook National University
Daegu, South Korea
Email: ijlee@knu.ac.kr

2

Milk and dairy products: good or bad for human health? An assessment of the totality of scientific evidence

Tanja Kongerslev Thorning[1], Anne Raben[1], Tine Tholstrup[1], Sabita S. Soedamah-Muthu[2], Ian Givens[3] and Arne Astrup[1]*

[1]Department of Nutrition, Exercise and Sports, Faculty of Science, University of Copenhagen, Copenhagen, Denmark; [2]Division of Human Nutrition, Wageningen University, Wageningen, The Netherlands; [3]Centre for Food, Nutrition and Health, University of Reading, Reading, UK

Abstract

Background: There is scepticism about health effects of dairy products in the public, which is reflected in an increasing intake of plant-based drinks, for example, from soy, rice, almond, or oat.
Objective: This review aimed to assess the scientific evidence mainly from meta-analyses of observational studies and randomised controlled trials, on dairy intake and risk of obesity, type 2 diabetes, cardiovascular disease, osteoporosis, cancer, and all-cause mortality.
Results: The most recent evidence suggested that intake of milk and dairy products was associated with reduced risk of childhood obesity. In adults, intake of dairy products was shown to improve body composition and facilitate weight loss during energy restriction. In addition, intake of milk and dairy products was associated with a neutral or reduced risk of type 2 diabetes and a reduced risk of cardiovascular disease, particularly stroke. Furthermore, the evidence suggested a beneficial effect of milk and dairy intake on bone mineral density but no association with risk of bone fracture. Among cancers, milk and dairy intake was inversely associated with colorectal cancer, bladder cancer, gastric cancer, and breast cancer, and not associated with risk of pancreatic cancer, ovarian cancer, or lung cancer, while the evidence for prostate cancer risk was inconsistent. Finally, consumption of milk and dairy products was not associated with all-cause mortality. Calcium-fortified plant-based drinks have been included as an alternative to dairy products in the nutrition recommendations in several countries. However, nutritionally, cow's milk and plant-based drinks are completely different foods, and an evidence-based conclusion on the health value of the plant-based drinks requires more studies in humans.
Conclusion: The totality of available scientific evidence supports that intake of milk and dairy products contribute to meet nutrient recommendations, and may protect against the most prevalent chronic diseases, whereas very few adverse effects have been reported.

Keywords: *obesity*; *type 2 diabetes*; *cardiovascular disease*; *osteoporosis*; *cancer*; *mortality*

Several media stories and organisations claim that dairy increases risk of chronic diseases including obesity, type 2 diabetes, cardiovascular disease, osteoporosis, and cancer. Therefore, there is an increasing scepticism among the general consumers about the health consequences of eating dairy products. This is reflected in an increasing consumption of plant-based drinks, for example, based on soy, rice, almond, or oats. Dairy is an essential part of the food culture in the Nordic countries; thus, inclusion of milk and dairy products in the diet may be natural for many Nordic individuals. The major causes of loss of disease-free years in the Nordic countries today are type 2 diabetes, cardiovascular diseases, and cancers. Moreover, the increasing prevalence of obesity greatly increases the risk of these chronic diseases. Given the increasing prevalence of these chronic diseases, it is critically important to understand the health effects of milk and dairy products in the diet. Accordingly, this narrative review presents the latest evidence from meta-analyses and systematic reviews of observational studies and randomised controlled trials on dairy intake (butter excluded) and risk of obesity, type 2 diabetes, cardiovascular disease, osteoporosis, and cancer as well as all-cause mortality.

We aim to answer the key questions: 1) For the general consumer, will a diet with milk and dairy products overall provide better or worse health, and increase or decrease risk of major diseases and all-cause mortality than a diet with no or low content of milk and dairy products? 2) Is it justified to recommend the general lactose-tolerant population to avoid consumption of milk and dairy products? 3) Is there scientific evidence to substantiate that replacing milk with plant-based drinks will improve health?

Obesity and type 2 diabetes

A large share of the on-going increase in prevalence of type 2 diabetes is driven by the obesity epidemic (1, 2), and it is therefore relevant to assess the role of milk and dairy products for body weight control. Childhood overweight and obesity worldwide is a major contributor to the current obesity epidemic, and childhood obesity frequently tracks into adulthood (3). Therefore, early prevention of childhood obesity is important. A meta-analysis showed that among children in the pre-school and school age, there was no association between dairy intake and adiposity (4). However, there was a modestly protective effect in adolescence. A recent meta-analysis by Lu et al. (5) found that children in the highest dairy intake group were 38% less likely to be overweight or obese compared to those in the lowest dairy intake group. An increase in dairy intake of one serving per day was associated with a 0.65% lower body fat and a 13% lower risk of overweight or obesity.

Milk and dairy products are good sources of high-quality protein. Protein is important during weight loss and subsequent weight maintenance due to the high satiating effect which helps to prevent over-consumption of energy and thereby reduces body fat stores (6, 7). Furthermore, dairy protein is a good source of essential amino acids for muscle protein synthesis and thus helps to maintain the metabolically active muscle mass during weight loss (8). Meta-analyses support that in adults, dairy products facilitate weight loss and improve body composition, that is, reduce body fat mass and preserve lean body mass during energy restriction and in short-term studies (9–11). The effect of an increased dairy consumption on body weight in long-term studies (>1 year) and in energy balance studies is less convincing (10, 11). This is likely due to the opposing effects of dairy on body composition, that is, reduction of fat mass and preservation of lean body mass.

Meta-analyses assessing the role of intake of milk and dairy products on risk of type 2 diabetes have consistently found no or a slight beneficial effect of dairy intake on diabetes risk (12–15). This is consistent with a Mendelian randomisation study using genetic polymorphisms for the lactase gene, which showed that milk intake assessed by lactose tolerance was not associated with risk of type 2 diabetes or obesity (16). The most recent meta-analysis on dairy intake and diabetes incidence included 22 cohort studies with a total of 579,832 subjects and 43,118 type 2 diabetes cases (17). An inverse association between total dairy and yoghurt intake and risk of type 2 diabetes was reported although there was no association with milk intake. The benefits of fermented dairy products (cheese and yoghurt) in relation to type 2 diabetes may be due to their effect on the gut microbiota (18, 19). Other studies have identified that whey protein (primarily in milk and yoghurt) can reduce postprandial plasma glucose concentration in type 2 diabetic subjects (20). This effect may be due to the branched chain amino acids in the whey protein fraction, particularly leucine which has been shown to induce a greater stimulation of glucose-dependent insulinotropic polypeptide (GIP), but not glucagon like peptide 1 (GLP-1), compared to other amino acids (21). The GIP response is possibly a key factor in the higher insulin response and the subsequent lowering of blood glucose seen after whey ingestion, at least in healthy subjects. In addition to the insulinotropic effect of milk, a recent study has indicated that dairy may also improve insulin sensitivity (22).

Conclusion on obesity and type 2 diabetes

A diet high in milk and dairy products reduces the risk of childhood obesity and improves body composition in adults. This likely contributes to lower the risk of developing type 2 diabetes. Additionally, dairy product consumption during energy restriction facilitates weight loss, whereas the effect of dairy intake during energy balance is less clear. Finally, there is increasing evidence suggesting that especially the fermented dairy products, cheese and yoghurt, are associated with a reduced risk of type 2 diabetes.

Cardiovascular disease

Low-fat, calcium-rich dairy products are generally considered to lower blood pressure. This was supported by a meta-analysis of six observational studies, whereas no association was found with intake of high-fat dairy products (23). High-fat dairy products are known to increase high density lipoprotein (HDL)- and low density lipoprotein (LDL)-cholesterol concentrations. The latter normally predicts risk of cardiovascular disease (24), but this may depend on the size of the LDL-cholesterol particles. Small, dense LDL particles are more atherogenic than their larger counterparts (25–28) due to their lower affinity for the LDL-receptor and higher susceptibility to oxidation (29). In agreement, some of the fatty acids typically found in milk and dairy products have been associated with less small, dense LDL particles (4:0–10:0 and 14:0 in the diet, and 15:0 and 17:0 in serum phospholipids) (30). In addition, the minerals in milk and dairy products have been shown to attenuate the LDL-response to high-fat dairy intake (31, 32).

Among high-fat dairy products, cheese in particular does not seem to increase LDL-cholesterol to the extent expected, based on the high content of saturated fat (33). When compared to habitual diet with a lower total and saturated fat content (33), or compared to diets with lower total fat content but higher content of high-GI carbohydrates (34, 35), a high intake of cheese was found not to increase LDL-cholesterol. A meta-analysis of randomised controlled trials studying the effect of cheese consumption compared with other foods on blood lipids and lipoproteins showed that cheese caused lower total cholesterol, LDL-cholesterol, and HDL-cholesterol concentrations compared with butter (36). Compared with milk, however, there was no statistically significant difference in blood lipids (32, 37). Several meta-analyses have been conducted on the relationship between intake of milk and dairy products and risk of developing cardiovascular disease. There was no consistent association between milk or dairy intake and cardiovascular disease, coronary heart disease or stroke in a meta-analysis by Soedamah-Muthu et al. (38). In a recent update, including a higher number of prospective cohort studies, there was a significant inverse association between milk intake and stroke, with a 7% lower risk of stroke per 200 ml milk/day, but considerable heterogeneity. Further, stratification for Asian and Western countries showed a more marked reduction in risk in Asian than in Western countries. This is consistent with a previous meta-analysis by Hu et al. (39) showing a non-linear dose–response relationship between milk intake and risk of stroke, with the highest risk reduction of 7–8% with a milk intake of 200–300 ml/day. Also, the meta-analyses by Hu et al. (39) and de Goede et al. (40) both showed an inverse association between cheese intake and stroke, however only borderline significant in the latter. Accordingly, another meta-analysis on dairy and cardiovascular disease found that intake of cheese and milk as well as yoghurt was inversely associated with cardiovascular disease risk (41). A later meta-analysis by Qin et al. (42) found that dairy intake was associated with a 12% lower risk of cardiovascular disease, and 13% lower risk of stroke as compared to individuals with no or a low dairy consumption (42). Likewise, a recent and comprehensive meta-analysis, including 31 cohort studies, suggested that a high dairy intake was associated with a 9% lower risk of stroke, whereas no association was found with total cardiovascular disease or coronary heart disease (43). Moreover, a high intake of cheese was associated with an 8% lower risk of coronary heart disease and a 13% lower risk of stroke. In addition, high plasma levels of the saturated fatty acid C 17:0, which primarily originates from dairy, were found to be associated with a reduced risk of coronary heart disease (44). Finally, a meta-analysis by O'Sullivan et al. (45) found no indication of total dairy intake or any specific dairy product being associated with an increased cardiovascular mortality. Studies are emerging showing that dairy products, particularly the low-fat types, cluster within a healthy dietary pattern (46), and therefore, the risk of residual confounding in the observational studies cannot be ruled out.

In accordance with the latest meta-analyses presented above, the latest Nordic Nutrition Recommendations have concluded that high consumption of low-fat milk products is associated with reduced risk of hypertension and stroke (47).

Conclusion on cardiovascular disease

The overall evidence indicates that a high intake of milk and dairy products, that is, 200–300 ml/day, does not increase the risk of cardiovascular disease. Specifically, there is an inverse association with risk of hypertension and stroke.

Bone health and osteoporosis

Milk and dairy products contain a number of nutrients that are required for building strong bones in childhood and for their maintenance during adulthood with the aim to reduce osteoporosis and bone fractures in older age (48). The European Commission has concluded that protein, calcium, phosphorus, magnesium, manganese, zinc, vitamin D, and vitamin K are necessary for maintaining normal bones (European Commission regulation 2012). With the exception of vitamin D, these nutrients are all present in significant amounts in milk and dairy products.

Osteoporosis has been described as a 'paediatric disease with geriatric consequences' as low milk, and hence, low mineral intake during childhood and adolescence has been associated with significantly increased risk of osteoporotic fractures in middle and older age, particularly in women (49, 50). A recent study indicated that in children and adolescents, except for those with very low calcium intakes, magnesium intake may be more important than calcium in relation to bone development (51). Calcium intake was found not to be significantly associated with total bone mineral content or density, whereas intake of magnesium and the amount absorbed were key predictors of bone mass. The extent to which these results can be extrapolated to the general population is uncertain, but milk and dairy products are important sources of magnesium and hence important supporters of bone growth during adolescence. In a meta-analysis by Huncharek et al. (52), dairy products, with or without vitamin D supplementation, increased total body and lumbar spine bone mineral content in children with low baseline dairy intake, whereas no effect was found for children with a high baseline dairy intake. Thus, there may be a threshold above which increasing intake of dairy products or dairy-calcium does not additionally benefit bone mineral content or density in children.

In adults, interactions between calcium, phosphorus, protein and vitamin D reduce bone resorption and increase bone formation, thereby attenuating age-related bone loss (53). Possibly due to the complex interaction between nutrients and the multifactorial nature of bone fractures, it has been difficult to establish whether or not a low intake of milk and dairy in adulthood increases the risk of osteoporosis and bone fractures. Hence, to date, meta-analyses have not supported a protective effect of milk and dairy intake in adulthood on risk of osteoporosis and bone fractures (54, 55). Nevertheless a recent systematic review concluded that calcium and dairy are important contributors to bone health in adults (56).

In the 2015–2020 Dietary Guidelines for Americans, it was stated that 'Healthy eating patterns include fat-free and low-fat (1%) dairy, including milk, yoghurt, cheese, or fortified soy beverages (commonly known as "soymilk"). Those who are unable or choose not to consume dairy products should consume foods that provide the range of nutrients generally obtained from dairy, including protein, calcium, potassium, magnesium, vitamin D, and vitamin A (e.g. fortified soy beverages)'. Although the focus is on achieving the nutrient requirements by foods rather than supplements, plant-based beverages typically contain inorganic chemical forms of calcium, which may actually increase cardiovascular risk (56, 57). As calcium in dairy is organic, milk and dairy products should still be considered the superior sources of calcium (58). Yet, future studies need to address whether or not vitamin D fortification of dairy products is crucial for these to have a positive effect on bone fracture risk.

Conclusion on bone health and osteoporosis

The present evidence suggests a positive effect of milk and dairy intake on bone health in childhood and adolescence, but with only limited evidence on bone health in adulthood and on the risk of bone fractures in older age.

Cancer

In population studies, dairy has been associated positively and negatively with various cancers, but most have been based on limited evidence and very few findings remain robust. Dairy products contain a variety of bioactive compounds that could exert both positive and negative effects on carcinogenesis. The positive effects may be related to the content of calcium, lactoferrin, and fermentation products, whereas the negative effects could be linked to the content of insulin-like growth factor I (IGF-1) (59). The World Cancer Research Fund (WCRF) continuously and systematically reviews the evidence on diet and physical activity in relation to prevention of cancer, and specific areas are updated when new evidence has emerged.

Colorectal cancer is the second most common cause of death among cancers in developed countries. Even though colorectal tumourigenesis is a complex process, epidemiological and experimental data indicate that milk and dairy products have a chemopreventive role in the pathogenesis. In the 2011 WCRF report on colorectal cancer, it was concluded that consumption of milk and calcium probably reduces the risk of this cancer (60). Likewise, in meta-analyses, dairy intake has consistently been associated with a decreased risk of colorectal cancer (61, 62) and colon cancer (63). The most recent meta-analysis by Ralston et al. (64) reported 26% lower colon cancer risk in males consuming 525 g of milk per day, whereas no association was found in females.

The link between dairy intake and colorectal cancer is considered to be mainly due to the calcium derived from dairy, with a 24% risk reduction with a dairy-calcium intake of 900 mg/day (65). The proposed mechanisms behind this are calcium binding to secondary bile acids and ionised fatty acids, thereby reducing their proliferative effects in the colorectal epithelium (66). Also, calcium may influence multiple intracellular pathways leading to differentiation in normal cells and apoptosis in transformed cells (67). Accordingly, a number of studies have reported reduced cell proliferation in the colon and rectum with intake of calcium and dairy products (68–72).

In the 2010 WCRF report on breast cancer, it was concluded that the evidence for dairy intake and risk of breast cancer is non-conclusive (73). In accordance with a meta-analysis from 2011 on prospective cohort studies (74), a recent meta-analysis by Zang et al. (75), however, suggested that a high (>600 g/d) and modest (400–600 g/d) dairy intake was associated with a reduced risk of breast cancer (10% and 6%, respectively) compared with a low dairy intake (<400 g/d). Within dairy subgroups, particularly yoghurt and low-fat dairy were found to be inversely associated with the risk of developing breast cancer. As calcium and vitamin D supplementation was previously shown to reduce risk of breast cancer in the Women's Health Initiative (76), these nutrients could be involved in the underlying mechanisms.

According to the 2014 WCRF report on prostate cancer, dairy may be associated with a limited-suggestive increased risk of prostate cancer, but the current evidence is limited (77). However, this conclusion was substantiated by the most recent meta-analysis by Aune et al. (78), which suggested that a high intake of dairy products, milk, low-fat milk, cheese, and calcium were associated with a 3–9% increased risk of prostate cancer. The mechanism behind this was suggested to be an increased circulating concentration of IGF-1, which has been previously shown to be associated with an increased prostate cancer risk (79).

The 2015 WCRF report on bladder cancer suggested that the evidence for milk and dairy on bladder cancer risk was inconsistent and inconclusive (80). Two meta-analyses on milk intake and bladder cancer risk have suggested a decreased risk of bladder cancer with a high intake of milk (61, 81). Others have found no association between milk and dairy intake and risk of bladder cancer risk (82), but none have suggested an adverse effect.

Of the cancer types for which the associations with dairy intake were not presented in the WCRF reports, recent meta-analyses have suggested no association between dairy intake and risk of ovarian cancer (83), lung cancer (84, 85), or pancreatic cancer (86) and an inverse association between dairy intake and risk of gastric cancer in Europe and the United States (87).

Studies in lactose-intolerant individuals

In a limited number of subjects, potential differences in cancer risk and mortality between lactose-tolerant and lactose-intolerant individuals (self-reported or assessed by polymorphisms for the lactase gene) have been reported under the assumption that lactose-intolerant individuals consume less milk. However, there may also be other differences between these two groups that need to be taken into consideration, for example, genetics, ethnicity, other dietary habits, smoking, physical activity, and socio-economic factors.

Bácsi et al. (88) examined the role of genetically determined differences in the ability to degrade lactose and showed that subjects with deficiencies in the genes coding for lactase (i.e. subjects not drinking milk due to intolerance) had an increased risk of colorectal cancer. This supports the ability of dairy products to reduce colorectal cancer risk and the causality of this relation. In the European EPIC study, the hypothesis that the genetically determined lactose tolerance was associated with elevated dairy product intake and increased prostate cancer risk was examined (89). The study included 630 men with prostate cancer and 873 matched control participants. Dairy product consumption was assessed by diet questionnaires, and intake of milk and total dairy products varied significantly by lactase genotype, with an almost twofold higher intake in lactose-tolerant compared to lactose-intolerant subjects. However, the lactase variant was not found to be significantly associated with prostate cancer risk. This indicates that residual confounding may have biased the associations observed between milk and dairy intake and prostate cancer risk in the observational studies included in a previous meta-analysis (78).

Ji et al. (90) investigated Swedish subjects with self-reported lactose intolerance and found a lower risk of lung, breast, and ovarian cancers compared to lactose-tolerant subjects. Unfortunately, no information about milk intake, or other genetic, ethnic, lifestyle (diet, smoking and physical activity), and behavioural characteristics were reported. Also, self-reported lactose intolerance may not be comparable to genetically determined lactose intolerance. Due to potential bias in the design and the lack of control for known confounders, it is impossible to conclude about the relationship with dairy intake. Also, these findings are in contrast with the additional literature suggesting no or an inverse association between dairy intake and risk of breast cancer (74, 75), ovarian cancer (83, 91), and lung cancer (84, 85).

Conclusion on cancer

According to WCRF reports and the latest meta-analyses, consumption of milk and dairy products probably protects against colorectal cancer, bladder cancer, gastric cancer, and breast cancer. Dairy intake does not seem to be associated with risk of pancreatic cancer, ovarian cancer, or lung cancer, whereas the evidence for prostate cancer risk is inconsistent. In women, dairy offers significant and robust health benefits in reducing the risk of the common and serious colorectal cancer and, possibly, also the risk of breast cancer. In men, the benefit of the protective effect of milk and dairy on the common and serious colorectal cancer is judged to outweigh a potentially increased risk of prostate cancer.

All-cause mortality

In medical research, the term 'all-cause mortality' implies all causes of death. There are many individual studies reporting that a high consumption of milk and dairy products is associated with decreased mortality (92), unchanged mortality (93), or even increased mortality (94). However, based on meta-analyses of observational cohort studies, there is no evidence to support the view that milk and dairy product intake is associated with all-cause mortality (45, 95). In a meta-analysis, O'Sullivan et al. (45) studied whether intake of milk and dairy products as food sources of saturated fat was related to all-cause mortality, cancer mortality, and cardiovascular mortality. Neither total dairy intake nor intake of any specific dairy products was found to be associated with all-cause mortality. In the most recent meta-analysis including 12 observational studies of milk intake and mortality, there were no consistent associations between milk intake and all-cause or cause-specific mortality (95).

Conclusion on all-cause mortality

The evidence from observational studies confirms that there is no association between consumption of milk and dairy products and all-cause mortality.

Comparison of nutrient content and health aspects of milk and plant-based drinks

In recent decades, the market for milk and dairy substitute drinks based on, for example, soy, rice, oats, or almonds has expanded, and calcium-fortified plant-based drinks have become part of the nutrition recommendations as alternatives to milk in several countries, such as the United States, Sweden, Australia, and Brazil. Among the plant-based milk substitutes, soy drink dominates the market in the Western world, but the emerging of other plant-based drinks has influenced the market for soy drink (96).

The nutrient density of plant-based milk substitutes varies considerably between and within types, and their nutritional properties depend on the raw material used, the processing, the fortification with vitamins and minerals, and the addition of other ingredients such as sugar and oil. Soy drink is the only plant-based milk substitute that approximates the protein content of cow's milk, whereas the protein contents of the drinks based on oat, rice, and almonds are extremely low, and the recent review of Mäkinen et al. (96) emphasises the importance of consumer awareness of such low-protein contents. Moreover, there are now cases of severe nutritional deficiencies in children being reported as a result of inappropriate consumption of plant-based drinks (97, 98).

Despite the fact that most of the plant-based drinks are low in saturated fat and cholesterol, some of these products have higher energy contents than whole milk due to a high content of oil and added sugar. Some plant-based drinks have a sugar content equal to that of sugar-sweetened beverages, which have been linked to obesity, reduced insulin sensitivity (99), increased liver, muscle, and visceral fat content as well as increased blood pressure, and increased concentrations of triglyceride and cholesterol in the blood (100, 101). Analyses of several commercially available plant-based drinks carried out at the Technical University of Denmark showed a generally higher energy content and lower contents of iodine, potassium, phosphorus, and selenium in the plant-based drinks compared to semi-skimmed milk (102). Also, rice drinks are known to have a high content of inorganic arsenic, and soy drinks are known to contain isoflavones with oestrogen-like effects. Consequently, The Danish Veterinary and Food Administration concluded that the plant-based drinks cannot be recommended as full worthy alternatives to cow's milk (102), which is consistent with the conclusions drawn by the Swedish National Food Agency (103).

The importance of studying whole foods instead of single nutrients is becoming clear as potential nutrient–nutrient interactions may affect the metabolic response to the whole food compared to its isolated nutrients. As the plant-based drinks have undergone processing and fortification, any health effects of natural soy, rice, oats, and almonds cannot be directly transferred to the drinks, but need to be studied directly. Only a few studies have compared the effects of cow's milk with plant-based drinks as whole foods on disease risk markers (104–108). However, none of these have included commercially available drinks or disease endpoints. Therefore, the evidence is currently insufficient to conclude that plant-based drinks possess health benefits above those of milk and dairy products. Until more research has been conducted and a scientifically sound conclusion can be drawn, health authorities should be cautious about recommending plant-based drinks as acceptable substitutes to cow's milk for the general population.

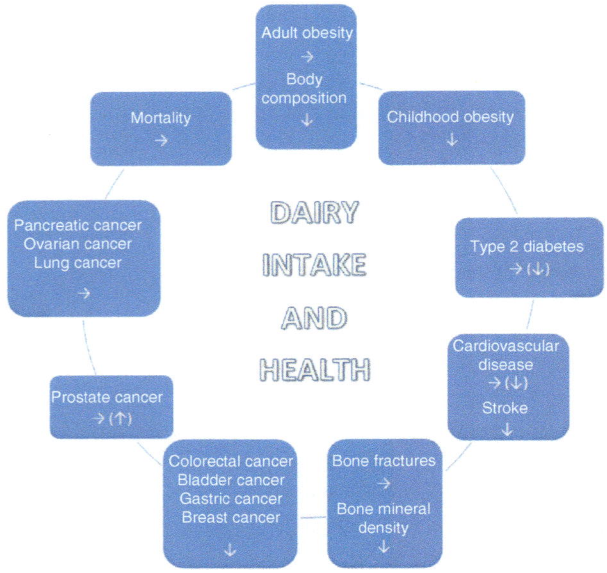

Fig. 1. Overall effect/association between dairy product intake and health outcomes. ↓ favourable effect/association; ↑adverse effect/association; → no effect/association.

Conclusion on nutrient content and health aspects of milk and plant-based drinks

Cow's milk and plant-based drinks are completely different products, both regarding nutrient content and presumably also health effects. Although there are concerns about children consuming the low-protein drinks, further evidence-based assessment of the nutritional and health value of the plant-based drinks must await more studies in humans.

Answers to the key questions

Key question 1: For the general consumer, will a diet with milk and dairy products overall provide better or worse health, and increase or decrease risk of major diseases and all-cause mortality than a diet with no or low content of milk and dairy products?

Consumption of dairy products is associated with an overall reduced risk of cardiometabolic diseases and some cancers, whereas only very few adverse effects have been reported (Fig. 1). Dairy products may therefore have the potential to reduce the burden of the most prevalent chronic diseases in the population and to substantially reduce the health care costs for society (109). Consumption of dairy products is part of the dietary recommendations in several nations, for example, Sweden, Denmark, and United States. A general recommendation to reduce the intake of dairy products in individuals who actually tolerate them may be counterproductive for health and could therefore increase health care expenses. However, more emphasis should be on the foods which dairy replaces in the diet. In addition, as most of the conducted meta-analyses are on observational data, residual confounding cannot be ruled out, and it is also possible that milk and dairy intake in these studies could be just a marker of diets of higher nutritional quality.

Key question 2: Is it justified to recommend the general lactose-tolerant population to avoid the consumption of milk and dairy products?

In the Nordic countries, as few as 2% of the population has primary lactase deficiency and can be classified as lactose-intolerant individuals (110). Yet, most lactose-intolerant adults can tolerate one glass of milk or a scoop of ice cream. Cheeses have negligible lactose contents, and the lactose in yoghurt is digested more efficiently than other dairy sources due to the bacterial lactase present in yoghurt which facilitates lactose digestion (111). Therefore, fermented dairy products, that is, yoghurt and most cheeses (cottage cheese, as well as soft and hard cheeses), can be tolerated by lactose-intolerant individuals without symptoms (111, 112).

The same applies to cow's milk protein allergy that typically occurs in 0.1–2.0% of children in the Nordic countries and Europe (113). Among children with verified cow's milk-specific IgE who were re-evaluated 1 year after diagnosis, 69% tolerated cow's milk at re-evaluation (114). Thus, the condition is generally seen to resolve in children. To warn the general population against dairy consumption based on rare milk allergies would be equivalent to warn against foods, such as peanuts or seafood due to the fact that a small subset of the population is allergic to these foods.

Key question 3: Is there scientific evidence to substantiate that replacing milk and dairy products with plant-based drinks will improve health?

Cow's milk and plant-based drinks are not nutritionally comparable foods. As only a few studies have investigated the health effects of replacing cow's milk with plant-based drinks and none have focused on commercially available drinks or on disease endpoints, the effect of this replacement can only be speculated on. There have, however, been individual cases reporting illness in children consuming low-protein plant-based drinks, but an evidence-based final assessment of the health value of plant-based drinks compared to cow's milk must await more studies in humans.

Overall conclusions regarding intake of milk and dairy products and health

Our review of the totality of available scientific evidence supports that intake of milk and dairy products contributes to meeting nutrient recommendations and may protect against the most prevalent, chronic non-communicable diseases, whereas very few adverse effects have been reported.

Conflicts of interest and funding

Tanja Kongerslev Thorning has no conflicts of interest to declare. Anne Raben is recipient of research funding from the Dairy Research Institute, Rosemont, IL, USA and the Danish Agriculture & Food Council.Tine Tholstrup is recipient of research grants from the Danish Dairy Research Foundation and the Dairy Research Institute, Rosemont, IL. The sponsors had no role in design and conduct of the studies, data collection and analysis, interpretation of the data, decision to publish, or preparation of the manuscripts. Sabita S. Soedamah-Muthu received funding from the Global Dairy Platform, Dairy Research Institute and Dairy Australia for meta-analyses on cheese and blood lipids and on dairy and mortality. The sponsors had no role in design and conduct of the meta-analyses, data collection and analysis, interpretation of the data, decision to publish, or preparation of the manuscripts. Ian Givens is recipient of research grants from UK Biotechnology and Biological Sciences Research Council (BBSRC), UK Medical Research Council (MRC), Arla Foods UK, AAK-UK (both in kind), The Barham Benevolent Foundation, Volac UK, DSM Switzerland and Global Dairy Platform. He is a consultant for The Bio-competence Centre of Healthy Dairy Products, Tartu, Estonia, and in the recent past for The Dairy Council (London). Arne Astrup is recipient of research grants from Arla Foods, DK; Danish Dairy Research Foundation; Global Dairy Platform; Danish Agriculture & Food Council; GEIE European Milk Forum, France. He is member of advisory boards for Dutch Beer Knowledge Institute, NL; IKEA, SV; Lucozade Ribena Suntory Ltd, UK; McCain Foods Limited, USA; McDonald's, USA; Weight Watchers, USA. He is a consultant for Nestlé Research Center, Switzerland; Nongfu Spring Water, China. Astrup receives honoraria as Associate Editor of *American Journal of Clinical Nutrition*, and for membership of the Editorial Boards of *Annals of Nutrition and Metabolism* and *Annual Review of Nutrition*. He is recipient of travel expenses and/or modest honoraria (<$2,000) for lectures given at meetings supported by corporate sponsors. He received financial support from dairy organisations for attendance at the Eurofed Lipids Congress (2014) in France and the meeting of The Federation of European Nutrition Societies (2015) in Germany.

References

1. Park YW, Zhu S, Palaniappan L, Heshka S, Carnethon MR, Heymsfield SB. The metabolic syndrome: prevalence and associated risk factor findings in the US population from the Third National Health and Nutrition Examination Survey, 1988–1994. Arch Intern Med 2003; 163(4): 427–36.
2. Laaksonen MA, Knekt P, Rissanen H, Harkanen T, Virtala E, Marniemi J, et al. The relative importance of modifiable

potential risk factors of type 2 diabetes: a meta-analysis of two cohorts. Eur J Epidemiol 2010; 25(2): 115–24.
3. Dietz WH, Gortmaker SL. Preventing obesity in children and adolescents. Annu Rev Public Health 2001; 22: 337–53.
4. Dror DK. Dairy consumption and pre-school, school-age and adolescent obesity in developed countries: a systematic review and meta-analysis. Obes Rev 2014; 15(6): 516–27.
5. Lu L, Xun P, Wan Y, He K, Cai W. Long-term association between dairy consumption and risk of childhood obesity: a systematic review and meta-analysis of prospective cohort studies. Eur J Clin Nutr 2016; 70(4): 414–23.
6. Gilbert JA, Bendsen NT, Tremblay A, Astrup A. Effect of proteins from different sources on body composition. Nutr Metab Cardiovasc Dis 2011; 21(Suppl 2): B16–31.
7. Bendtsen LQ, Lorenzen JK, Bendsen NT, Rasmussen C, Astrup A. Effect of dairy proteins on appetite, energy expenditure, body weight, and composition: a review of the evidence from controlled clinical trials. Adv Nutr 2013; 4(4): 418–38.
8. Astrup A, Raben A, Geiker N. The role of higher protein diets in weight control and obesity-related comorbidities. Int J Obes (Lond) 2015; 39(5): 721–6.
9. Abargouei AS, Janghorbani M, Salehi-Marzijarani M, Esmaillzadeh A. Effect of dairy consumption on weight and body composition in adults: a systematic review and meta-analysis of randomized controlled clinical trials. Int J Obes (Lond) 2012; 36(12): 1485–93.
10. Chen M, Pan A, Malik VS, Hu FB. Effects of dairy intake on body weight and fat: a meta-analysis of randomized controlled trials. Am J Clin Nutr 2012; 96(4): 735–47.
11. Booth AO, Huggins CE, Wattanapenpaiboon N, Nowson CA. Effect of increasing dietary calcium through supplements and dairy food on body weight and body composition: a meta-analysis of randomised controlled trials. Br J Nutr 2015; 114(7): 1013–25.
12. Maghsoudi Z, Ghiasvand R, Salehi-Abargouei A. Empirically derived dietary patterns and incident type 2 diabetes mellitus: a systematic review and meta-analysis on prospective observational studies. Public Health Nutr 2016; 19(2): 230–41.
13. Gao D, Ning N, Wang C, Wang Y, Li Q, Meng Z, et al. Dairy products consumption and risk of type 2 diabetes: systematic review and dose-response meta-analysis. PLoS One 2013; 8(9): e73965.
14. Aune D, Norat T, Romundstad P, Vatten LJ. Dairy products and the risk of type 2 diabetes: a systematic review and dose-response meta-analysis of cohort studies. Am J Clin Nutr 2013; 98(4): 1066–83.
15. Tong X, Dong JY, Wu ZW, Li W, Qin LQ. Dairy consumption and risk of type 2 diabetes mellitus: a meta-analysis of cohort studies. Eur J Clin Nutr 2011; 65(9): 1027–31.
16. Bergholdt HK, Nordestgaard BG, Ellervik C. Milk intake is not associated with low risk of diabetes or overweight-obesity: a Mendelian randomization study in 97,811 Danish individuals. Am J Clin Nutr 2015; 102(2): 487–96.
17. Gijsbers L, Ding EL, Malik VS, de Goede J, Geleijnse JM, Soedamah-Muthu SS. Consumption of dairy foods and diabetes incidence: a dose-response meta-analysis of observational studies. Am J Clin Nutr 2016; 103(4): 1111–24.
18. Astrup A. A changing view on saturated fatty acids and dairy: from enemy to friend. Am J Clin Nutr 2014; 100(6): 1407–8.
19. Zheng H, Yde CC, Clausen MR, Kristensen M, Lorenzen J, Astrup A, et al. Metabolomics investigation to shed light on cheese as a possible piece in the French paradox puzzle. J Agr Food Chem 2015; 63(10): 2830–9.
20. Frid AH, Nilsson M, Holst JJ, Bjorck IM. Effect of whey on blood glucose and insulin responses to composite breakfast and lunch meals in type 2 diabetic subjects. Am J Clin Nutr 2005; 82(1): 69–75.
21. Nilsson M, Stenberg M, Frid AH, Holst JJ, Bjorck IM. Glycemia and insulinemia in healthy subjects after lactose-equivalent meals of milk and other food proteins: the role of plasma amino acids and incretins. Am J Clin Nutr 2004; 80(5): 1246–53.
22. Rideout TC, Marinangeli CP, Martin H, Browne RW, Rempel CB. Consumption of low-fat dairy foods for 6 months improves insulin resistance without adversely affecting lipids or bodyweight in healthy adults: a randomized free-living cross-over study. Nutr J 2013; 12: 56.
23. Soedamah-Muthu SS, Verberne LD, Ding EL, Engberink MF, Geleijnse JM. Dairy consumption and incidence of hypertension: a dose-response meta-analysis of prospective cohort studies. Hypertension 2012; 60(5): 1131–7.
24. Huth PJ, Park KM. Influence of dairy product and milk fat consumption on cardiovascular disease risk: a review of the evidence. Adv Nutr 2012; 3(3): 266–85.
25. Musunuru K, Orho-Melander M, Caulfield MP, Li S, Salameh WA, Reitz RE, et al. Ion mobility analysis of lipoprotein subfractions identifies three independent axes of cardiovascular risk. Arterioscler Thromb Vasc Biol 2009; 29(11): 1975–80.
26. St-Pierre AC, Cantin B, Dagenais GR, Mauriege P, Bernard PM, Despres JP, et al. Low-density lipoprotein subfractions and the long-term risk of ischemic heart disease in men: 13-year follow-up data from the Quebec Cardiovascular Study. Arterioscler Thromb Vasc Biol 2005; 25(3): 553–9.
27. Mora S, Buring JE, Ridker PM, Cui Y. Association of high-density lipoprotein cholesterol with incident cardiovascular events in women, by low-density lipoprotein cholesterol and apolipoprotein B100 levels: a cohort study. Ann Intern Med 2011; 155(11): 742–50.
28. Krauss RM. Lipoprotein subfractions and cardiovascular disease risk. Curr Opin Lipidol 2010; 21(4): 305–11.
29. Berneis KK, Krauss RM. Metabolic origins and clinical significance of LDL heterogeneity. J Lipid Res 2002; 43(9): 1363–79.
30. Sjogren P, Rosell M, Skoglund-Andersson C, Zdravkovic S, Vessby B, de Faire U, et al. Milk-derived fatty acids are associated with a more favorable LDL particle size distribution in healthy men. J Nutr 2004; 134(7): 1729–35.
31. Lorenzen JK, Astrup A. Dairy calcium intake modifies responsiveness of fat metabolism and blood lipids to a high-fat diet. Br J Nutr 2011; 105: 1–10.
32. Soerensen KV, Thorning TK, Astrup A, Kristensen M, Lorenzen JK. Effect of dairy calcium from cheese and milk on fecal fat excretion, blood lipids, and appetite in young men. Am J Clin Nutr 2014; 95(5): 984–91.
33. Hjerpsted J, Leedo E, Tholstrup T. Cheese intake in large amounts lowers LDL-cholesterol concentrations compared with butter intake of equal fat content. Am J Clin Nutr 2011; 94(6): 1479–84.
34. Thorning TK, Raziani F, Bendsen NT, Astrup A, Tholstrup T, Raben A. Diets with high-fat cheese, high-fat meat, or carbohydrate on cardiovascular risk markers in overweight postmenopausal women: a randomized crossover trial. Am J Clin Nutr 2015; 102(3): 573–81.
35. Raziani F, Tholstrup T, Kristensen MD, Svanegaard ML, Ritz C, Astrup A, et al. High intake of regular-fat cheese compared with reduced-fat cheese does not affect LDL cholesterol or risk markers of the metabolic syndrome: a randomized controlled trial. Am J Clin Nutr 2016; 104(4): 973–981.
36. de Goede J, Geleijnse JM, Ding EL, Soedamah-Muthu SS. Effect of cheese consumption on blood lipids: a systematic

review and meta-analysis of randomized controlled trials. Nutr Rev 2015; 73(5): 259–75.
37. Tholstrup T, Hoy CE, Andersen LN, Christensen RD, Sandstrom B. Does fat in milk, butter and cheese affect blood lipids and cholesterol differently? J Am Coll Nutr 2004; 23(2): 169–76.
38. Soedamah-Muthu SS, Ding EL, Al-Delaimy WK, Hu FB, Engberink MF, Willett WC, et al. Milk and dairy consumption and incidence of cardiovascular diseases and all-cause mortality: dose-response meta-analysis of prospective cohort studies. Am J Clin Nutr 2011; 93(1): 158–71.
39. Hu D, Huang J, Wang Y, Zhang D, Qu Y. Dairy foods and risk of stroke: a meta-analysis of prospective cohort studies. Nutr Metab Cardiovasc Dis 2014; 24(5): 460–9.
40. de Goede J, Soedamah-Muthu SS, Pan A, Gijsbers L, Geleijnse JM. Dairy consumption and risk of stroke: a systematic review and updated doseresponse meta-analysis of prospective cohort studies. J Am Heart Assoc 2016; 5(5): e002787, doi: http://dx.doi.org/10.1161/JAHA.115.002787
41. Rice BH. Dairy and cardiovascular disease: a review of recent observational research. Curr Nutr Rep 2014; 3: 130–8.
42. Qin LQ, Xu JY, Han SF, Zhang ZL, Zhao YY, Szeto IM. Dairy consumption and risk of cardiovascular disease: an updated meta-analysis of prospective cohort studies. Asia Pac J Clin Nutr 2015; 24(1): 90–100.
43. Alexander DD, Bylsma LC, Vargas AJ, Cohen SS, Doucette A, Mohamed M, et al. Dairy consumption and CVD: a systematic review and meta-analysis. Br J Nutr 2016; 115(4): 737–50.
44. Chowdhury R, Warnakula S, Kunutsor S, Crowe F, Ward HA, Johnson L, et al. Association of dietary, circulating, and supplement fatty acids with coronary risk: a systematic review and meta-analysis. Ann Intern Med 2014; 160(6): 398–406.
45. O'Sullivan TA, Hafekost K, Mitrou F, Lawrence D. Food sources of saturated fat and the association with mortality: a meta-analysis. Am J Public Health 2013; 103(9): e31–42.
46. Mursu J, Steffen LM, Meyer KA, Duprez D, Jacobs DR Jr. Diet quality indexes and mortality in postmenopausal women: the Iowa Women's Health Study. Am J Clin Nutr 2013; 98(2): 444–53.
47. Nordic Council of Ministers (2014). Nordic nutrition recommendations 2012–integrating nutrition and physical activity, 5th edition. Copenhagen, DK: Nordic Council of Ministers.
48. Rizzoli R. Dairy products, yogurts, and bone health. Am J Clin Nutr 2014; 99(5 Suppl): 1256S–62S.
49. Kalkwarf HJ, Khoury JC, Lanphear BP. Milk intake during childhood and adolescence, adult bone density, and osteoporotic fractures in US women. Am J Clin Nutr 2003; 77(1): 257–65.
50. Power ML, Heaney RP, Kalkwarf HJ, Pitkin RM, Repke JT, Tsang RC, et al. The role of calcium in health and disease. Am J Obstet Gynecol 1999; 181(6): 1560–9.
51. Abrams SA, Chen Z, Hawthorne KM. Magnesium metabolism in 4-year-old to 8-year-old children. J Bone Miner Res 2014; 29(1): 118–22.
52. Huncharek M, Muscat J, Kupelnick B. Impact of dairy products and dietary calcium on bone-mineral content in children: results of a meta-analysis. Bone 2008; 43(2): 312–21.
53. Bonjour JP, Kraenzlin M, Levasseur R, Warren M, Whiting S. Dairy in adulthood: from foods to nutrient interactions on bone and skeletal muscle health. J Am Coll Nutr 2013; 32(4): 251–63.
54. Bischoff-Ferrari HA, Dawson-Hughes B, Baron JA, Kanis JA, Orav EJ, Staehelin HB, et al. Milk intake and risk of hip fracture in men and women: a meta-analysis of prospective cohort studies. J Bone Miner Res 2011; 26(4): 833–9.
55. Kanis JA, Johansson H, Oden A, De Laet C, Johnell O, Eisman JA, et al. A meta-analysis of milk intake and fracture risk: low utility for case finding. Osteoporos Int 2005; 16(7): 799–804.
56. Weaver CM. Calcium supplementation: is protecting against osteoporosis counter to protecting against cardiovascular disease? Curr Osteoporos Rep 2014; 12(2): 211–18.
57. Bolland MJ, Grey A, Reid IR. Calcium supplements and cardiovascular risk: 5 years on. Ther Adv Drug Saf 2013; 4(5): 199–210.
58. Astrup A. Yogurt and dairy product consumption to prevent cardiometabolic diseases: epidemiologic and experimental studies. Am J Clin Nutr 2014; 99(5 Suppl): 1235S–42S.
59. Latino-Martel P, Cottet V, Druesne-Pecollo N, Pierre FH, Touillaud M, Touvier M, et al. Alcoholic beverages, obesity, physical activity and other nutritional factors, and cancer risk: a review of the evidence. Crit Rev Oncol Hematol 2016; 99: 308–23.
60. World Cancer Research Fund/American Institute for Cancer Research (2011). Food, nutrition, physical activity, and the prevention of colorectal cancer. London, UK: WCRF International.
61. Lampe JW. Dairy products and cancer. J Am Coll Nutr 2011; 30(5 Suppl 1): 464S–70S.
62. Aune D, Lau R, Chan DS, Vieira R, Greenwood DC, Kampman E, et al. Dairy products and colorectal cancer risk: a systematic review and meta-analysis of cohort studies. Ann Oncol 2012; 23(1): 37–45.
63. Huncharek M, Muscat J, Kupelnick B. Colorectal cancer risk and dietary intake of calcium, vitamin D, and dairy products: a meta-analysis of 26,335 cases from 60 observational studies. Nutr Cancer 2009; 61(1): 47–69.
64. Ralston RA, Truby H, Palermo CE, Walker KZ. Colorectal cancer and nonfermented milk, solid cheese, and fermented milk consumption: a systematic review and meta-analysis of prospective studies. Crit Rev Food Sci Nutr 2014; 54(9): 1167–79.
65. Keum N, Aune D, Greenwood DC, Ju W, Giovannucci EL. Calcium intake and colorectal cancer risk: dose-response meta-analysis of prospective observational studies. Int J Cancer 2014; 135(8): 1940–8.
66. Newmark HL, Wargovich MJ, Bruce WR. Colon cancer and dietary fat, phosphate, and calcium: a hypothesis. J Natl Cancer Inst 1984; 72(6): 1323–5.
67. Lamprecht SA, Lipkin M. Cellular mechanisms of calcium and vitamin D in the inhibition of colorectal carcinogenesis. Ann N Y Acad Sci 2001; 952: 73–87.
68. Holt PR, Atillasoy EO, Gilman J, Guss J, Moss SF, Newmark H, et al. Modulation of abnormal colonic epithelial cell proliferation and differentiation by low-fat dairy foods: a randomized controlled trial. JAMA 1998; 280(12): 1074–9.
69. Holt PR, Wolper C, Moss SF, Yang K, Lipkin M. Comparison of calcium supplementation or low-fat dairy foods on epithelial cell proliferation and differentiation. Nutr Cancer 2001; 41(1–2): 150–5.
70. Karagas MR, Tosteson TD, Greenberg ER, Rothstein RI, Roebuck BD, Herrin M, et al. Effects of milk and milk products on rectal mucosal cell proliferation in humans. Cancer Epidemiol Biomarkers Prev 1998; 7(9): 757–66.
71. Rozen P, Lubin F, Papo N, Knaani J, Farbstein H, Farbstein M, et al. Calcium supplements interact significantly with long-term diet while suppressing rectal epithelial proliferation of adenoma patients. Cancer 2001; 91(4): 833–40.
72. Ahearn TU, McCullough ML, Flanders WD, Long Q, Sidelnikov E, Fedirko V, et al. A randomized clinical trial of the effects of supplemental calcium and vitamin D3 on markers of their metabolism in normal mucosa of colorectal adenoma patients. Cancer Res 2011; 71(2): 413–23.

73. World Cancer Research Fund/American Institute for Cancer Research (2010). Food, nutrition, physical activity, and the prevention of breast cancer. London, UK: WCRF International.
74. Dong JY, Zhang L, He K, Qin LQ. Dairy consumption and risk of breast cancer: a meta-analysis of prospective cohort studies. Breast Cancer Res Treat 2011; 127(1): 23–31.
75. Zang J, Shen M, Du S, Chen T, Zou S. The association between dairy intake and breast cancer in western and Asian populations: a systematic review and meta-analysis. J Breast Cancer 2015; 18(4): 313–22.
76. Cauley JA, Chlebowski RT, Wactawski-Wende J, Robbins JA, Rodabough RJ, Chen Z, et al. Calcium plus vitamin D supplementation and health outcomes five years after active intervention ended: the women's health initiative. J Womens Health (Larchmt) 2013; 22(11): 915–29.
77. World Cancer Research Fund International/American Institute for Cancer Research (2014). Diet, nutrition, physical activity, and prostate cancer. London, UK: WCRF International.
78. Aune D, Navarro Rosenblatt DA, Chan DS, Vieira AR, Vieira R, Greenwood DC, et al. Dairy products, calcium, and prostate cancer risk: a systematic review and meta-analysis of cohort studies. Am J Clin Nutr 2015; 101(1): 87–117.
79. Roddam AW, Allen NE, Appleby P, Key TJ, Ferrucci L, Carter HB, et al. Insulin-like growth factors, their binding proteins, and prostate cancer risk: analysis of individual patient data from 12 prospective studies. Ann Intern Med 2008; 149(7): 461–71, W83–8.
80. World Cancer Research Fund International/American Institute for Cancer Research (2015). Diet, nutrition, physical activity and bladder cancer. London, UK: WCRF International.
81. Mao QQ, Dai Y, Lin YW, Qin J, Xie LP, Zheng XY. Milk consumption and bladder cancer risk: a meta-analysis of published epidemiological studies. Nutr Cancer 2011; 63(8): 1263–71.
82. Li F, An SL, Zhou Y, Liang ZK, Jiao ZJ, Jing YM, et al. Milk and dairy consumption and risk of bladder cancer: a meta-analysis. Urology 2011; 78(6): 1298–305.
83. Hou R, Wu QJ, Gong TT, Jiang L. Dietary fat and fatty acid intake and epithelial ovarian cancer risk: evidence from epidemiological studies. Oncotarget 2015; 6(40): 43099–119.
84. Yu Y, Li H, Xu K, Li X, Hu C, Wei H, et al. Dairy consumption and lung cancer risk: a meta-analysis of prospective cohort studies. Onco Targets Ther 2015; 9: 111–16.
85. Yang Y, Wang X, Yao Q, Qin L, Xu C. Dairy product, calcium intake and lung cancer risk: a systematic review with meta-analysis. Sci Rep 2016; 6: 20624.
86. Genkinger JM, Wang M, Li R, Albanes D, Anderson KE, Bernstein L, et al. Dairy products and pancreatic cancer risk: a pooled analysis of 14 cohort studies. Ann Oncol 2014; 25(6): 1106–115.
87. Guo Y, Shan Z, Ren H, Chen W. Dairy consumption and gastric cancer risk: a meta-analysis of epidemiological studies. Nutr Cancer 2015; 67(4): 555–68.
88. Bácsi K, Hitre E, Kosa JP, Horvath H, Lazary A, Lakatos PL, et al. Effects of the lactase 13910 C/T and calcium-sensor receptor A986S G/T gene polymorphisms on the incidence and recurrence of colorectal cancer in Hungarian population. BMC Cancer 2008; 8: 317.
89. Travis RC, Appleby PN, Siddiq A, Allen NE, Kaaks R, Canzian F, et al. Genetic variation in the lactase gene, dairy product intake and risk for prostate cancer in the European prospective investigation into cancer and nutrition. Int J Cancer 2013; 132(8): 1901–10.
90. Ji J, Sundquist J, Sundquist K. Lactose intolerance and risk of lung, breast and ovarian cancers: aetiological clues from a population-based study in Sweden. Br J Cancer 2015; 112(1): 149–52.
91. Merritt MA, Poole EM, Hankinson SE, Willett WC, Tworoger SS. Dairy food and nutrient intake in different life periods in relation to risk of ovarian cancer. Cancer Causes Control 2014; 25(7): 795–808.
92. Wang C, Yatsuya H, Tamakoshi K, Iso H, Tamakoshi A. Milk drinking and mortality: findings from the Japan collaborative cohort study. J Epidemiol 2015; 25(1): 66–73.
93. Paganini-Hill A, Kawas CH, Corrada MM. Non-alcoholic beverage and caffeine consumption and mortality: the Leisure World Cohort Study. Prev Med 2007; 44(4): 305–10.
94. Michaelsson K, Wolk A, Langenskiold S, Basu S, Warensjo Lemming E, Melhus H, et al. Milk intake and risk of mortality and fractures in women and men: cohort studies. BMJ 2014; 349: g6015.
95. Larsson SC, Crippa A, Orsini N, Wolk A, Michaelsson K. Milk consumption and mortality from all causes, cardiovascular disease, and cancer: a systematic review and meta-analysis. Nutrients 2015; 7(9): 7749–63.
96. Mäkinen OE, Wanhalinna V, Zannini E, Arendt EK. Foods for special dietary needs: non-dairy plant based milk substitutes and fermented dairy type products. Crit Rev Food Sci Nutr 2016; 56(3): 339–49.
97. Ellis D, Lieb J. Hyperoxaluria and genitourinary disorders in children ingesting almond milk products. J Pediatr 2015; 167(5): 1155–8.
98. Le Louer B, Lemale J, Garcette K, Orzechowski C, Chalvon A, Girardet JP, et al. Severe nutritional deficiencies in young infants with inappropriate plant milk consumption. Arch Pediatr 2014; 21(5): 483–8.
99. Jakobsen MU, Dethlefsen C, Joensen AM, Stegger J, Tjonneland A, Schmidt EB, et al. Intake of carbohydrates compared with intake of saturated fatty acids and risk of myocardial infarction: importance of the glycemic index. Am J Clin Nutr 2010; 91(6): 1764–8.
100. Maersk M, Belza A, Stodkilde-Jorgensen H, Ringgaard S, Chabanova E, Thomsen H, et al. Sucrose-sweetened beverages increase fat storage in the liver, muscle, and visceral fat depot: a 6-mo randomized intervention study. Am J Clin Nutr 2012; 95(2): 283–9.
101. Raben A, Moller BK, Flint A, Vasilaris TH, Christina Moller A, Juul Holst J, et al. Increased postprandial glycaemia, insulinemia, and lipidemia after 10 weeks' sucrose-rich diet compared to an artificially sweetened diet: a randomised controlled trial. Food Nutr Res 2011; 55. doi: http://dx.doi.org/10.3402/fnr.v55i0.5961
102. Fødevarestyrelsen (2015). Slutrapport: Næringsstofindhold i ris-, havre-, mandel- og sojadrikke. Glostrup, Denmark: Ministry of Environment and Food of Denmark.
103. Konde ÅB, Bjerselius R, Haglund L, Jansson A, Pearson M, Färnstrand JS, et al. Råd om bra matvanor - risk- och nyttohanteringsrapport. Uppsala, Sweden: Livsmedelsverket; 2015, Rapport 5.
104. Gardner CD, Messina M, Kiazand A, Morris JL, Franke AA. Effect of two types of soy milk and dairy milk on plasma lipids in hypercholesterolemic adults: a randomized trial. J Am Coll Nutr 2007; 26(6): 669–77.
105. Beavers KM, Serra MC, Beavers DP, Cooke MB, Willoughby DS. Soymilk supplementation does not alter plasma markers of inflammation and oxidative stress in postmenopausal women. Nutr Res 2009; 29(9): 616–22.
106. Beavers KM, Serra MC, Beavers DP, Hudson GM, Willoughby DS. The lipid-lowering effects of 4 weeks of daily soymilk or dairy milk ingestion in a postmenopausal female population. J Med Food 2010; 13(3): 650–6.

107. Onning G, Akesson B, Oste R, Lundquist I. Effects of consumption of oat milk, soya milk, or cow's milk on plasma lipids and antioxidative capacity in healthy subjects. Ann Nutr Metab 1998; 42(4): 211–20.
108. Lindstrom C, Voinot A, Forslund A, Holst O, Rascon A, Oste R, et al. An oat bran-based beverage reduce postprandial glycaemia equivalent to yoghurt in healthy overweight subjects. Int J Food Sci Nutr 2015; 66(6): 700–5.
109. Doidge JC, Segal L, Gospodarevskaya E. Attributable risk analysis reveals potential healthcare savings from increased consumption of dairy products. J Nutr 2012; 142(9): 1772–80.
110. Heyman MB, Committee on Nutrition. Lactose intolerance in infants, children, and adolescents. Pediatrics 2006; 118(3): 1279–86.
111. Savaiano DA. Lactose digestion from yogurt: mechanism and relevance. Am J Clin Nutr 2014; 99(5 Suppl): 1251S–5S.
112. Sieber R, Stransky M, de Vrese M. Lactose intolerance and consumption of milk and milk products. Z Ernahrungswiss 1997; 36(4): 375–93.
113. Schoemaker AA, Sprikkelman AB, Grimshaw KE, Roberts G, Grabenhenrich L, Rosenfeld L, et al. Incidence and natural history of challenge-proven cow's milk allergy in European children – EuroPrevall birth cohort. Allergy 2015; 70(8): 963–72.
114. Host A, Halken S, Jacobsen HP, Christensen AE, Herskind AM, Plesner K. Clinical course of cow's milk protein allergy/intolerance and atopic diseases in childhood. Pediatr Allergy Immunol 2002; 13(Suppl 15): 23–8.

*Arne Astrup
Department of Nutrition, Exercise and Sports
Faculty of Science, University of Copenhagen
Noerre Alle 51, DK-2200 Copenhagen N
Denmark
Email: ast@nexs.ku.dk

3

Effects of cereal fiber on leptin resistance and sensitivity in C57BL/6J mice fed a high-fat/cholesterol diet

Ru Zhang[1], Jun Jiao[1], Wei Zhang[1], Zheng Zhang[1], Weiguo Zhang[2], Li-Qiang Qin[1]* and Shu-Fen Han[1]*

[1]Jiangsu Key Laboratory of Preventive and Translational Medicine for Geriatric Disease, Department of Nutrition and Food Hygiene, School of Public Health, Soochow University, Suzhou, China; [2]DSM Nutritional Products Human Nutrition and Health, Beijing, China

Abstract

Background: Cereal fiber is reported to be associated with obesity and metabolic diseases. However, whether cereal fiber improves leptin resistance and sensitivity remains unclear.
Design: For 24 weeks, 48 male C57BL/6J mice were randomly given a normal chow diet (Chow), high-fat/cholesterol diet (HFD), HFD with 0.8% oat fiber (H-oat) or HFD with 0.8% wheat bran fiber (H-wheat). At the end of feeding period, both the serum insulin and leptin levels were determined by ELISA kits. Western blotting was used to assess the protein expressions of the leptin receptor (LepR) and the leptin-signaling pathway in the adipose tissues.
Results: Our results suggested that mice fed oat or wheat bran fiber exhibited lower body weight, serum lipids, as well as insulin and leptin levels. The two cereal fibers potently increased the protein expressions of LepR in the adipose tissue. In addition, protein expressions of Janus kinase 2 (JAK2) and transcription 3 (STAT3) (induced by LepR), which enhances leptin signaling, were significantly higher and the expression of cytokine signaling-3 (SOCS3), which inhibits leptin signaling, was significantly lower in the two cereal fiber groups than in the HFD group.
Conclusion: Taken together, our findings suggest that cereal fiber can improve leptin resistance and sensitivity by the JAK2/STAT3 pathway in C57BL/6J mice fed a HFD; furthermore, oat fiber is more effective in the improvement of leptin sensitivity than wheat bran fiber, in this murine model.

Keywords: *cereal fiber*; *leptin resistance*; *leptin signaling*; *high-fat/cholesterol diet*

Responsible Editor: Per Ole Iversen, University of Oslo, Norway.

Leptin, a peptide hormone mainly secreted by adipocytes, plays a vital role in body weight regulation by suppressing food intake and increasing energy expenditure (1). The effect of leptin on food intake is mediated in part via leptin receptors (LepRs) presented in the hypothalamus. Peripherally applied leptin in rodents induces a central neuronal signaling pathway that involves the activation of a signal transducer and activator of transcription 3 (STAT3) (2). The requirement of this pathway to prevent severe hyperphagia and obesity was recently demonstrated in mice specifically lacking the STAT3-binding site of the LepR (3). After binding to the long LepR, STAT3 becomes phosphorylated by Janus kinase 2 (JAK2) and acts in the nucleus to regulate transcription (4). On the other hand, signaling molecules, such as cytokine signaling-3 (SOCS3), mitigate leptin actions via tyrosine 1,138 of LepR in hypothalamic neurons (5). Thus, a negative feedback mechanism exists in leptin-induced STAT3 signaling, through the induction of SOCS3 (6). Exogenous leptin administration failed as an effective approach to manage obesity, even though therapies that improve leptin sensitivity have become one of the developing alternative approaches to treat obesity and related comorbidities (7, 8).

Cereal fiber has been linked to the prevention of a number of obesity-associated diseases and disorders by decreasing appetite and weight gain (9, 10). Recently, several studies have focused on the metabolic benefits of cereal fiber supplementation, such as body weight management and the improvement of insulin resistance (11, 12). Animal and population studies have demonstrated that fiber can reduce plasma leptin and fiber intake and is inversely associated with plasma leptin concentrations (13, 14). However, the effects of cereal fiber supplementation on leptin resistance and leptin sensitivity remain unclear. Therefore, the aim of the present study was to explore the effects of cereal fiber, including those of oat and wheat bran, on leptin sensitivity by the mechanism of the JAK2/STAT3 signaling pathway in the adipose tissue of mice.

Materials and methods

The treatment of the animals and experiment design

A total of 48 7-week-old male C57BL/6J mice were obtained from SLAC Laboratory Animal Company and housed in an air-conditioned environment (22 ± 2°C) with 60% humidity and a 12-h light–dark cycle. After 14 days of acclimatization, animals were randomly allocated to the following four dietary groups (12 mice in each group): the chow diet (Chow) group, the high-fat/cholesterol diet (HFD) group, the HFD plus 0.8% oat fiber (H-oat) group, and the HFD plus 0.8% wheat bran fiber (H-wheat) group. Chow (3.90 kcal/g) was purchased from Research diets Inc., which contained 11.5% fat, 67.7% carbohydrates, and 20.8% protein. HFD (4.77 kcal/g) was also obtained from Research diets Inc., which contained 46% fat, 34.4% carbohydrates, and 19.6% protein. Oat fiber (OatWell®22) was granted from DSM Nutritional Products Ltd. Wheat bran fiber was obtained from Shanxi Aote Food Science and Technology Company. Dietary fiber was directly mixed with HFD according the above recipe. The animals were allowed access to food and water during the whole experiment *ad lib.* The experiment lasted for 24 weeks. All of the animal studies were treated in accordance with the Guidelines in the Care and Use of Animals and with the approval of the Soochow University Animal Welfare Committee. All possible efforts were made to minimize the suffering and the number of animals used in the present study.

Body weight, serum lipids, and insulin and leptin levels

During the whole experiment, body weights and food intake were recorded weekly. Energy intake was calculated according to food intake and calories content. Blood samples were taken from the retrobulbar vein of fasted mice (12–14 h) at the start, 8th, 16th and 24th week of the diet study. Serum was separated by centrifugation, and stored at -80°C freezer until assayed. After the mice were sacrificed, epididymal adipose tissues were quickly removed and stored at -80°C freezer for further analysis. Serum total cholesterol and triglycerides were determined by enzymatic methods using commercial kits (Applygen Technologies Inc., Beijing, China). Serum insulin and leptin levels were measured by commercial ELISA kits, according to strict specifications (Mercodia, Sweden and Merck Millipore Bioscience, CA, USA). The appropriate detection range for insulin and leptin assay was, respectively, 0.2 μg/L to 6.5 μg/L, 0.23 ng/mL to 30 ng/mL, and the lowest detection level was, respectively, 0.2 μg/L and 0.05 ng/mL.

Western blot analysis in the adipose tissues

Epididymal adipose tissue samples were homogenized in lysis buffer (Beyotime Institute of Biotechnology, Nantong, China) and centrifuged at 13,000 g for 15 min. After collecting the supernatants, the protein concentration was determined, according to the BCA protein assay (Beyotime Institute of Biotechnology, Nantong, China). Equal amounts of protein (50–100 μg) were loaded into 12% sodium dodecyl sulfate-polyacrylamide gel and then transferred to a polyvinylidene difluoride membrane by electrophoretic transfer. Blots were incubated overnight at 4°C with the following primary antibodies: leptin (1:2,000, Abcam), LepR (1:2,000, ImmunoWay), JAK2 (1:1,000, Cell Signaling Technology), STAT3 (1:1,000, Cell Signaling Technology), and SOCS3 (1:1,000, Cell Signaling Technology). Subsequently, blots were washed three times and antigen-antibody complexes were incubated for 1 h at room temperature with Peroxidase AffiniPure goat anti-mouse or anti-rabbit IgG antibody (1:2,000, Jackson ImmunoResarch Laboratories). Antibody reactivity was detected by chemiluminescene ECL Detection Systems (EMD Millipore). To confirm the reproducibility of results, each blot was performed at least three times. The intensity of the bands was normalized, using each corresponding β-actin density as an internal control.

Statistical analysis

All statistical parameters were calculated using an SPSS version 17.0 statistical analysis package (SPSS Inc., Chicago, IL, USA) and expressed as a mean and standard deviation (SD). One-way ANOVA was used to analyze differences among groups, followed by the LSD post hoc test. A $p < 0.05$ was considered statistically significant.

Results

After 24 weeks' feeding, a trend of increasing body weights was observed in the four different diet groups. At the end of the 24 weeks' feeding experiment, body weights did not differ between the two groups of H-oat and H-wheat, but were much lower in the HFD group ($p < 0.01$) (Fig. 1a). Interestingly, the H-wheat group tended to have higher average food intake and energy intake compared with the two HFD and H-oat groups during the whole experiment (all $p < 0.05$) (Fig. 1b and c).

Ten animals from 48 mice were randomly selected to measure serum total cholesterol and triglycerides as a baseline. After 24 weeks' feeding, compared with the HFD group, H-oat and H-wheat decreased the serum total cholesterol and triglycerides concentration (all $p < 0.05$)

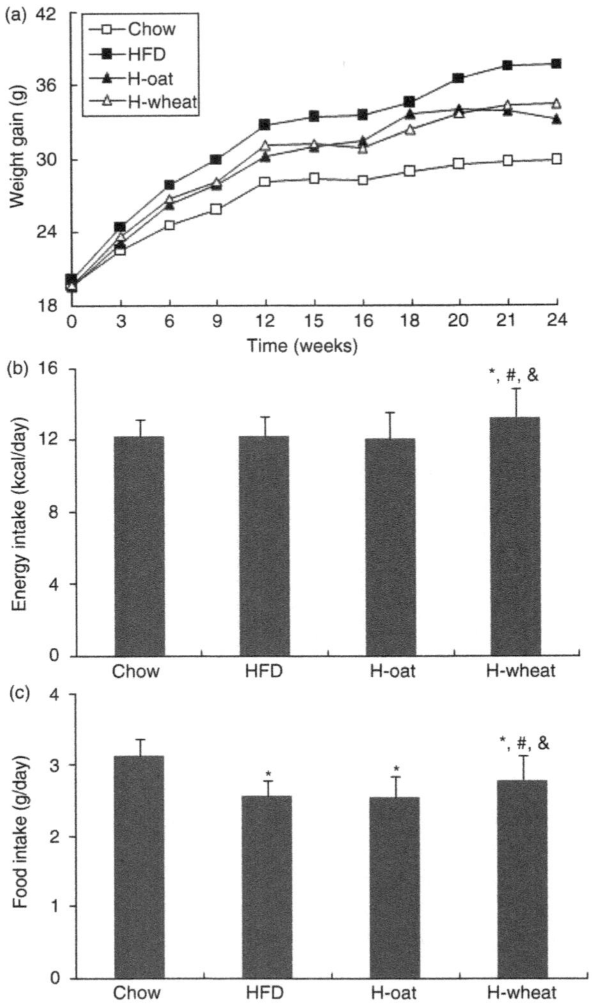

Fig. 1. Changes in body weights (a), the food intake (b), and the energy intake (c) of mice in the four diet groups during the whole experiment. Data are means for 12 mice with SD represented by vertical bars. The mean value was significantly different from that of the chow group at $^{*}p < 0.05$, from that of the HFD group at $^{\#}p < 0.05$, and from that of the H-oat group at $^{\&}p < 0.05$. HFD, high-fat diet; H-oat, high-fat diet supplemented with 0.8% oat fiber; H-wheat, high-fat diet supplemented with 0.8% wheat bran fiber.

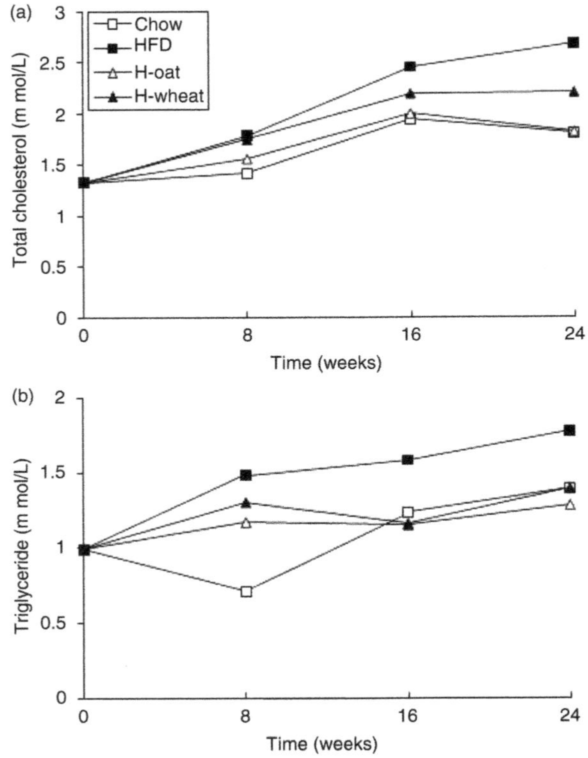

Fig. 2. Changes in the total cholesterol (a) and triglycerides (b) of mice in the four diet groups during the whole experiment. Data are the means for 10 ~ 12 mice with SD represented by vertical bars. HFD, high-fat diet; H-oat, high-fat diet supplemented with 0.8% oat fiber; H-wheat, high-fat diet supplemented with 0.8% wheat bran fiber.

(Fig. 2a and b). As shown in Fig. 3, serum insulin and leptin levels were also measured. Compared with the Chow-fed mice, the HFD-fed mice exhibited a significant increase in serum insulin and leptin levels. Compared with the HFD group, the serum insulin level was significantly lower in the H-oat group, and serum leptin levels were significantly lower in the two fiber groups of H-oat and H-wheat (all $p < 0.05$). No significant difference was observed in the serum insulin of the HFD and H-wheat groups ($p > 0.05$). Compared with the H-wheat group, concentrations of serum insulin or leptin showed a decreasing trend in the H-oat group, but there were no significant differences in the two groups (all $p > 0.05$).

Figure 4 shows the effects of oat fiber and wheat bran fiber on the leptin-signaling pathway in adipose tissues. Compared with the HFD group, the protein expression of leptin, LepR, and STAT3 was higher and that of SOCS3 was lower in the two groups of H-oat and H-wheat (all $p < 0.05$), and JAK2 was higher in the H-oat group. In addition, there were significant differences in the expression of these proteins, except LepR, in the two groups of H-oat and H-wheat (all $p < 0.05$).

Discussion

A high cereal fiber intake is emphasized in the recommendations of most nutritional and metabolic associations. In the present study, we found that cereal fiber from oat or wheat bran improved leptin resistance and sensitivity by increasing the protein expressions of JAK2 and STAT3 (which sensitizes the leptin signaling), and by decreasing the protein expression of SOCS3 (which blunts the leptin signaling). In addition, the effects of oat fiber on JAK2/STAT3 signaling were more significant than those of wheat bran fiber.

Our present findings showed that long-term HFD resulted in additional body weight gain, and increased

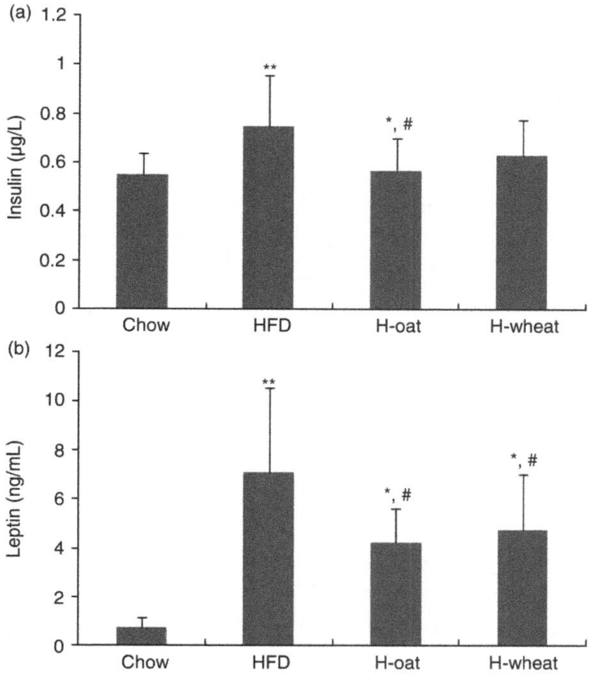

Fig. 3. Changes in the serum leptin (a) and insulin (b) of mice in the four diet groups during the whole experiment. Data are means for 12 mice with SD represented by vertical bars. The mean value was significantly different from that of the Chow group at $^{**}p < 0.01$, and from that of the HFD group at $^{\#}p < 0.05$. HFD, high-fat diet; H-oat, high-fat diet supplemented with 0.8% oat fiber; H-wheat, high-fat diet supplemented with 0.8% wheat bran fiber.

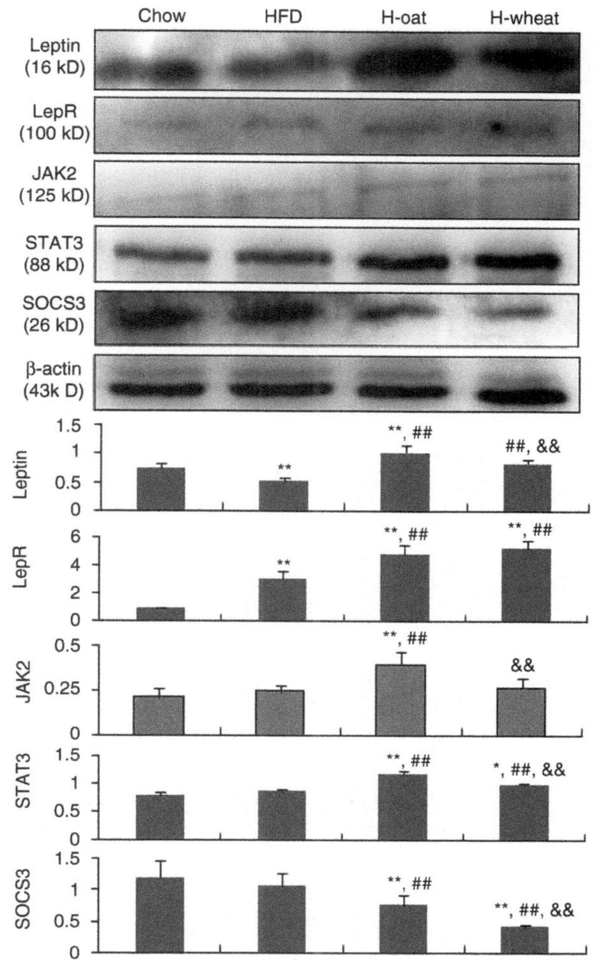

Fig. 4. The relative protein expression of leptin, LepR, JAK2, STAT3, and SOCS3 in the four diet groups. The intensity of the bands was quantified by densitometric analysis and normalized with corresponding β-actin. Data are means for six mice with SD represented by vertical bars. The mean value was significantly different from that of the Chow group at $^{*}p < 0.05$ or $^{**}p < 0.01$, from that of the HFD group at $^{\#\#}p < 0.01$, and from that of the H-oat group at $^{\&\&}p < 0.01$. HFD, high-fat diet; H-oat, high-fat diet supplemented with 0.8% oat fiber; H-wheat, high-fat diet supplemented with 0.8% wheat bran fiber. HFD, high-fat diet; H-oat, high-fat diet supplemented with 0.8% oat fiber; H-wheat, high-fat diet supplemented with 0.8% wheat bran fiber; LepR, leptin receptor; JAK2, Janus kinase 2; STAT3, transcription 3; SOCS3, cytokine signaling-3.

serum total cholesterol and triglycerides levels in the C57BL/6J mice, which were similar to the results of previous studies by our laboratory and others (15, 16). These metabolic abnormalities were blunted in the same animals receiving supplementation with oat or wheat bran fiber. Most animal studies also demonstrated the effect of fiber on weight/fat loss and lipid lowering in diet-induced obese mice (12, 15, 16). Interestingly, the averages of both food intake and energy intake in the H-wheat group were much higher than those in the H-oat group, although there was no significant difference in the final body weights between the two groups. These data suggested that wheat bran fiber, rich in insoluble fiber, may have more effect on body weight management than bran fiber, rich in soluble fiber. Isken found that insoluble fiber was more effective than soluble fiber in controlling body weights (15), which is consistent with our current result. Through a dynamic observation, we found a significantly lower effect on serum lipids in the two cereal fiber groups, compared with the effect on the HFD group, after 16 weeks' feeding. This suggested that a long-time cereal fiber supplementation was positive in its effect on serum lipids, including total cholesterol and triglycerides. This is consistent with the results of animal studies, however, population studies demonstrated that soluble fiber only lowered plasma total cholesterol (17). This decrease may be accounted for a mechanism by which soluble fiber is fermented by intestinal microflora, such that the fermentation could then modify the production of short chain fatty acids, thereby reducing the acetate and increasing the propionate synthesis.

Population studies demonstrated that high fiber intake, particularly soluble fiber, is significantly related to reducing insulin resistance (18). Animal studies demonstrated that soluble fiber decreases the postprandial glucose curve and possibly ameliorates both the resistance and sensitivity to insulin in Zucker Diabetic Fatty rats (11). Our result also showed that a cereal fiber supplement decreased the levels of serum insulin, and oat fiber, rich in soluble fiber, may be better for insulin resistance than wheat bran fiber, rich in insoluble fiber. Serum leptin, which is a cytokine-like hormone predominantly produced in the white adipose tissue and secreted into the systemic circulation, was positively correlated with markers of insulin resistance. Leptin suppresses energy intake and stimulates energy expenditure, leading to a reduction in stored body fat. Some studies indicated that diet-induced obesity may induce leptin resistance, a phenomenon characterized by elevated circulating leptin levels and decreased leptin sensitivity (19). Our results showed that the serum leptin level in the HFD group was the highest, however, after 24-weeks' feeding with HFD-supplemented cereal fiber, while serum leptin levels were significantly inhibited and leptin resistance and sensitivity improved. Several studies observed the effect of fiber-rich diets on modulating leptin secretion and ameliorating leptin resistance in high-fat-diet-fed mice (12, 16). All in all, these results, based on circulating parameters, suggest that cereal fiber has beneficial metabolic health effects via improving leptin resistance and sensitivity.

Leptin exerts its regulatory effects on energy homeostasis through its receptors (LepR) present in the hypothalamus and corresponding signaling pathways. JAK2/STAT3 signaling is a representative signaling pathway through which leptin regulates food intake and energy homeostasis (3, 20). Our results showed that cereal fiber significantly increased the protein expression of leptin and LepR in the adipose tissues. Besides that, our study also showed that cereal fiber increased the protein expression of JAK2 and STAT3 in the adipose tissues. Leptin can bind to its receptors (LepR) and initiate downstream signaling through the sequential phosphorylation of the tyrosine kinase JAK2 and the transcription factor signal transducer and activators of STAT3. Then the phosphorylation STAT binds DNA and modulates the transcription of genes involved in food intake and energy homeostasis (21). SOCS3 is known to inhibit leptin activities. Thus, a negative feedback mechanism exists in leptin-induced STAT3 signaling, through the induction of SOCS3 (6). A recent research that investigated the role of SOCS3 in the regulation of leptin sensitivity indicated that the inactivation of SOCS3 in LepR-expressing cells protected mice from leptin resistance induced by a high-fat diet (7). In the present study, the protein expression of SOCS3 was dramatically down-regulated by cereal fiber. The results suggested that cereal fiber can improve leptin resistance and sensitivity through the JAK2/STAT3 pathway, which may be vital for the maintenance of energy homeostasis through the fine-tuning of a modulatory loop in the molecular network of leptin action. As far as we know, our study is one of the first to explore the effect of cereal fiber on the JAK2/STAT3 pathway. Considering the differences among cereal fiber types on JAK2/STAT3 pathway, we found that oat fiber was more effective than wheat bran fiber. The difference may result from the differences of molecular structure of cereal fiber. Cereal fiber can be considered a 'black box' since its molecular structure can vary significantly (22). The physiological effects of cereal fiber may be related to its molecular structure. However, this issue remains to be elucidated.

In the present study, we did not specifically investigate whether cereal fiber improved leptin resistance in the central nervous system (CNS) and skeletal muscle. However, most of the potential mechanisms underlying leptin resistance have been explored in the CNS (23, 24), and very little has been published regarding leptin resistance in peripheral tissues. It is still controversial whether leptin resistance resides mainly in the CNS or in peripheral tissues (25). Thus, further studies are needed to elucidate whether cereal fiber also effectively improves leptin resistance and sensitivity in the CNS. In addition, the signaling pathways known to mediate the actions of leptin resistance also include PI3K–Akt–FoxO1 signaling, AMP-activated protein kinase (AMPK) signaling, and mTOR–S6K signaling. The precise molecular mechanisms of cereal fiber on leptin resistance and sensitivity in-depth remain to be elucidated, in order to promote the proof that cereal fiber prevents obesity-associated diseases.

In conclusion, the present study suggests that a high cereal-fiber intake can improve HFD-induced leptin resistance and sensitivity through the leptin signal pathway in the adipose tissue. Specifically, cereal fiber increases leptin signaling by enhancing the expression of JAK2 and STAT3 (induced by LepR), and inhibiting the expression of SOCS3. In addition, oat fiber is more effective in the improvement of leptin resistance and sensitivity than wheat bran fiber.

References

1. Ahima RS, Flier JS. Leptin. Annu Rev Physiol 2000; 62: 413–37.
2. Vaisse C, Halaas JL, Horvath CM, Darnell JE, Jr., Stoffel M, Friedman JM. Leptin activation of STAT3 in the hypothalamus of wild-type and ob/ob mice but not db/db mice. Nat Genet 1996; 14: 95–7.
3. Bates SH, Stearns WH, Dundon TA, Schubert M, Tso AWK, Wang YP, et al. STAT3 signalling is required for leptin regulation of energy balance but not reproduction. Nature 2003; 421: 856–9.
4. Bjorbaek C, Kahn BB. Leptin signaling in the central nervous system and the periphery. Recent Prog Horm Res 2004; 59: 305–31.
5. Howard JK, Flier JS. Attenuation of leptin and insulin signaling by SOCS proteins. Trends Endocrinol Metab 2006; 17: 365–71.

6. Starr R, Willson TA, Viney EM, Murray LJL, Rayner JR, Jenkins BJ, et al. A family of cytokine-inducible inhibitors of signalling. Nature 1997; 387: 917–21.
7. Pedroso JA, Buonfiglio DC, Cardinali LI, Furigo IC, Ramos-Lobo AM, Tirapegui J, et al. Inactivation of SOCS3 in leptin receptor-expressing cells protects mice from diet-induced insulin resistance but does not prevent obesity. Mol Metab 2014; 3: 608–18.
8. Myers MG, Jr., Heymsfield SB, Haft C, Kahn BB, Laughlin M, Leibel RL, et al. Challenges and opportunities of defining clinical leptin resistance. Cell Metab 2012; 15: 150–6.
9. Cho SS, Qi L, Fahey GC, Jr., Klurfeld DM. Consumption of cereal fiber, mixtures of whole grains and bran, and whole grains and risk reduction in type 2 diabetes, obesity, and cardiovascular disease. Am J Clin Nutr 2013; 98: 594–619.
10. Wanders AJ, van den Borne JJ, de Graaf C, Hulshof T, Jonathan MC, Kristensen M, et al. Effects of dietary fibre on subjective appetite, energy intake and body weight: a systematic review of randomized controlled trials. Obes Rev 2011; 12: 724–39.
11. Brockman DA, Chen X, Gallaher DD. Hydroxypropyl methylcellulose, a viscous soluble fiber, reduces insulin resistance and decreases fatty liver in Zucker Diabetic Fatty rats. Nutr Metab (Lond) 2012; 9: 100.
12. Wang ZQ, Zuberi AR, Zhang XH, Macgowan J, Qin J, Ye X, et al. Effects of dietary fibers on weight gain, carbohydrate metabolism, and gastric ghrelin gene expression in mice fed a high-fat diet. Metabolism 2007; 56: 1635–42.
13. Islam A, Civitarese AE, Hesslink RL, Gallaher DD. Viscous dietary fiber reduces adiposity and plasma leptin and increases muscle expression of fat oxidation genes in rats. Obesity (Silver Spring) 2012; 20: 349–55.
14. Kuroda M, Ohta M, Okufuji T, Takigami C, Eguchi M, Hayabuchi H, et al. Frequency of soup intake and amount of dietary fiber intake are inversely associated with plasma leptin concentrations in Japanese adults. Appetite 2010; 54: 538–43.
15. Isken F, Klaus S, Osterhoff M, Pfeiffer AF, Weickert MO. Effects of long-term soluble vs. insoluble dietary fiber intake on high-fat diet-induced obesity in C57BL/6J mice. J Nutr Biochem 2010; 21: 278–84.
16. Han SF, Jiao J, Zhang W, Xu JY, Wan ZX, Zhang WG, et al. Dietary fiber prevents obesity-related liver lipotoxicity by modulating sterol-regulatory element binding protein pathway in C57BL/6J mice fed a high-fat/cholesterol diet. Sci Rep 2015; 5: 15256.
17. Brown L, Rosner B, Willett WW, Sacks FM. Cholesterol-lowering effects of dietary fiber: a meta-analysis. Am J Clin Nutr 1999; 69: 30–42.
18. Breneman CB, Tucker L. Dietary fibre consumption and insulin resistance – the role of body fat and physical activity. Br J Nutr 2013; 110: 375–83.
19. Friedman JM, Halaas JL. Leptin and the regulation of body weight in mammals. Nature 1998; 395: 763–70.
20. Kwon O, Kim KW, Kim MS. Leptin signalling pathways in hypothalamic neurons. Cell Mol Life Sci 2016; 73: 1457–77.
21. Akira S. Functional roles of STAT family proteins: lessons from knockout mice. Stem Cells 1999; 17: 138–46.
22. Gemen R, De Vries JF, Slavin JL. Relationship between molecular structure of cereal dietary fiber and health effects: focus on glucose/insulin response and gut health. Nutr Rev 2011; 69: 22–33.
23. Howard JK, Cave BJ, Oksanen LJ, Tzameli I, Bjorbaek C, Flier JS. Enhanced leptin sensitivity and attenuation of diet-induced obesity in mice with haploinsufficiency of Socs3. Nat Med 2004; 10: 734–8.
24. Myers MG, Jr. Leptin receptor signaling and the regulation of mammalian physiology. Recent Prog Horm Res 2004; 59: 287–304.
25. Ceddia RB. Direct metabolic regulation in skeletal muscle and fat tissue by leptin: implications for glucose and fatty acids homeostasis. Int J Obes (Lond) 2005; 29: 1175–83.

***Li-Qiang Qin**
Department of Nutrition and Food Hygiene
School of Public Health
Soochow University
199 Renai Road
Suzhou 215123, China
Email: qinliqiang@suda.edu.cn

***Shu-Fen Han**
Department of Nutrition and Food Hygiene
School of Public Health
Soochow University
199 Renai Road
Suzhou 215123, China
Email: sfhan@suda.edu.cn

4

Hypolipidemic effects of chitosan and its derivatives in hyperlipidemic rats induced by a high-fat diet

Haitao Pan[1†], Qingyun Yang[1†], Guidong Huang[1], Chen Ding[1], Peiqiu Cao[1], Lanlan Huang[1], Tiancun Xiao[2,3], Jiao Guo[1]* and Zhengquan Su[1]*

[1]Key Research Center of Liver Regulation for Hyperlipidemia SATCM/Class III Laboratory of Metabolism SATCM, Guangdong TCM Key Laboratory for Metabolic Diseases, Guangdong Pharmaceutical University, Guangzhou, China; [2]Inorganic Chemistry Laboratory, Oxford University, Oxford, United Kingdom; [3]Guangzhou Boxabio Ltd, D-106 Guangzhou International Business Incubator, Guangzhou Science City, Guangzhou, China

Abstract

Background: Hyperlipidemia (HLP) is the primary risk factor of cardiovascular disease (CVD). Various factors, including genetics, physical inactivity, and daily nutritional habits, affect the prevalence of HLP. Recently, it was revealed that dietary fibers, such as pectin, psyllium, and especially chitosan (CTS), may play important roles in hypolipidemic management. Thus, this study aims to determine the hypolipidemic effect and mechanism of CTS and its water-soluble derivatives, chitosan oligosaccharides ($M_N \leq 1{,}000$ Da (COSI) and $M_N \leq 3{,}000$ Da (COSIII)), in male hyperlipidemic rats induced by a high-fat diet (HFD).

Design: After the model creation, 120 Sprague-Dawley (SD) rats were equally assigned to 12 groups fed various diets as follows: the normal group with basic diet, an HFD group, an HFD group supplemented with three doses of CTS, COSI and COSIII groups, and an HFD group treated with simvastatin (7 mg/kg·d). After 6 weeks, body weight, fat/body ratio, and the relevant biomarkers of serum, liver, and feces were measured. Additionally, the histological analysis of liver and adipose tissue was performed, and the mRNA expressions of liver peroxisome proliferator-activated receptor-α (PPARα) and hepatic lipase (HL) were examined.

Results: Compared with HFD group, rats fed CTS, COSI, and COSIII showed a better ability to regulate their body weight, liver and cardiac indices, fat/body ratio, as well as serum, liver, and fecal lipids, and simultaneously to maintain the appropriate activity of liver and serum superoxide dismutase (SOD), alanine aminotransferase (ALT), aspartate aminotransferase (AST), as well as liver and fecal total bile acids (TBA). Simultaneously, there had been a higher mRNA expression of PPARα and HL in the treatment groups.

Conclusion: The obtained results suggested that these three function foods can effectively improve liver lipid metabolism by normalizing the expressions of PPARα and HL, and protect liver from the oxidized trauma by enhancing hepatic function, which could be potentially used to remedy hyperlipidemia.

Keywords: *chitosan*; *chitosan oligosaccharides*; *hypolipidemic effect*; *high-fat diet*; *PPARα*

Hyperlipidemia (HLP), characterized by abnormal levels of serum lipids and the dysregulation of lipid metabolism, is the primary risk factor contributing to the formation and progression of atherosclerosis (AS) and subsequent cardiovascular disease (CVD) (1, 2). Recently, increasing studies have focused on how to improve serum lipid concentrations and the absorption of fat in the gastrointestinal tract to remit diet-related chronic diseases, some of which indicated that dietary fibers, such as pectin, psyllium, and chitosan, may display potent hypolipidemic effects (3, 4).

Chitosan (CTS), a kind of de-acetylated derivative of chitin, is a natural polymer of glucosamine derived from the cell walls of some fungi and the exoskeleton of crustaceans, including shrimps, crabs, lobsters, and prawns (5, 6). CTS has beneficial effects on serum lipids, including total cholesterol (TC), triglyceride (TG), and low-density lipoprotein cholesterol (LDL-C), as well as body weight gain (7–9). As the small molecular derivatives of CTS, chitosan oligosaccharides (COS) have shown the better water-solubility and thus can be digested and absorbed more easily by the gastrointestinal tract in animals and

[†]These authors have equally contributed to this work.

humans, which may make them more efficient hypolipidemic and weight-lowering functional food especially in western countries (10–12). Notably in Japan, as the dietary supplements, CTS and COS are the only function foods can be disseminated in public. In this study, we compared the hypolipidemic and hepatoprotective functions of CTS and its derivatives (COSI and COSIII) for the very first time. Additionally, we testified that whether CTS and COS can effectively better the process that liver cholesterol are translated into bile acid, which is useful for improving hyperlipidemia.

To further explore the in-depth molecular mechanisms of CTS and COS regulating the process above, we examined the mRNA expressions of two important regulating factors in the liver: peroxisome proliferator-activated receptor-α (PPARα), a ligand-activated transcription factor involved in the regulation of various aspects of liver lipid metabolisms (13, 14), and its target regulatory proteins, hepatic lipase (HL), which can catalyze TG hydrolysis in chylomicrons (CM) and VLDL-C for tissue use in the form of free fatty acid (FFA) and monoacylglycerol, and provide high-density lipoprotein (HDL) with apolipoproteins and phospholipids for the reverse cholesterol transport (RCT) process (15, 16). Therefore, we speculated about the regulating function of CTS and its derivatives for lipid metabolism via up-regulating the expressions of liver PPARα and HL mRNA levels, which further contributes to the RCT process.

In the present study, we first testified that CTS, COSI, and COSIII can really improve the hepatic cholesterol metabolism by up-regulating the expression levels of liver PPARα and HL mRNA in male hyperlipidemic SD rats induced by HFD. In addition, we also confirmed that the hepatoprotective effects of these foods can significantly contribute to the improvement of liver lipid metabolism in the hyperlipidemic rats.

Materials and methods

Materials and regents

CTS (Lot, 10321A; viscosity, >200 mP/s; degree of deacetylation, 96.2%) was purchased from Shandong Aokang Biotech Ltd. (Shandong, China). COSI (Lot, HL130813G; $M_N \leq 1{,}000$ g.mol^{-1}; degree of deacetylation, 95.6%) and COSIII (Lot, HL130921G; $M_N \leq 3{,}000$ g.mol^{-1}; degree of deacetylation, 91.1%) were obtained from Shandong Laizhou Highly Bio-Products Co., Ltd. (Shandong, China). Simvastatin tablets were supplied from Merck Sharp & Dohme Pharmaceutical Company Limited (Hangzhou, Zhejiang, China). Triacylglycerol (TG), total cholesterol (TC), HDL cholesterol (HDL-C), LDL-C, and total bile acid (TBA) kits were purchased from BioSino Biotechnology and Science Inc. (Beijing, China). Superoxide dismutase (SOD), alanine aminotransferase (ALT), and aspartate aminotransferase (AST) assay kits were purchased from the Nanjing Jiancheng Bioengineering Institute (Nanjing, China). All other reagents and solvents were of analytical grade.

Animals and diets

One-hundred twenty male SPF Sprague–Dawley (SD) rats (weight, 200±20 g; age, 8 weeks) were used for animal experiments. The rats were supplied by the Guangdong Medical Laboratory Animal Center (GMLAC, Guangzhou, China). All animal experimental protocols were approved by the Institutional Animal Care and Use Committee of Guangdong Pharmaceutical University (Guangzhou, China). The rats were maintained in a SPF room at a temperature of 23–25°C, related humidity of 40–70%, and a differential pressure no less than 10 Pa under a constant day-night rhythm. Rats were given water ad libitum throughout the experiments. All animals were provided standard rodent chow (Guangdong Pharmaceutical University Laboratory Animal Center, Guangzhou, China) for 1 week. Then, the 120 rats were divided into two groups: the normal group (NF, $n = 10$) fed randomly with the basic diet and the HFD group ($n = 110$) were fed an HFD to obtain the hyperlipidemic model.

The basic diet was composed of 20.0% total crude protein, 4.3% total crude fat, 4.8% total crude fiber, 9.7% moisture, 1.19% calcium, 0.77% phosphorus, $Ca^{2+}/P^{5-} = 1.55$, 6.6% crude ash. The test results showed that total bacterial count (<10 cfu/g), the *Escherichia coli* count (<3.0 MPN/100 g), total molds and yeasts (<10 cfu/g), and salmonella (not detected) all met the stipulated standards. The HFD was composed of 52.6% basic feed, 20.0% sucrose, 15.0% lard, 1.2% cholesterol, 0.2% bile salts, 10% casein, 0.6% calcium hydrophosphate, and 0.4% mountain flour in SPF packaging (provided by GMLAC (No. 20130823)). After 2 weeks, blood samples were collected from the orbital vein using a capillary under ether anesthesia. The blood samples were centrifuged (4°C, 3,500 r·min^{-1}, 15 min) to obtain plasma samples to determine serum TC, TG, and LDL-C levels, which were the basis of the desired HLP model.

The 110 model rats were randomly divided into 11 groups for the additional feeding study: (1) HFD group (HF) fed with HFD ad libitum only; (2) HFD group treated with simvastatin (7 mg/kg·d) (SV); (3) HFD supplemented with high (1,000 mg/kg·d), middle (500 mg/kg·d), and low (250 mg/kg·d) dose CTS groups (CTS-H, CTS-M, and CTS-L, respectively); (4) HFD supplemented with high (1,000 mg/kg·d), middle (500 mg/kg·d), and low (250 mg/kg·d) dose COSI groups (COSI-H, COSI-M, and COSI-L, respectively); (5) HFD supplemented with high (1,000 mg/kg·d), middle (500 mg/kg·d), and low (250 mg/kg·d) dose COSIII groups (COSIII-H, COSIII-M, and COSIII-L, respectively). The high, middle, and low doses of CTS, COSI, and COSIII were carried out according to reference (17). Each group consisted of 10 animals. The corresponding foods were administered orally by gavage at a dose of 1 mL/100 g per day at the same time for 6 weeks until the study ended. As the control animals, the rats in the HF and NF groups were simultaneously administered with 1 mL/100 g distilled water by the same way above. All rats, including the NF group were sacrificed at 16 weeks old.

Experimental design

Measurement of food intake and body weight gain

The 24 h food intake of rats were recorded every day, body weight, body length, and abdominal girth were measured every week during the experimental period.

Measurement of fecal TC, TG and TBA

Three days before the end of the experiments, 72 h feces were collected from each group and dried to a constant weight for smashing and blending. Then, 3.0 mL of 95% ethyl alcohol was used to dissolve 0.25 g of the resulting powder. This suspension was placed in a water bath for three times for 30 min at 60°C until ethyl alcohol volatilization. Then, the solution was transferred to 10 mL of 60% acetic acid to measure TC, TG, and TBA using the respective commercial assay kits.

Determination of serum lipids, ALT and AST

Serum was prepared from blood by centrifugation at 3,000 rpm for 15 min at 4°C, and stored at –70°C until the analysis of the lipid parameters. Plasma TC, TG, HDL-C, and LDL-C levels were measured with commercial assay kits using an Automated Biochemistry Analyzer BC200 (Beijing Precil Instrument Co. Ltd, Beijing, China). The activity of plasma ALT and AST were analyzed with ALT and AST assay kits, respectively, using a Mithras LB 940 Multimode Microplate Reader (Berthold Technologies GmBH & Co. KG, Germany).

Measurement of fat/body ratio and visceral indices

Rats were subjected to ether anesthesia, sacrificed, and necropsied after serum preparation. The heart, liver, kidney, perirenal white adipose tissue, and epididymal white adipose tissue were quickly removed and weighed on ice. A picture was taken of the whole liver from each animal, and the total weight of the perirenal and epididymal white adipose tissues were used to determine the fat/body ratio (Fat/body ratio = fat mass/body mass). We also measured the wet weight of the heart, liver, and kidneys for each visceral index. Tissues were immediately stored at −80°C following the biopsy for further analysis.

Determination of liver lipids, TBA, and SOD

The liver lipid contents were measured as follows: a piece (approximately 0.1 g) of liver tissue was homogenized in chloroform-methanol (1:1, v/v, 2 mL) and the homogenate was extracted with the extracting solution described above (3 mL) by shaking the tubes horizontally for 24 h. The lipid mixtures were centrifuged at 3,000 rpm for 5 min, and the upper aqueous phase was aspirated to determine the liver lipid content using commercial assay kits.

Rat liver TBA contents were determined using the following methods: 0.5 g of liver tissue was homogenized in sodium chloride solution (0.9%, 2 mL) in an ice-water bath, the resulting homogenate (1 mL) was homogenized three times in acetic acid (60%, 9 mL) and the final homogenate was extracted by shaking the tubes horizontally for 10 min. The mixtures were centrifuged at 4,000 rpm for 10 min, and the upper aqueous phase was used to measure liver TBA contents using commercial assay kits.

Liver SOD activity was measured as follows: approximately 0.1 g of liver tissue was homogenized in a sodium chloride solution (0.9%, 0.9 mL) in an ice-water bath. The homogenate was centrifuged at 2,500 rpm for 10 min, and the upper aqueous phase was diluted 10 times to determine liver SOD activity using commercially available analytical kits and the Mithras LB 940 Multimode Microplate Reader.

Quantitative RT-PCR analysis

Total RNA was isolated from rat livers using TRIzol reagent (Invitrogen, Inc., USA). Single-stranded cDNA was synthesized from 1 μg of total RNA using the PrimeScript^{TM} RT reagent kit with gDNA Eraser (TaKaRa, Code NO. RR047A, Japan) using the following conditions: 37°C for 15 min, 85°C for 5 s, and storage at 4°C. cDNA products were quantified by real-time RT-PCR using a TaKaRa SYBR Premix EX Taq^{TM} kit (TaKaRa, Code NO. RR420A, Japan) and Bio-Rad IQ5 real-time PCR system and analysis software (Applied Biosystems, Canada). The primer sequences used for PCR were designed and synthesized by Sangon Biotech (Shanghai) Co., Ltd. Glyceraldehyde-3-phosphate Dehydrogenase (GAPDH) was used as internal control (Housekeeping gene). The sequences of the forward and reverse primers used for amplification were as follows:

PPARα: Forward: 5′-GAGGTCCGATTCTTCCACTG-3′
Reverse: 5′-GCATCCCGTCTTTGTTCATC-3′
HL: Forward: 5′-AAATCTCCGTTTCCCTGGTG-3′
Reverse: 5′-GGCGGTCACTTTCATCTTTG-3′
GAPDH: Forward: 5′-ACAGCAACAGGGTGGTGGAC-3′
Reverse: 5′-TTTGAGGGTGCAGCGAACTT-3′.

PCR protocols were performed as follows: 95°C for 30 s (initial denaturation), followed by 39–40 cycles at 95°C for 5 s and 60°C for 30 s. Melt curve analyses were performed with each series to confirm the specificity of the primers and amplified products using the following parameters: heated the amplified products from 65°C to 95°C at 0.5°C steps for 5 s. Relative quantification of mRNA expression was analyzed by the $2^{-\Delta\Delta Ct}$ method.

Histology of different tissues

The liver, white subcutaneous, and mesenteric adipose tissues were cut into 0.5 cm^3, washed with saline, and placed in the tissue cassette. The cassettes were marked with a pencil, and then placed into 12% formaldehyde solution to fix for 24 h. Residual fixative was washed away by the distilled water. These tissues were dehydrated by 30, 50, 70, 80, 90, 95, and 100% ethanol, embedded in paraffin (BMJ-III embedding machine, Changzhou Electronic Instrument Factory, Jiangsu, China), and then cut into 5 μm thick sections using a the slicing instrument (Leica RM2235; Leica, Heidelberg, Germany). The tissues were stained with hematoxylin and eosin (H&E) and observed under a microscope with 200 magnifications.

Statistical analysis

All data are expressed as the mean ± SE. Differences between groups were determined by one-way ANOVA using SPSS for Windows, version 19.0 (SPSS Inc., Chicago, IL, USA). Significant differences among means were determined using Student–Newman–Keuls multiple range tests, and a $p < 0.05$ was considered statistically significant.

Results and discussion

Food intake, body weight gain, fat/body ratio, and visceral indices

Six-week food intake, body weight gain, and fat/body ratio of rats are shown in Fig. 1a–c, respectively. The food intake in the HF group was slightly higher than that of the NF and treatment groups during the experimental period, but the difference was not very significant (Figs. 1a and 2a), which indicates that the lipid- and weight-lowering function of CTS and COS is unrelated to appetite suppression, and the minor decrease of food intake in the treatment groups is due to the fact that the rats generated a slight anorectic effect during the long-term HFD intake, and additionally that the very minimum side effects of CTS and COS, including nausea, vomiting, and constipation, also contributed to the reduced food intake (18).

CTS, COSI, and COSIII can lower body weight gains (Fig. 1b, $p < 0.05$) and fat/body ratio (Fig. 1c, $p < 0.05$) of rats dose-dependently to the normal range when compared with that in the NF and HF groups.

Figure 1d and e displays the visceral (liver and cardiac) indices (visceral index = visceral mass × 100/body mass). The liver index of HF group was clearly higher than that of NF group that is due to the high fat content in HF livers. Treatment experiments revealed that CTS, COSI, and COSIII consistently reduced the liver index in dose-dependent manner ($p < 0.05$). Similarly, cardiac indices in the NF, SV, and all treatment groups were remarkably inferior to that of the HF group ($p < 0.05$), because these foods effectively suppressed the HFD-induced increase in cardiac fat mass and cardiomyocyte hypertrophy. In addition, COSI showed the best decreases of liver

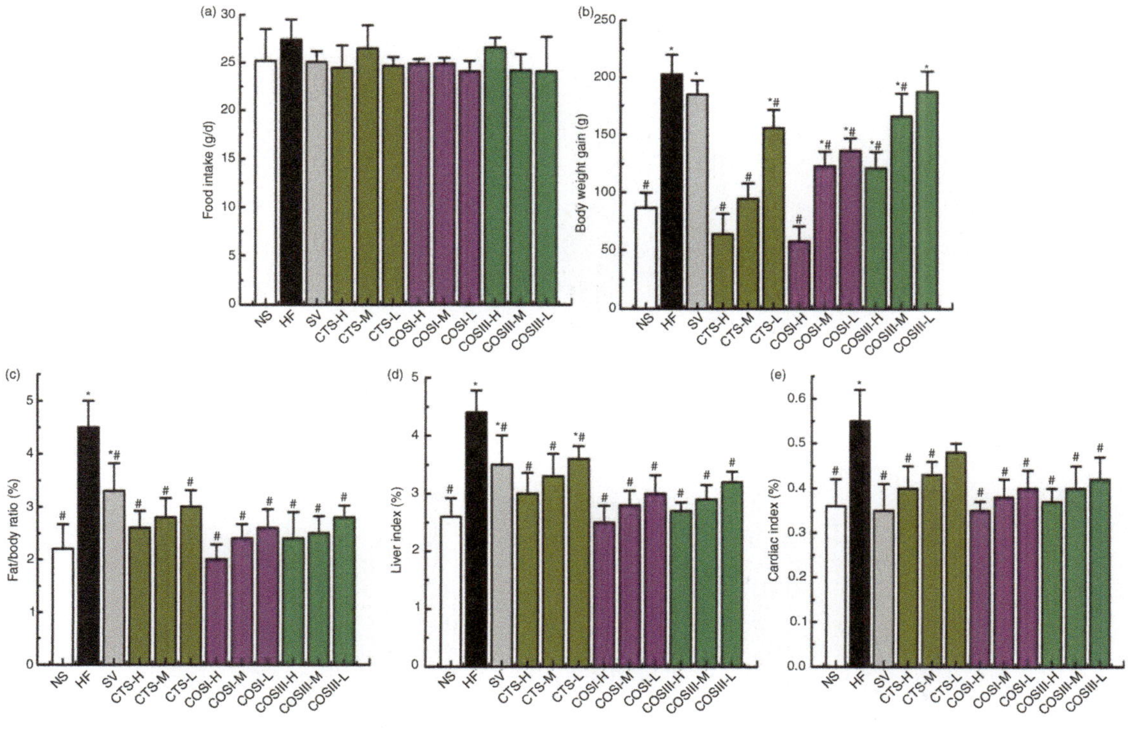

Fig. 1. Changes in food intake (a), body weight gain (b), fat/body ratio (c), liver (d), and cardiac (e) indices in hyperlipidemic rats during the treatment (*$p < 0.05$, significant difference when compared with rats in the NF group; #$p < 0.05$, significant difference when compared with rats in the HF group; same as Figs. 3, 5, 7, and 10). The data are expressed as means ± SD ($n = 10$).

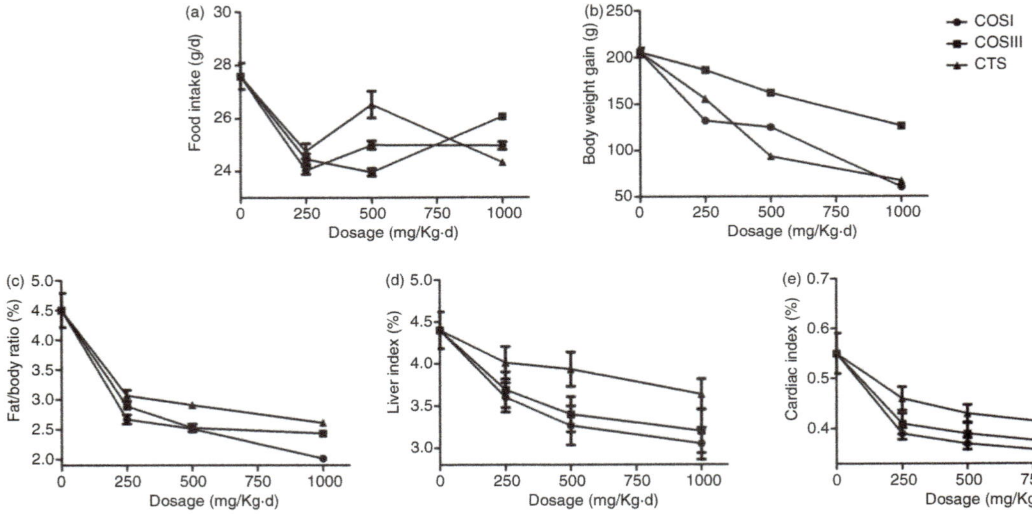

Fig. 2. Comparison of different dose COSI, COSIII, and CTS (HFD only, HFD supplemented with low (250 mg/kg·d), middle (500 mg/kg·d), and high (1,000 mg/kg·d) dose COSI, COSIII, and CTS, respectively) in food intake (a), body weight gain (b), fat/body ratio (c), liver (d), and cardiac (e) indices in hyperlipidemic rats during the treatment.

(Fig. 2d) and cardiac (Fig. 2e) indices compared with other treatment groups. However, there was no reduction in the kidney index of each treatment group (data not shown).

Serum lipids

Currently, statins (i.e. simvastatin) are the most commonly used drugs for treating CHC, especially widely used to lower cholesterol and LDL-C levels, and simultaneously simvastatin can effectively increase levels of PPARα in some recent studies, which are the reasons for choosing simvastatin as the positive control material in this study (19). During the experimental period, serum TC, TG, HDL-C, and LDL-C levels were determined after 2 weeks. TC, TG, and LDL-C concentrations increased significantly in all 11 HFD groups ($p < 0.05$), which became the selective criterion of HLP rats for the next treatment experiment. Figure 3 displays rat plasma lipids levels after

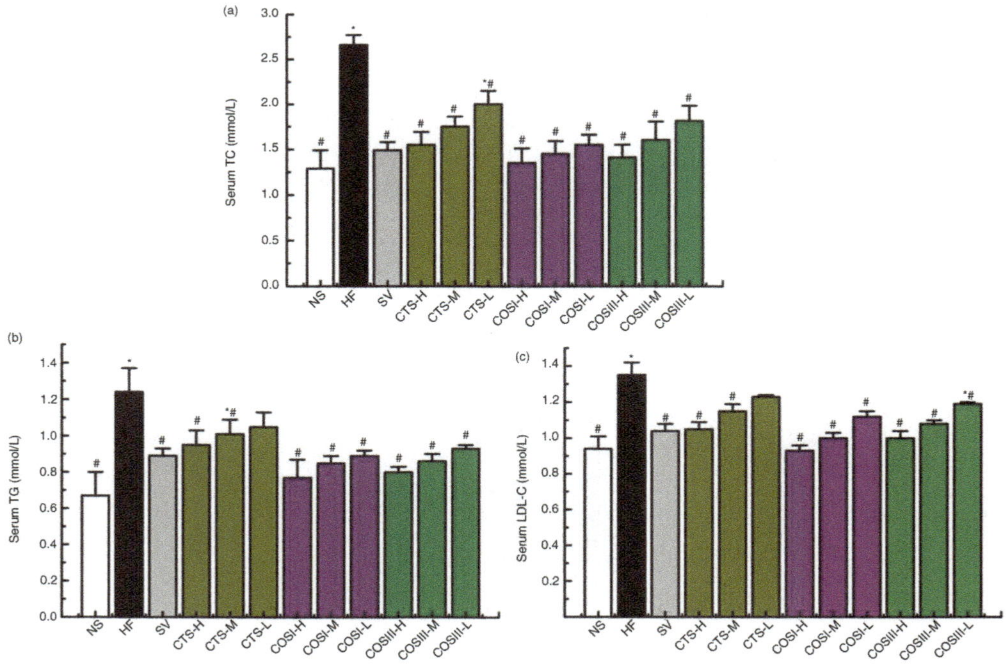

Fig. 3. Effects of CTS, COSI, and COSIII on serum TC (a), TG (b), and LDL-C (c) in hyperlipidemic rats during the treatment. The data are expressed as means ± SD ($n = 10$).

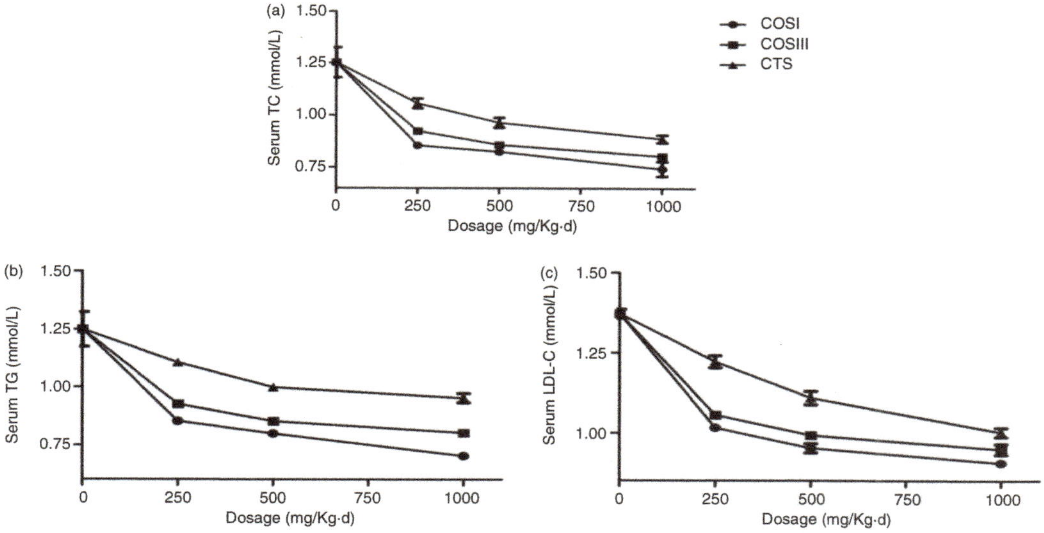

Fig. 4. Comparison of COSI, COSIII, and CTS in serum TC (a), TG (b), and LDL-C (c) in hyperlipidemic rats during the treatment.

an additional 6 weeks. The HF group displayed significantly higher serum TC, TG, and LDL-C compared with the NF group ($p < 0.05$). The high serum TC levels in the CTS, COSI, and COSIII treated groups were significantly reversed in a dose-dependent compared to the HFD group ($p < 0.05$), and the therapeutic effects of COSI and COSIII were equivalent to that of SV. Similar changes were also observed for serum TG concentrations, especially for rats fed with COSI and COSIII, which had lower serum TG levels that were similar to the SV group. CTS, COSI, and COSIII also dramatically improved the high plasma LDL-C levels induced by HFD accompanied by not changing the HDL levels.

In a word, this project successfully established a HLP rat model by feeding an optimized HFD, which displayed remarkably increased serum TC, TG, and LDL-C concentrations, as well as relative indices, including liver index, cardiac index, body weight gain, and fat/body ratio,

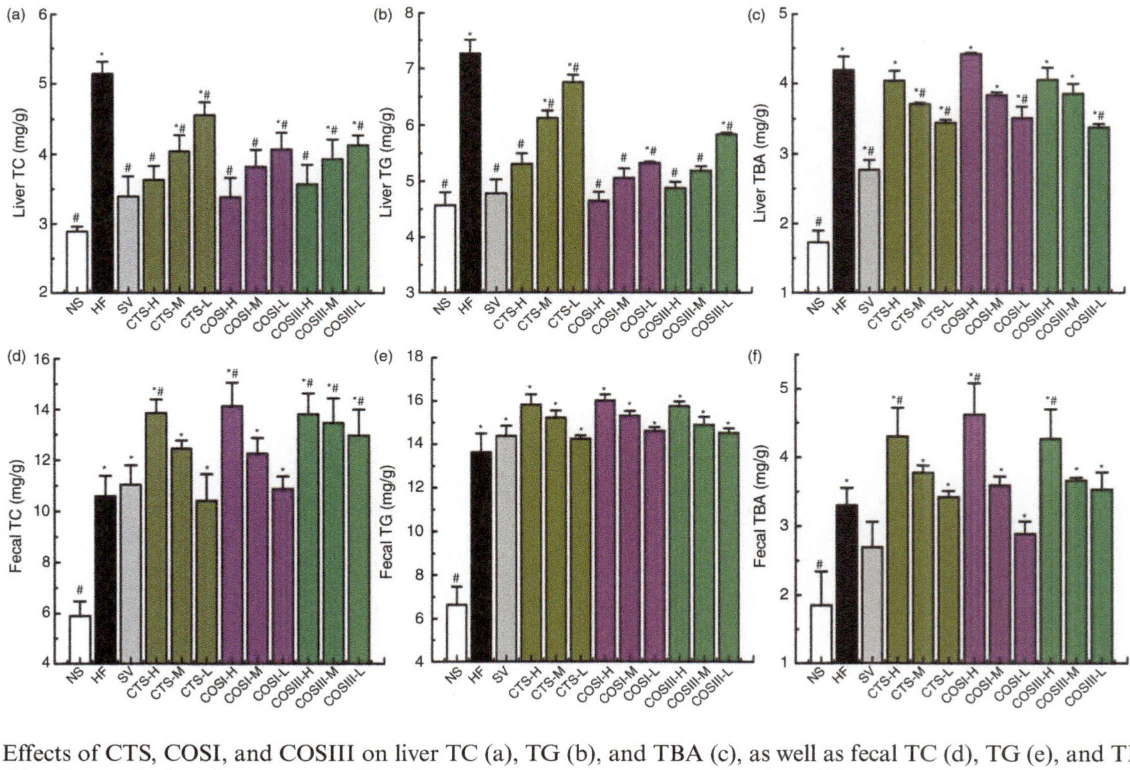

Fig. 5. Effects of CTS, COSI, and COSIII on liver TC (a), TG (b), and TBA (c), as well as fecal TC (d), TG (e), and TBA (f) in hyperlipidemic rats during the treatment. The data are expressed as means ± SD ($n = 10$).

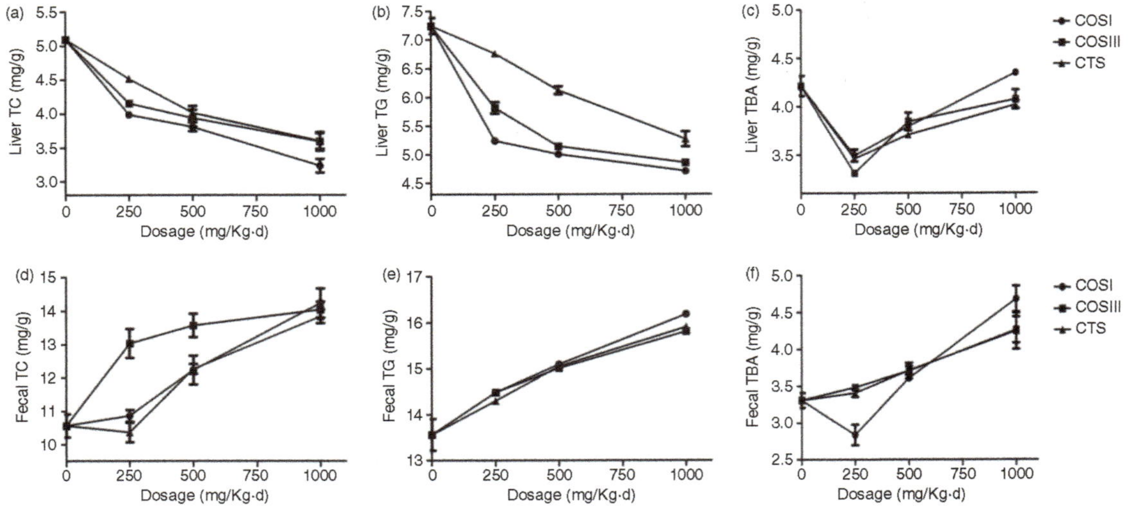

Fig. 6. Comparison of COSI, COSIII, and CTS in liver TC (a), TG (b), and TBA (c), as well as fecal TC (d), TG (e), and TBA (f) in hyperlipidemic rats during the treatment.

when compared with the normal peers. After the 6-week preventative treatment, these indices above were improved in rats fed with different doses of CTS, COSI, and COSIII, which indicated that CTS and its relative derivatives play the vital role in preventing the invasion of HLP with no effect on the appetite of rats (20). Therein, compared with the SV, CTS, and COSIII groups, the three doses of COSI groups showed the better inhibition of increases in rat body weight gain (Fig. 2b), fat/body ratio (Fig. 2c), especially liver index (Fig. 2d), serum TC, TG, and LDL-C levels (Fig. 4a–c). Given its smaller molecular weight, COSI has the better water-solubility and can be digested and absorbed more easily by the gastrointestinal tract in animals and humans.

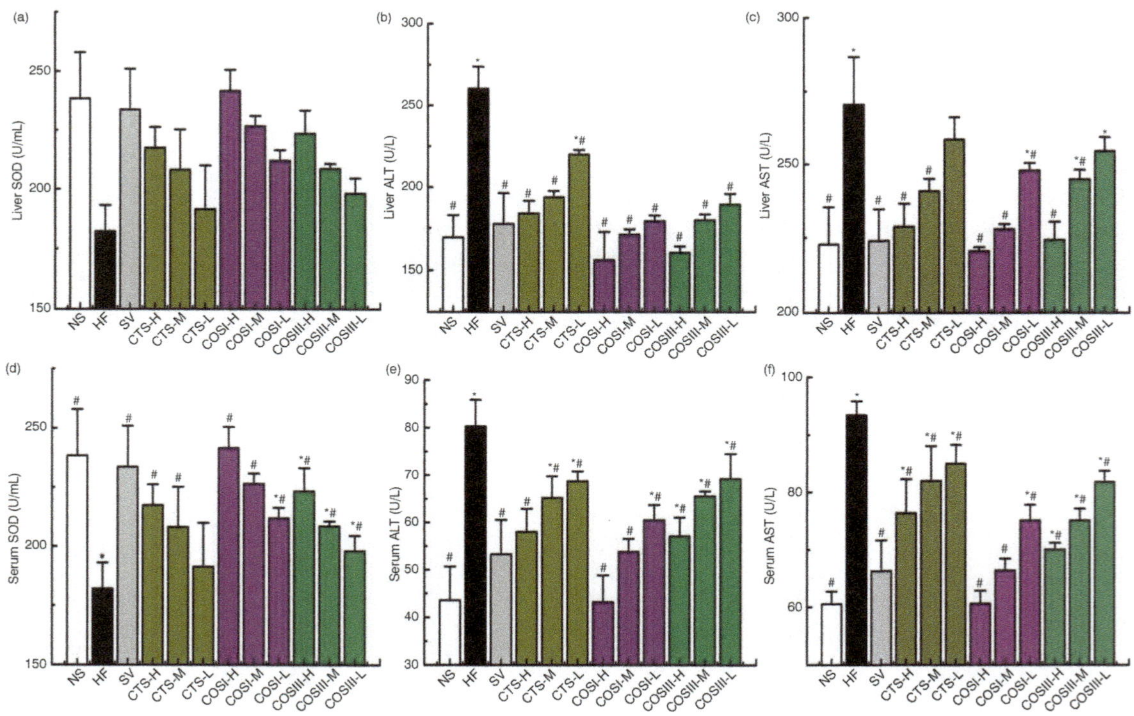

Fig. 7. The hepatoprotective effects of CTS, COSI, and COSIII on hyperlipidemic rats. The liver function test, including the determinations of liver (a) and serum SOD (d), serum ALT (e) and AST (f), liver ALT (b) and AST (c), shows that the three compounds can rectify these indices which contribute to normalizing the liver physiological function. The data are expressed as means ± SD ($n = 10$).

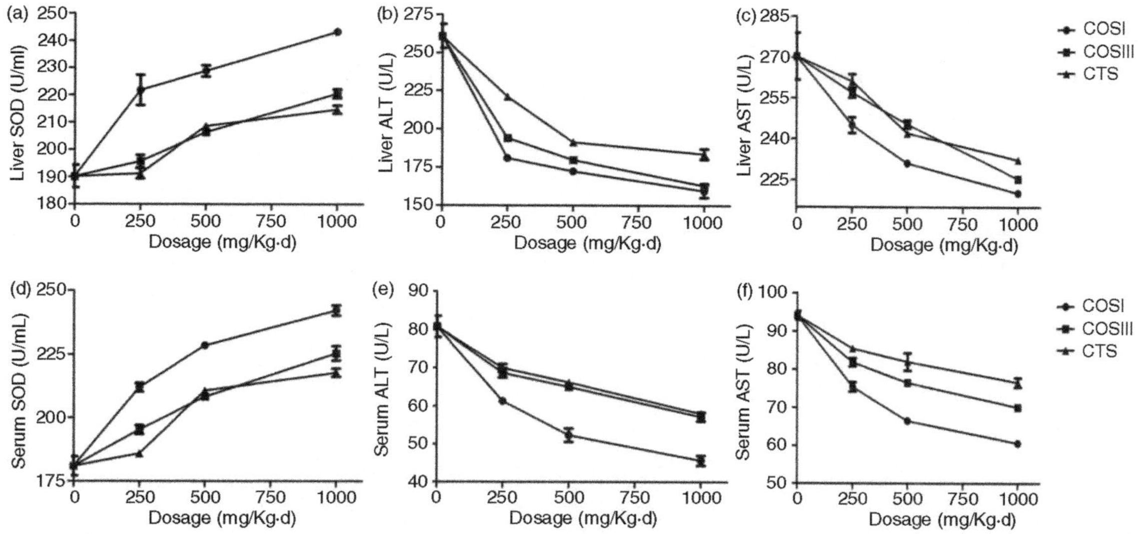

Fig. 8. Comparison of COSI, COSIII, and CTS in liver (a) and serum SOD (d), serum ALT (e) and AST (f), liver ALT (b) and AST (c) in hyperlipidemic rats during the treatment.

Liver and fecal TC, TG and TBA

It is generally accepted that the positive charge in the structure of CTS and COS can vigorously absorb fat, fatty acids (FA) and bile acids (BA), containing a negative charge, which contributes to lowering serum TC and TG (21). Nonetheless, several studies have described the mechanism by which CTS, COSI, and COSIII reduce lipid levels are related to charge as well as the regulation of liver lipid metabolism (3, 8, 9, 17). To remove excess cholesterol, it must be transported from the peripheral tissues to the liver and intestine, where it is finally excreted in the form of BA via the feces. The metabolic pathway is traditionally considered the RCT or centripetal cholesterol flux pathway (22). In order to determine the effects of the three compounds on the RCT process, we investigated the changes in liver and fecal lipids and BA levels after the administration of these foods.

The liver TC, TG, and TBA levels of tested rats are shown in Fig. 5a–c. TC and TG concentrations in rats fed different doses of CTS, COSI, and COSIII decreased dose-dependently when compared with that in the HF groups, which were consistent with changes in serum TC and TG ($p < 0.05$). The results indicated that CTS, COSI, and COSIII can effectually reduce lipid concentration by accelerating the synthesis of TBA in liver and promoting the excretion of cholesterol.

In the following experiments, we determined the concentrations of TC, TG, and TBA in rats' feces. Figure 5d–f demonstrates that fecal TC, TG, and TBA concentrations of the HF group were higher than that of the NF group ($p < 0.05$). After 6 weeks of treatment, fecal TC, TG, and TBA levels in the treatment groups were elevated in a dose-dependent manner compared with the NF and HF groups ($p < 0.05$).

Therefore, the decreased liver and increased fecal TC, TG, and TBA in the treatment groups indicated that CTS, COSI, and COSIII can promote the RCT process for the excretion of TC, TG, and TBA in hyperlipidemic rats. Specifically, the liver and fecal TBA contents of the HF group were significantly higher than the NF group, because the rise in liver TC and TG contributes to the BA synthesis in the liver, which promotes the excretion of TC and TG in the form of BA via feces. CTS, COSI, and COSIII effectively accelerate the RCT process in HLP rats, as liver BA was markedly higher than the NF group, and BA excretion via feces was greatly increased compared to the HF and NF groups. As we expected that COSI also had a better improvements of lipids and TBA in rat livers (Fig. 6a–c), but the ability to increase fecal lipids and TBA levels was similar with that of CTS and COS (Fig. 6d–f). The reason for that is the three foods share the common excretion pathway, namely feces, although the smaller molecular weight material, COSI, is more apt to improve the RCT process.

Hepatoprotective effects

Liver injury, or hepatotoxicity, is the main relative factor of HLP (23). Increased serum ALT and AST damages the structural integrity of the liver because they are located in the cytoplasm and are released into the circulation after hepatocyte damage (24, 25). Elevated liver SOD was accompanied by a decrease in superoxide radicals and further suppression of LDL oxidation, which delays the occurrence and development of AS and HLP (26). The previous research significantly indicated that CTS and its relative derivatives showed antioxidant and hepatoprotective activity *in vivo* and *in vitro* (27, 28). To determine the mechanism underlying the hepatoprotective and antioxidant effects of CTS, COSI, and COSIII, we measured

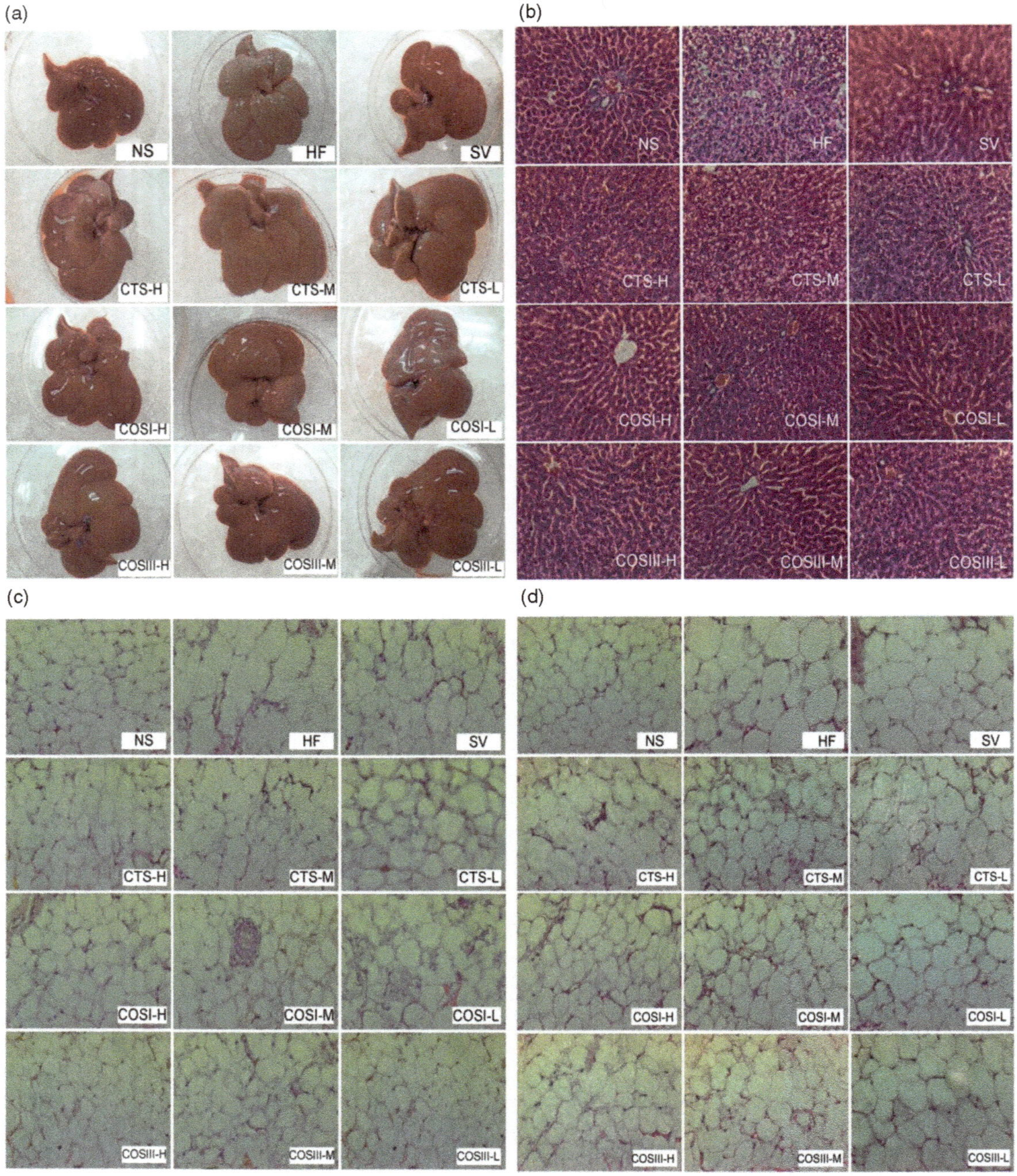

Fig. 9. The whole liver (a), slices of liver (b), white subcutaneous, (c) and mesenteric adipose tissues (d) obtained from different groups of SD rats (200 ×). Tissue sections were stained with hematoxylin and eosin (H&E).

the levels of liver and serum factors regarding liver function and antioxidant properties, including the activities of ALT, AST, and SOD (Fig. 7).

As shown in Fig. 7b, c, e, and f, rats fed HFD displayed a remarkable increase of ALT and AST in either serum or liver ($p < 0.05$) when compared with the NF group. Different doses of COSI, COSIII, and CTS significantly lowered the activities of ALT and AST in serum and liver to the normal range, and particularly the effects of COSI and COSIII in high and middle dose were equivalent to that of SV ($p < 0.05$), suggesting that they play an important role in protecting liver function. Meanwhile, liver and serum SOD (Fig. 7a and d) were significantly increased in the SV and treatment groups compared with that in the NF and HF groups, especially in response to different doses of COSI ($p < 0.05$) (Fig. 8),

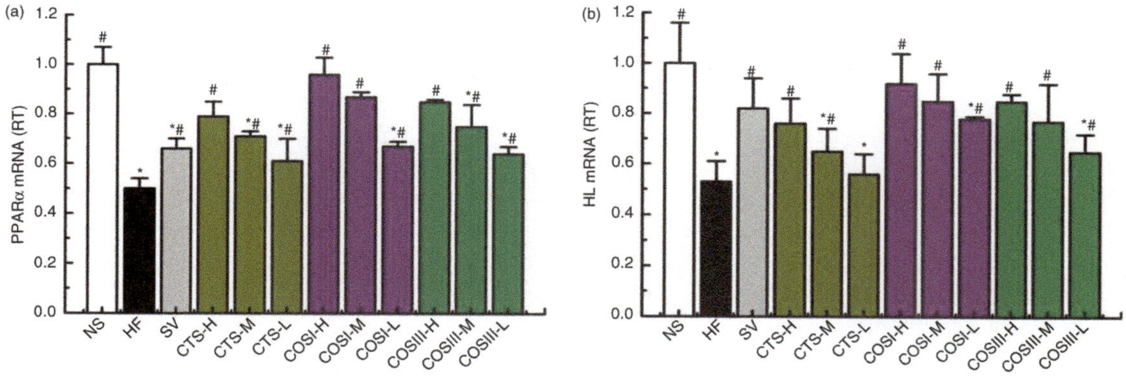

Fig. 10. The mRNA expression levels of liver PPARα (a) and HL (b) in the different group. The level of mRNA was detected by Q-PCR. ΔCt is the average value of 10 samples in the formulation (average mRNA expression of experiment groups/average mRNA expression of NF groups) $= 2^{-\Delta\Delta Ct} = 2^{(-\Delta Ct\ \text{control}\ -\Delta Ct\ \text{FF})}$. If $2^{-\Delta\Delta Ct} < 1$, the average mRNA expression of the experiment groups is lower than that in the NF group. If this value is higher than 1, the average mRNA expression of the experiment groups is higher than that in the NF group.

which suggests that the antioxidant activity of CTS, COSI, and COSIII contributes to the hepatoprotective effects described previously.

The expected results clearly demonstrate that CTS, COSI, and COSIII play important roles in preventing liver lipid-oxidation, which contributes to protecting HLP rats' liver function. Therefore, the hepatoprotective and antioxidant role as well as the cholesterol lowering effects of the three foods could contribute to maintain normal liver function and thus remit the development and/or progression of HLP (29).

Histopathological responses of liver and adipose tissues

As shown in Fig. 9a, the livers of the NF group were sharp red in color and characterized by being soft, supple, and small in volume, whereas livers in the HF group became dull pale, slightly soft, rich to the touch and swollen, indicating that rats eating the HFD developed serious fatty-liver-like illness. The color of rat livers in the treatment and SV groups was between sharp red and dull pale, specifically in the CTS group. Additionally, the liver morphology of the SV group was similar to that of the NF group, and apart from the three CTS groups, different doses of COSI and COSIII relieved fatty liver to varying degrees.

Tissue sections, including white subcutaneous adipose tissue, mesenteric adipose tissue, and the right lobe of liver tissue, were stained with H&E (Fig. 9b–d). In the NF group, rat livers presented the integrated hepatic lobule and distinct liver sinusoid, and liver cells were neatly distributed around the central vein in a radial pattern. Excess adipose cells were observed in the ampliative central vein surroundings the livers of rats in the HF group. Hepatocytes contained a pale, watery cytoplasm, a cell nucleus that extended to the edge of cytoplasm, and several different shaped lipid droplets in the cytoplasm. Spotty and focal necrosis was observed in hepatic cells from the HF group, and an inflammatory cell infiltrate was observed. Simvastatin effectively reversed the physiological states listed above: the size of liver cells and liver adipose levels returned to normal, and a healthy nucleus was located in the center of sufficient cytoplasm.

The significant decrease of adipocytes and swelling of liver cells in the COSI treatment groups, especially the

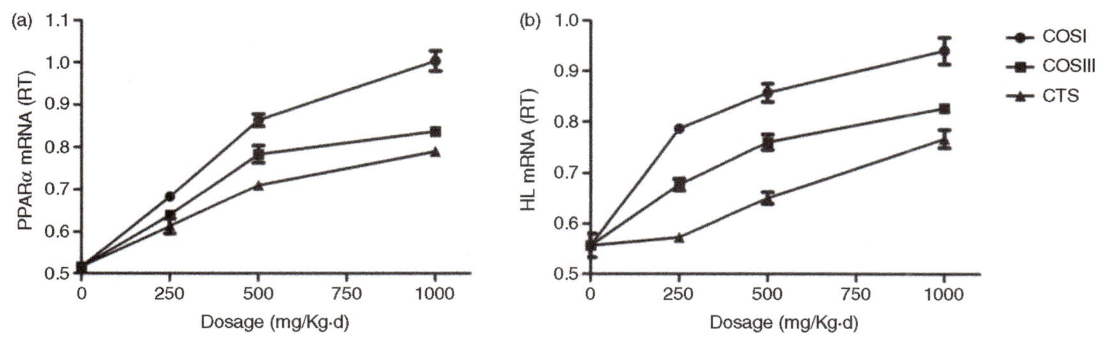

Fig. 11. Comparison of COSI, COSIII, and CTS in improvement the mRNA expression levels of liver PPARα (a) and HL (b) in hyperlipidemic rats during the treatment.

COSI-H group, suggests that COSI can effectually improve liver lesions. However, the improvements of COSIII and CTS were pale in comparison to COSI. Additionally, CTS, COSI, and COSIII can significantly inhibit the growth of white subcutaneous and mesenteric adipose tissues dose-dependently; this effect was stronger in the COSIII-H group and the three COSI groups.

Expression of liver PPARα and HL mRNA

Liver lipid metabolism, especially the RCT process, is modulated by various regulatory enzymes, of which HL is the most important. HL can catalyze TG hydrolysis into CM and VLDL-C for tissue use in the form of FFA and monoacylglycerol, and also provide HDL with apolipoproteins and phospholipids for the RCT. Cenarro et al. (30) demonstrated a negative correlation between the development of HLP and liver HL levels. PPARα, a transcription factor for various aspects of liver lipid metabolism, including the uptake, activation, trafficking, β-oxidation, and ketogenesis of FA, and the metabolism of lipoproteins, TG, and TBA can govern the hepatic lipid metabolic processes by increasing the expression of liver HL for the uptake and transportation of FA, which also contributes to the RCT process (31, 32). A number of studies reported that the expression of liver PPARα is down-regulated in hyperlipidemic rats, especially in the hypercholesterolemic rats (33–35). The facts that CTS can reduce the expression and activities of liver HL and PPARα in hyperlipidemic rats compared to controls, and that increased liver HL was invariably correlated with elevated PPARα, indicates the hypolipidemic mechanism of CTS and its derivatives (9).

In this study, we measured the expressions of rat liver PPARα and HL mRNA using real-time quantitative PCR. Figure 10a demonstrates that PPARα mRNA expression was increased in response to different doses of CTS, COSI, and COSIII, and these differences were statistically significant compared to the HF and NF groups ($p < 0.05$). Notably, the effect was stronger in the three COSI groups, especially in COSI-H group (Fig. 11a). As displayed in Fig. 10b, CTS, COSI, and COSIII effectively un-regulated the liver HL mRNA levels in rats fed a HFD, which is similar to liver PPARα mRNA levels changes with the stronger increase in the three COSI groups (Fig. 11b).

In consequence, the increased PPARα and HL are of the dominant factors in controlling the RCT process, which contributes to the improvement of RCT process in the HLP rat model. Simultaneously, we confirmed that simvastatin can also improve the down-regulated PPARα and HL mRNA expressions in liver.

Conclusions

The obtained results suggested that these three function foods, CTS, COSI, and COSIII, can effectively improve liver lipid metabolism by normalizing the expressions of PPARα and HL, and protect liver from the oxidized trauma by enhancing hepatic function, which could be potentially developed as future functional foods for remedying hyperlipidemia. However, the long-term clinical trials in humans are needed to investigate the hypolipidemic effects of the three function foods and their in-depth mechanisms of lipid-lowering and hepatoprotective effects should be further explored in the future.

Acknowledgements

This study was financially supported by the National Science Foundation of China (no. 81173107), the Science and Technology Planning Project of Guangdong, China (no: 2013B021100018, 2013B090600050, and 2015A010101318).

Conflict of interest and funding

The authors declare that they have no conflict of interest.

References

1. Navar-Boggan AM, Peterson ED, D'Agostino RB, Sr., Neely B, Sniderman AD, Pencina MJ. Hyperlipidemia in early adulthood increases long-term risk of coronary heart disease. Circulation 2015; 131: 451–8.
2. Ahmad S, Beg ZH. Hypolipidemic and antioxidant activities of thymoquinone and limonene in atherogenic suspension fed rats. Food Chem 2013; 138: 1116–24.
3. Zhang HL, Tao Y, Guo J, Hu YM, Su ZQ. Hypolipidemic effects of chitosan nanoparticles in hyperlipidemia rats induced by high fat diet. Int Immunopharmacol 2011; 11: 457–61.
4. Pan H, Guo J, Su Z. Advances in understanding the interrelations between leptin resistance and obesity. Physiol Behav 2014; 130: 157–69.
5. Zhang HL, Zhong XB, Tao Y, Wu SH, Su ZQ. Effects of chitosan and water-soluble chitosan micro- and nanoparticles in obese rats fed a high-fat diet. Int J Nanomed 2012; 7: 4069–76.
6. Tao Y, Zhang HL, Hu YM, Wan S, Su ZQ. Preparation of chitosan and water-soluble chitosan microspheres via spray-drying method to lower blood lipids in rats fed with high-fat diets. Int J Mol Sci 2013; 14: 4174–84.
7. Zhang W, Zhang J, Jiang Q, Xia W. The hypolipidemic activity of chitosan nanopowder prepared by ultrafine milling. Carbohydr Polym 2013; 95: 487–91.
8. Wang D, Han J, Yu Y, Li X, Wang Y, Tian H, et al. Chitosan oligosaccharide decreases very-low-density lipoprotein triglyceride and increases high-density lipoprotein cholesterol in high-fat-diet-fed rats. Exp Biol Med (Maywood) 2011; 236: 1064–9.
9. Tan S, Gao B, Tao Y, Guo J, Su ZQ. Antiobese effects of capsaicin-chitosan microsphere (CCMS) in obese rats induced by high fat diet. J Agric Food Chem 2014; 62: 1866–74.
10. Zou P, Yang X, Wang J, Li Y, Yu H, Zhang Y, et al. Advances in characterisation and biological activities of chitosan and chitosan oligosaccharides. Food Chem 2016; 190: 1174–81.
11. Choi EH, Yang HP, Chun HS. Chitooligosaccharide ameliorates diet-induced obesity in mice and affects adipose gene expression involved in adipogenesis and inflammation. Nutr Res 2012; 32: 218–28.
12. Alishahi A, Aider M. Applications of chitosan in the seafood industry and aquaculture: a review. Food Bioprocess Tech 2012; 5: 817–30.

13. Shiomi Y, Yamauchi T, Iwabu M, Okada-Iwabu M, Nakayama R, Orikawa Y, et al. A novel peroxisome proliferator-activated receptor (PPAR)alpha agonist and PPARgamma antagonist, Z-551, ameliorates high-fat diet-induced obesity and metabolic disorders in mice. J Biol Chem 2015; 290: 14567–81.
14. Usuda D, Kanda T. Peroxisome proliferator-activated receptors for hypertension. World J Cardiol 2014; 6: 744–54.
15. Kobayashi J, Miyashita K, Nakajima K, Mabuchi H. Hepatic Lipase: a comprehensive view of its role on plasma lipid and lipoprotein metabolism. J Atheroscler Thromb 2015; 22: 1001–11.
16. Yang P, Subbaiah PV. Regulation of hepatic lipase activity by sphingomyelin in plasma lipoproteins. Biochim Biophys Acta 2015; 1851: 1327–36.
17. Zong C, Yu Y, Song G, Luo T, Li L, Wang X, et al. Chitosan oligosaccharides promote reverse cholesterol transport and expression of scavenger receptor BI and CYP7A1 in mice. Exp Biol Med (Maywood) 2012; 237: 194–200.
18. Jull AB, Ni Mhurchu C, Bennett DA, Dunshea-Mooij CA, Rodgers A. Chitosan for overweight or obesity. Cochrane Database Syst Rev 2005; 20(3): CD003892.
19. Xu QY, Liu YH, Zhang Q, Ma B, Yang ZD, Liu L, et al. Metabolomic analysis of simvastatin and fenofibrate intervention in high-lipid diet-induced hyperlipidemia rats. Acta Pharmacol Sin 2014; 35: 1265–73.
20. Chen JK, Yeh CH, Wang LC, Liou TH, Shen CR, Liu CL. Chitosan, the marine functional food, is a potent adsorbent of humic acid. Mar Drugs 2011; 9: 2488–98.
21. Zhang J, Zhang W, Mamadouba B, Xia W. A comparative study on hypolipidemic activities of high and low molecular weight chitosan in rats. Int J Biol Macromol 2012; 51: 504–8.
22. van der Velde AE. Reverse cholesterol transport: from classical view to new insights. World J Gastroenterol 2010; 16: 5908–15.
23. Xia X, Ma Y, Xing X, Huang C, Li L, Gui G, et al. Antioxidant and hepatoprotective effect of different extracts of guizhencao (herba bidentis bipinnatae) against liver injury in hyperlipidemia rats. J Tradit Chin Med 2013; 33: 518–23.
24. Kang MY, Cho SH, Lim YH, Seo JC, Hong YC. Effects of environmental cadmium exposure on liver function in adults. Occup Environ Med 2013; 70: 268–73.
25. de Souza Predes F, da Silva Diamante MA, Foglio MA, Camargo Cde A, Aoyama H, Miranda SC, et al. Hepatoprotective effect of *Arctium lappa* root extract on cadmium toxicity in adult Wistar rats. Eur J Pharmacol 2014; 160: 250–7.
26. Kimura F, Hasegawa G, Obayashi H, Adachi T, Hara H, Ohta M, et al. Serum extracellular superoxide dismutase in patients with type 2 diabetes: relationship to the development of micro- and macrovascular complications. Diabetes Care 2003; 26: 1246–50.
27. Wan A, Xu Q, Sun Y, Li H. Antioxidant activity of high molecular weight chitosan and N,O-quaternized chitosans. J Agric Food Chem 2013; 61: 6921–8.
28. Jarmila V, Vavrikova E. Chitosan derivatives with antimicrobial, antitumour and antioxidant activities – A review. Curr Pharm Des 2011; 17: 3596–607.
29. Chung MJ, Sung NJ, Park CS, Kweon DK, Mantovani A, Moon TW, et al. Antioxidative and hypocholesterolemic activities of water-soluble puerarin glycosides in HepG2 cells and in C57 BL/6J mice. Eur J Pharmacol 2008; 578: 159–70.
30. Cenarro A, Artieda M, Gonzalvo C, Meriño-Ibarra E, Arístegui R, Gañán A, et al. Genetic variation in the hepatic lipase gene is associated with combined hyperlipidemia, plasma lipid concentrations, and lipid-lowering drug response. Am Heart J 2005; 150(6): 1154–62.
31. Chinetti G, Lestavel S, Bocher V, Remaley AT, Neve B, Torra IP, et al. PPAR-alpha and PPAR-gamma activators induce cholesterol removal from human macrophage foam cells through stimulation of the ABCA1 pathway. Nat Med 2001; 7: 53–8.
32. Lee CH, Olson P, Evans RM. Minireview: lipid metabolism, metabolic diseases, and peroxisome proliferator-activated receptors. Endocrinology 2003; 144: 2201–7.
33. Berger J, Leibowitz MD, Doebber TW, Elbrecht A, Zhang B, Zhou G, et al. Novel Peroxisome Proliferator-Activated Receptor (PPAR) gamma and PPARdelta ligands produce distinct biological effects. J Biol Chem 1999; 274: 6718–25.
34. Cholesterol Treatment Trialists C, Mihaylova B, Emberson J, Blackwell L, Keech A, Simes J, et al. The effects of lowering LDL cholesterol with statin therapy in people at low risk of vascular disease: meta-analysis of individual data from 27 randomised trials. Lancet 2012; 380: 581–90.
35. Swerdlow DI, Preiss D, Kuchenbaecker KB, Holmes MV, Engmann JE, Shah T, et al. HMG-coenzyme a reductase inhibition, type 2 diabetes, and bodyweight: evidence from genetic analysis and randomised trials. Lancet 2015; 385: 351–61.

*Zhengquan Su
Key Research Center of Liver Regulation for Hyperlipidemia SATCM/Class III Laboratory of Metabolism SATCM
Guangdong TCM Key Laboratory for Metabolic Diseases
Guangdong Pharmaceutical University
Guangzhou, 510006, China
Email: suzhq@scnu.edu.cn

*Jiao Guo
Key Research Center of Liver Regulation for Hyperlipidemia SATCM/Class III Laboratory of Metabolism SATCM
Guangdong TCM Key Laboratory for Metabolic Diseases
Guangdong Pharmaceutical University
Guangzhou, 510006, China
Email: wshxalb@163.com

5

Lipolysis stimulating peptides of potato protein hydrolysate effectively suppresses high-fat-diet-induced hepatocyte apoptosis and fibrosis in aging rats

Wen-Dee Chiang[1†], Chih Yang Huang[2,3,4†], Catherine Reena Paul[2,5], Zong-Yan Lee[5] and Wan-Teng Lin[5*]

[1]Department of Food Science, College of Agriculture, Tunghai University, Taichung, Taiwan; [2]Graduate Institute of Basic Medical Science, China Medical University, Taichung, Taiwan; [3]School of Chinese Medicine, China Medical University, Taichung, Taiwan; [4]Department of Health and Nutrition Biotechnology, Asia University, Taichung, Taiwan; [5]Department of Hospitality Management, College of Agriculture, Tunghai University, Taichung, Taiwan

Abstract

Background: Non-alcoholic fatty liver disease (NAFLD) is one of the most common outcomes of obesity and is characterized by the accumulation of triglycerides, increased tissue apoptosis, and fibrosis. NAFLD is more common among elderly than in younger age groups, and it causes serious hepatic complications.
Objective: In this study, alcalase treatment derived potato protein hydrolysate (APPH) with lipolysis-stimulating property has been evaluated for its efficiency to provide hepato-protection in a high-fat-diet (HFD)-fed aging rats.
Design: Twenty-four-month-old SD rats were randomly divided into six groups ($n = 8$): aged rats fed with standard chow, HFD-induced aged obese rats, HFD with low-dose (15 mg/kg/day) APPH treatment, HFD with moderate (45 mg/kg/day) APPH treatment, HFD with high (75 mg/kg/day) APPH treatment, and HFD with probucol.
Results: APPH was found to reduce the NAFLD-related effects in rat livers induced by HFD and all of the HFD-fed rats exhibited heavier body weight than those with control chow diet. However, the HFD-induced hepatic fat accumulation was effectively attenuated in rats administered with low (15 mg/kg/day), moderate (45 mg/kg/day), and high (75 mg/kg/day) doses of APPH. APPH oral administration also suppressed the hepatic apoptosis- and fibrosis-related proteins induced by HFD.
Conclusions: Our results thus indicate that APPH potentially attenuates hepatic lipid accumulation and anti-apoptosis and fibrosis effects in HFD-induced rats. APPH may have therapeutic potential in the amelioration of NAFLD liver damage.

Keywords: *apoptosis*; *fibrosis*; *high fat diet*; *lipolysis stimulating protein hydrolysates*; *obesity*; *APPH*

Aging is a biological process characterized by a progressive decrease in physiological capacity and increases in age-related diseases, and the process of aging is frequently associated with progressive insulin resistance and associated decline in blood sugar regulation, arising from deteriorated control of glucose production and triglyceride secretion in the liver (1). Aging therefore increases the occurrence of metabolic disorders such as dyslipidemia and hyperinsulinemia (2–4). Non-alcoholic fatty liver disease (NAFLD) is a common metabolic syndrome that progresses into chronic liver disease in obese adults (5, 6). Hypernutrition or insulin resistance potentially causes imbalance in the uptake and removal of lipids in the liver, leading to excess accumulation of hepatic triglycerides (7). NAFLD occurs more often in the middle-aged and in the elderly as the risk factors for NAFLD increases with aging (8). Hepatic apoptosis is one of the reasons for NAFLD-induced liver injury (9, 10). A higher incidence of apoptosis also leads to hepatic fibrosis. Therefore, inhibition of hepatic apoptosis is a potential approach in treating NAFLD. As there are no drugs so far that effectively treat NAFLD, diet control and diet-related treatment become more crucial in preventing NAFLD (7).

†These authors contributed equally to this work.

Potato (*Solanum tuberosum* L.) is an important food crop and a major source of high-quality proteins, minerals, and antioxidants, including vitamin C (11). Recent reports highlight the efficiency of the potato as an effective functional food with various health-promoting benefits such as protection from degenerative diseases, cancer, heart disease, and hypertension (11). Enzymatic hydrolysis of dietary proteins produces potential bioactive peptides with altered molecular size, hydrophobicity, and polar groups of peptides (12). Alcalase treatment–derived potato protein hydrolysate (APPH) with lipolysis-stimulating property was found to have the potential to act as an efficient anti-obesity diet ingredient (13–15). Recent in vitro studies on the stability of APPH against gastric proteases also show that APPH is highly resistant to proteolytic digestion (15).

In this study, we investigated the effect of APPH on fatty liver–associated hepatic apoptosis and fibrosis in aged obese rats. Twenty-four-month-old male SD rats that were fed with HFD for 60 days (HFD group) were found to develop symptoms of NAFLD with hepatic apoptosis and fibrosis. However, HFD-fed rats treated with different doses of APPH for the final 30 days showed a significant reduction in HFD-related apoptosis and fibrosis. The administration of APPH also protected the liver by reducing the accumulation of lipid droplets and regulating the level of apoptosis- and fibrosis-related events. APPH administration can therefore be considered as a potential therapeutic agent to ameliorate aging-associated NAFLD effects.

Materials and methods

APPH preparation

APPH was prepared, purified, and characterized as reported previously; the characteristics were consistent with the composition of APPH mentioned in earlier reports (13). Briefly, a reaction mixture containing 2.5% commercially purchased potato protein (Han-Sient Corporation, Taipei, Taiwan) and 1% alcalase enzyme (Nono Nodisk A/S, Bagsvaerd, Denmark) were used to produce potato protein hydrolysate (~81% protein) by subjecting it to alcalase enzyme hydrolysis for 2 h. The molecular size of the resultant APPH was determined using different membrane cut-off filters. It was confirmed, as in the previous report, that 5% of the content was >6,000 Da, 40% was between 1,000 and 6,000 Da, and 55% was <1,000 Da size. The hydrolysate was vacuum-dried and stored for future use. The degree of hydrolysis of the product was more than 9.5% and the hydrolysate was fractionated by reverse phase HPLC; characterized according to the methods reported previously (13, 16) by MS/MS/TIC and by analyzing the data with TurboSequest (Thermo Fisher Scientific, MA, USA) against protein database (UniProt, *Solanum tuberosum*) and the results revealed the presence of peptides with patatin sequences (Fig. 1).

Animal experiments

This study was conducted according to the IACUC-100-12 protocol after appropriate ethical approval from the Institutional Animal Care and Use Committee (IACUC) of the China Medical University, Taiwan. Five-week-old male SD rats were housed in cages maintained at 24±2°C and 55±10% humidity with a 12-h light cycle, and the rats were allowed to feed on normal laboratory chow for 22 months. The rats were randomly divided into six groups ($n = 8$): aged rats fed with standard chow, aged rats fed with HFD, aged rats with HFD and low-dose (15 mg/kg/day) APPH treatment, aged rats with HFD and moderate dose (45 mg/kg/day) APPH treatment, aged rats with HFD and high-dose (75 mg/kg/day) APPH treatment, and aged rats with HFD and probucol. The animals were fed with a standard laboratory diet (PMI Nutrition International, Brentwood, MO, USA) and provided with reverse osmosis–treated water *ad libitum*. In the next 8 weeks, obesity was induced by giving HFD (58Y1, LabDiet, Missouri, USA) containing 60% of energy as fat. The treatment was administrated orally using non-flexible needless feeding gavage simultaneously during the next 30 days of HFD feeding course. The probucol treatment group rats were fed with high fat diet and probucol (500 mg/kg/day).

Hematoxylin and eosin staining

The livers were excised; soaked in formalin; dehydrated by passing through 100, 95, and 75% alcohol sequentially and then embedded in paraffin wax. The embedded tissue blocks were cut into 0.2-μm-thick sections and de-paraffinized by soaking in xylene. The slices were stained using hematoxylin and eosin (H&E) and rinsed with water. Photomicrographs were obtained using Zeiss Axiophot microscopes (Carl Zeiss Microscopy, Thornwood, NY, USA).

Terminal deoxynucleotide transferase-mediated dUTP Nick End Labeling (TUNEL)

The tissue sections were incubated with proteinase K, washed in phosphate-buffered saline, incubated with permeabilization solution, blocking buffer, and then washed two times with PBS. The sections were stained with terminal deoxynucleotidyl transferase and fluorescein isothiocyanate- dUTP (Roche Applied Science, Indianapolis, IN, USA) for 60 min at 37°C in order to detect the number of apoptotic nuclei. The tissue sections were also stained with 0.1 μg/mL 4',6-diamidino-2-phenylindole (DAPI) for 5 min, and the nuclei were detected by UV light microscopy at 454 nm. Photomicrographs were obtained using a Zeiss Axiophot microscope. All counts were performed by at least three independent individuals in a blinded manner.

Masson's trichrome staining

Liver tissues were fixed in formalin, embedded in paraffin, and sectioned. Slides were hydrated through a series of

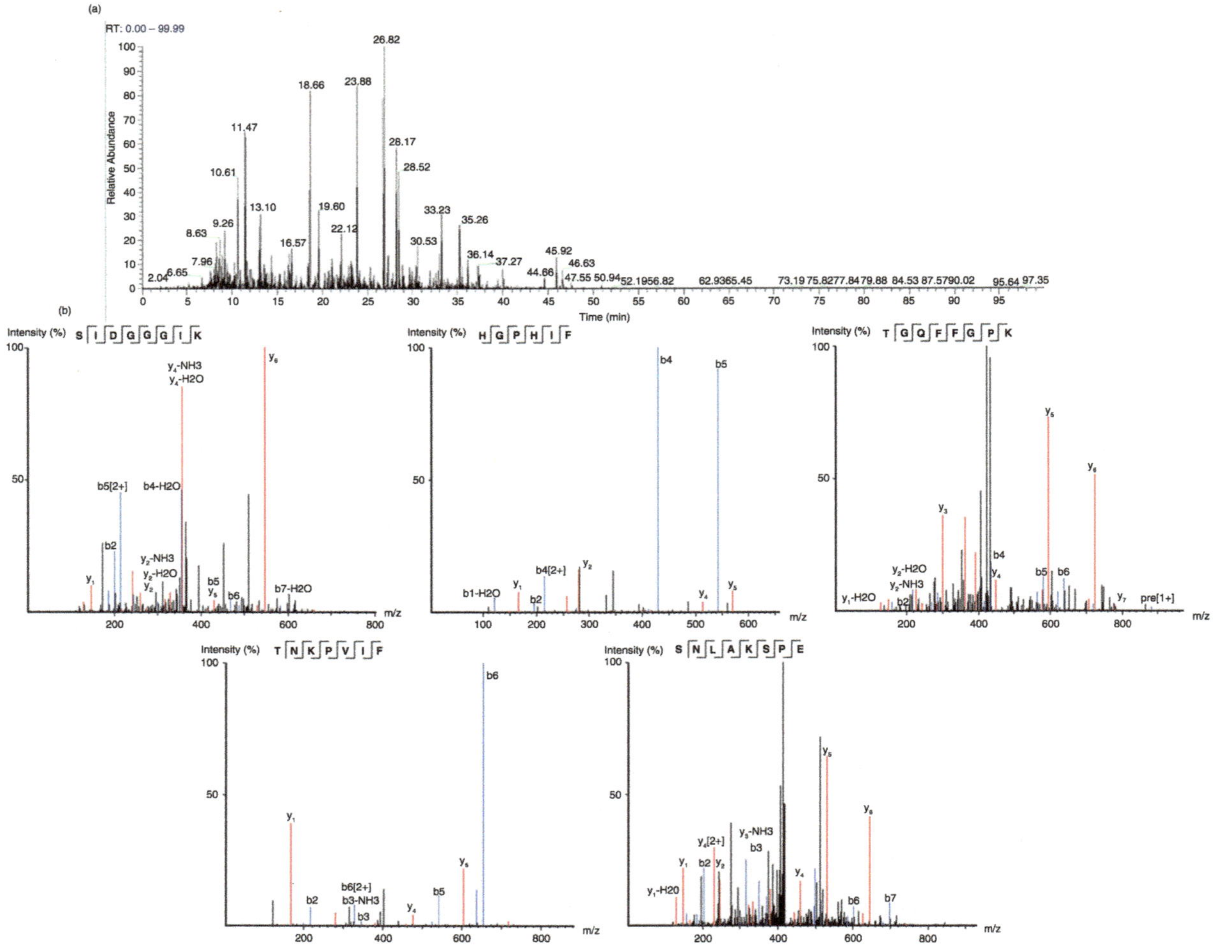

Fig. 1. Characterization of lipolysis stimulating APPH. (a) MS/MS/TIC chromatogram for APPH. (b) Ion series for chosen peptides from the MS/MS/TIC chromatogram showing sequence homogeneity with patatin.

graded alcohols (100, 95, and 75%), for 15 min each. The slides were then stained with Masson's trichrome dye. And photomicrographs were obtained using the Zeiss Axiophot microscopes.

Tissue protein extraction and western blotting

Proteins were obtained by homogenizing the liver tissue in lysis buffer (100 mg/mL). The homogenates were placed on ice and then centrifuged at 12,000 *g* for 40 min. The supernatants were collected and stored at −80°C for further experiments. The extract protein concentration was determined using the Lowry protein assay method. Protein samples were separated in a 12% SDS polyacrylamide gel electrophoresis (SDS-PAGE) using 75 V of constant power supply. Proteins were then transferred to PVDF (GE Healthcare Life Sciences, Pittsburgh, PA, USA) membranes using 50 V current for 3 h. The membranes were incubated in 3% bovine serum albumin (BSA) in TBS buffer and the primary antibodies (Santa Cruz Biotechnology, Santa Cruz, CA, USA) were added onto the membranes for conjugation with specific proteins. Horseradish peroxidase–labelled secondary antibodies were used for detection, and pictures were finally taken with Fujifilm LAS-3000 (GE Healthcare Life Sciences).

Statistical analysis

The results shown are the means ± SD of three independent experiments. Statistical analysis was performed by one-way analysis of variants. For paired samples, the Student's *t* test was used.

Results

APPH administration alleviated HFD-induced effects

The HFD intake induced several notable changes in the test rats. The rats fed with HFD showed significant increase in body weight compared to the control rats. Although some reduction in body weight was observed, the effect of APPH and probucol on the HFD induced increase in body weight was not statistically significant (Fig. 2). Massive fat accumulation in the livers of rats fed with HFD was also observed from H&E-stained liver sections (Fig. 3). However, APPH treatment effectively

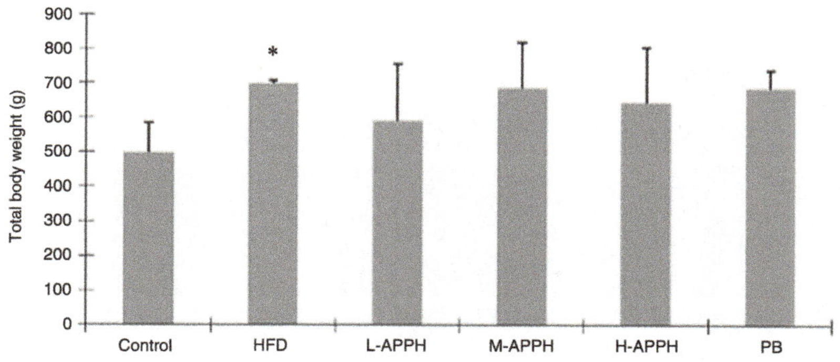

Fig. 2. Effect of APPH on total body weight changes. The changes in body weight (g) were measured in the controls and in the treatment groups were determined. The results represent mean ± SD ($n = 8$). *$P < 0.05$, when compared with control group (one-way ANOVA analysis).

reduced the fat accumulation in the liver tissue. Moderate and high dose of APPH were comparatively more effective in attenuating the fat accumulation than the probucol treatment group.

APPH administration supresses apoptosis

TUNEL and DAPI staining of the liver sections showed more number of TUNEL positive cells in HFD rat groups indicating a hepatotoxic effect caused by HFD feeding. However, treatment with low, moderate, and high levels of APPH supressed the number of apoptosis nuclei in a dose-dependent manner (Fig. 4).

APPH administration regulates apoptosis- and survival-related proteins

The protein expression in the HFD-fed rat livers, when analyzed by western blotting, revealed that the incidence of fatty liver in rats is correlated with suppression in the levels of activated phosphatidylinositol 3-kinase (p-PI3K) and serine–threonine kinase (p-Akt) and elevation in pro-apoptotic protein levels such as Fas receptor (Fas), Fas-Associated protein with Death Domain (FADD), Bcl-2 associated X protein (Bax), and activated caspase 3. However, in the rat groups administered with low, moderate, and high levels of APPH, the levels of survival proteins were elevated (Fig. 5) and the levels of apoptosis proteins were suppressed (Fig. 6).

Effect of APPH on liver fibrosis

Masson's trichrome staining of LV tissue sections revealed that HFD in aging rats induced liver fibrosis (Fig. 7). Tissue sections showed prominent blue staining in the HFD-fed rat liver sections. However, treatment with APPH effectively reduced the fibrosis effects induced by HFD. The results show that APPH has more potential than probucol to inhibit HFD associated liver fibrosis in hamster livers.

Discussion

Age-related disorders are widespread throughout the world and are the leading cause of death in developed countries. The deterioration of organ structure and function during aging is associated with oxidative stress, genetic instability,

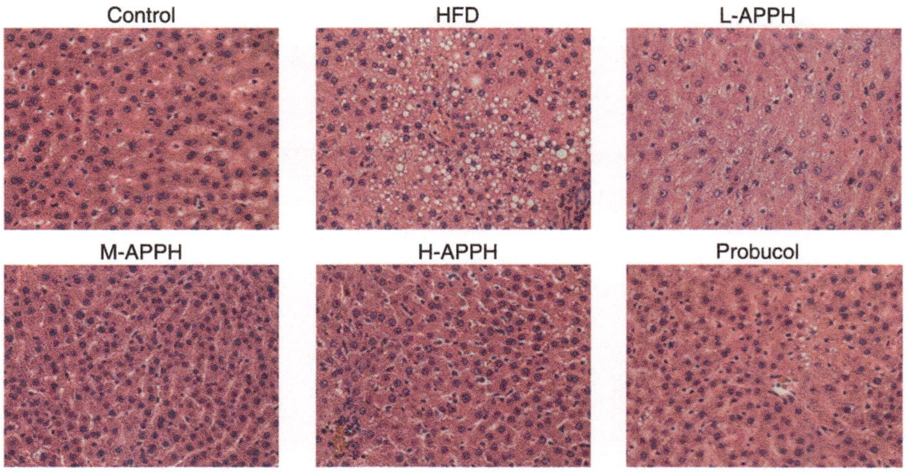

Fig. 3. Hematoxylin and eosin (H&E) staining of tissue sections showing the liver tissue architecture and lipid droplets. Histopathological analysis of hepatic sections of control rats, high-fat-diet-fed rats, and the treatment group rats was performed. Magnification 400x.

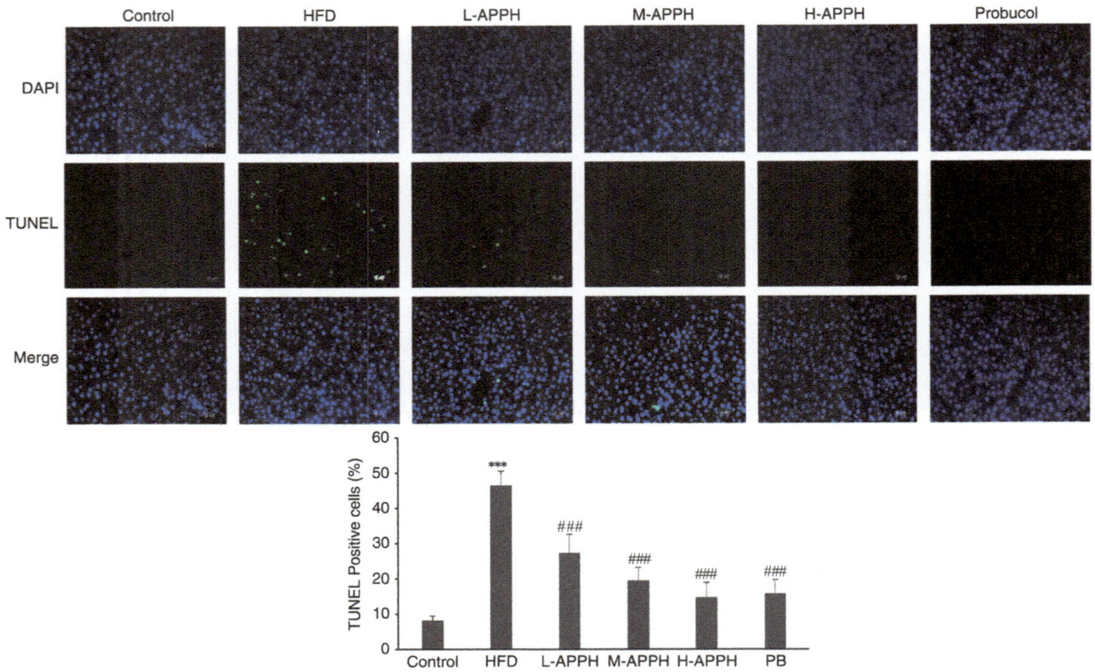

Fig. 4. Effect of APPH on cellular apoptosis. DAPI and TUNEL stained liver sections show the degree of apoptosis in control rats, high-fat-diet-fed rats, and the treatment group rats. Magnification 400x. $^{***}P < 0.001$, when compared with control group and $^{###}P < 0.001$ when compared with HFD group.

and the disruption of homeostatic pathways, resulting in metabolic syndromes such as obesity, insulin resistance, impaired glucose tolerance or overt diabetes, hypertension, dyslipidemia, and cardiovascular complications (16). Diabetes is also recognized to accelerate aging, but the mechanisms linking diabetes and aging are poorly understood (17).

Obesity is a major cause of insulin resistance and is linked to several common diseases such as type two diabetes, cardiovascular disease, NAFLD, and various cancers (18–20). The HFD-fed rats used in our experiments displayed liver apoptosis and fibrosis symptoms as determined from their liver histology. APPH effectively reduced the liver fat accumulation; however, this change

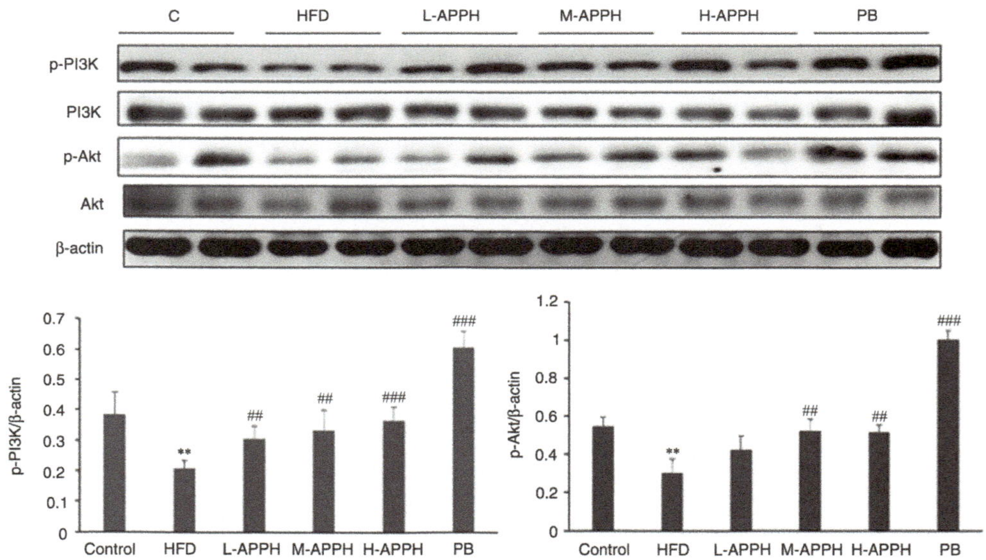

Fig. 5. Effect of APPH on survival proteins. The cell survival protein levels such as p-PI3K and p-Akt in the 24-month-old control rats, high-fat-diet-fed rats, and the treatment group rats. $^{**}P < 0.01$ and $^{***}P < 0.001$, when compared with control group $^{\#}P < 0.05$, $^{\#\#}P < 0.01$ and $^{\#\#\#}P < 0.001$ when compared with the HFD group.

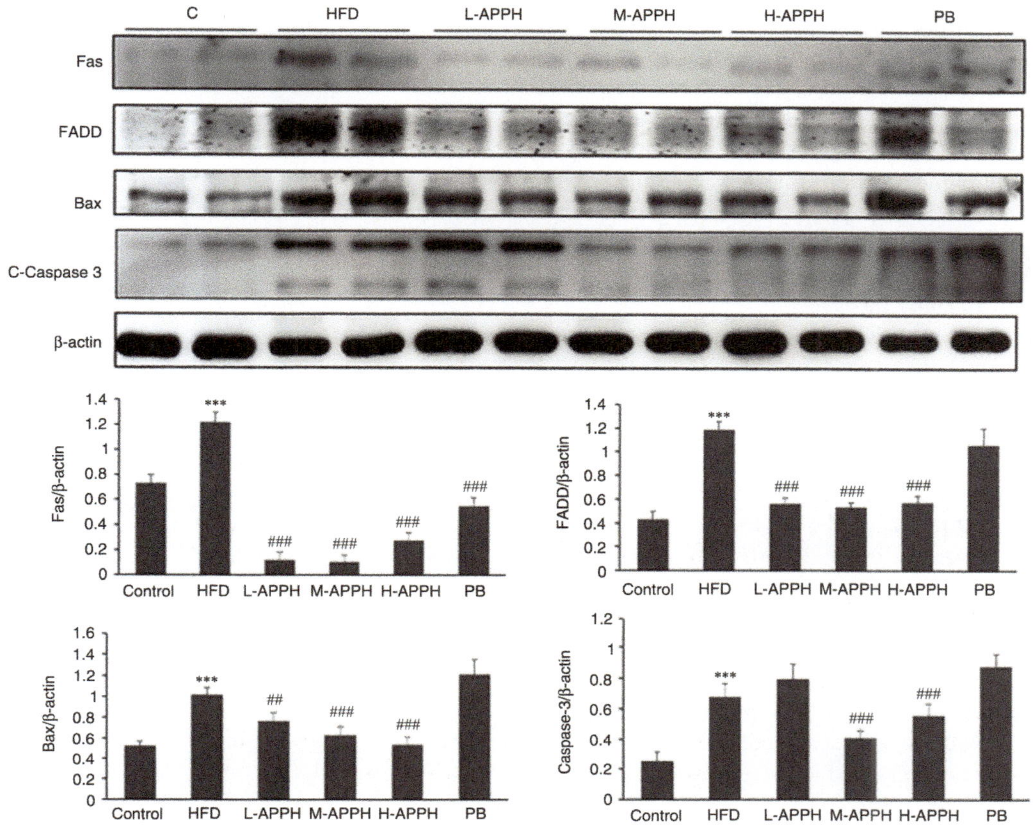

Fig. 6. Effect of APPH on apoptosis marker proteins. The levels of apoptosis protein such as Fas, FADD, Bax, and caspase 3 in the 24-month-old control rats, high-fat diet-fed rats, and the treatment group rats. $^{***}P < 0.001$, when compared with control group, $^{\#\#}P < 0.01$ and $^{\#\#\#}P < 0.001$ when compared with HFD group.

would have caused an increase in fat accumulation elsewhere in the form of visceral or the adipose fat. Therefore, changes in the liver lipid mass were not reflected on the total body weight differences post APPH treatment. The potato proteins have been classified tentatively into three classes: patatin family (41 kDa; ≈40% of total soluble protein), protease inhibitors (5–25 kDa; ≈50% of total soluble protein), and others (21). Patatin exhibits a known lipid acyl hydrolase (LAH) activity (21). APPH contains fragments of lipolysis stimulating peptides such as patatin

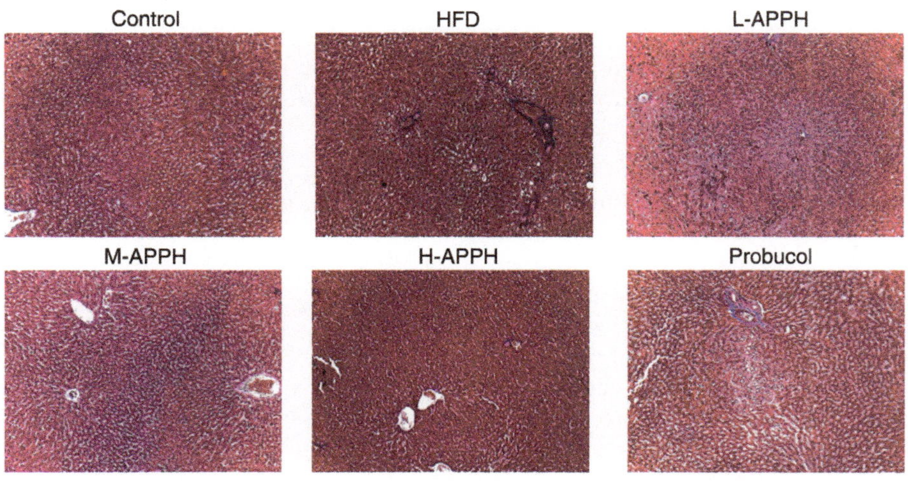

Fig. 7. Effect of APPH on fibrosis. Masson's trichrome staining in liver tissue sections from 24-month-old control rats, high-fat-diet-fed rats, and the treatment group rats. Magnification 400x.

that has proven anti-obesity effect in rodents. APPH administration is known to confer cardiac protection and improve heart function against HFD-induced effects by attenuating apoptosis and by improving cardiomyocyte survival mechanism (13). In aging rats, APPH administration efficiently reduces serum triacylglycerol and total cholesterol (TC) levels and provides cardio protection to the HFD-fed ailing rats (14). Our present study reveals the effect of APPH in preventing HFD-induced fatty liver and liver fibrosis in aging rats.

The causes of chronic liver diseases are known to be multifactorial, involving obesity, insulin resistance, inflammation, and oxidative stress. Targeting these pathways is considered a potential treatment approach but the strategy has either shown limited efficacy or an unfavorable safety profile (22). Increased hepatocyte apoptosis is a prominent feature of liver diseases leading to liver damage, severe inflammation, and fibrosis. Inflammatory cytokines from hepatocytes in response to liver injury may lead to NAFLD (23, 24). Two major cellular pathways are attributed to the induction and progression of apoptosis in response to different types of stimuli (25). The intrinsic pathway involves the disruption of mitochondrial membrane potential and release of cytochrome *c*, thereby triggering caspase 9. The extrinsic pathway involves activation of death receptors such as the Fas receptor, recruitment of the adaptor molecule FADD, and activation of caspase 8 (26). The members of the Bcl-2 family of proteins-Bcl-2 and Bax, that are, respectively, anti-apoptotic and pro-apoptotic factors, are crucial markers of the events in apoptosis (26). The results indicate that the extrinsic apoptosis pathway proteins that were elevated in HFD-fed rats were regulated when treated with APPH. The APPH also up-regulated Bax in the livers of HFD-fed rats. Therefore, our results indicate that HFD increases apoptosis in rat livers but is regulated when treated with APPH.

Obesity is known to be associated with PI3K/AKT pathway deregulation (27). The IGF1R mediated activation of PI3K and AKT prompts immune cell activation by regulating key inflammatory cytokines (28, 29). APPH treatment has also shown to compensatively enhance IGF1R-PI3K-Akt signaling to improve the cardiomyocyte viability in aging rat hearts (14). In this study, APPH administration increased the levels of PI3K and AKT in HFD-fed rats, indicating improvements in the hepatocyte survival condition. Further, as a consequence of apoptosis associated liver injury, hepatic stellate cells are known to migrate to the apoptosis site to engulf apoptotic bodies. In this process, hepatic stellates are activated to promote the deposition of extracellular matrix and scar formation in the liver (30).

Probucol is a potent antioxidative drug that has been used for the prevention and treatment of atherosclerotic cardiovascular diseases due to its lipid-lowering effects. Probucol decreases serum LDL-C by 10–20% and enhances the excretion of cholesterol into bile (31). Probucol has been known to be effective in attenuating biochemical and histological changes associated with NASH. Probucol treatment normalizes the serum aminotransferase levels and improves hepatic inflammation and fibrosis (32, 33). However, probucol also reduces serum HDL-cholesterol, thereby restricting its therapeutic usage (34). The APPH has shown superior activity compared to probucol and therefore APPH is potentially a valuable alternative to probucol.

In this study, the effect of APPH to attenuate HFD-related apoptosis and fibrosis was determined in HFD-fed aging rat livers. HFD induced changes in the rat bodyweight and expression levels of cellular apoptosis and fibrosis proteins; however, the modulations were found to be regulated when treated with APPH. Therefore, low, moderate, and high concentrations of APPH can potentially rescue rat livers from the effects of HFD.

Conflict of interest and funding

The authors declare no conflict of financial interest. This Research was financially supported by a grant from the Ministry of Science and Technology of Taiwan (MOST103-2410-H-029-037 and MOST104-2410-H-029-033-MY2).

References

1. Lee J, Cho JY, Kim WK. Anti-inflammation effect of exercise and Korean red ginseng in aging model rats with diet-induced atherosclerosis. Nutr Res Pract 2014; 8(3): 284–91.
2. Elahi D, Muller DC, Egan JM, Andres R, Veldhuist J, Meneilly GS. Glucose tolerance, glucose utilization and insulin secretion in ageing. Novartis Found Symp 2002; 242: 222–42; discussion 42–6.
3. Buettner R, Scholmerich J, Bollheimer LC. High-fat diets: modeling the metabolic disorders of human obesity in rodents. Obesity (Silver Spring) 2007; 15(4): 798–808.
4. Bravo E, Rivabene R, Bruscalupi G, Calcabrini A, Arancia G, Cantafora A. Age-related changes in lipid secretion of perfused livers from male Wistar rats donors. J Biochem 1996; 119(2): 240–5.
5. Yilmaz Y. Review article: is non-alcoholic fatty liver disease a spectrum, or are steatosis and non-alcoholic steatohepatitis distinct conditions? Aliment Pharmacol Ther 2012; 36(9): 815–23.
6. Bogdanova K, Poczatkova H, Uherkova L, Riegrova D, Rypka M, Feher J, et al. Non-alcoholic fatty liver disease (NAFLD) – a novel common aspect of the metabolic syndrome. Biomed Pap Med Fac Univ Palacky Olomouc Czech Repub 2006; 150(1): 101–4.
7. Kawano Y, Cohen DE. Mechanisms of hepatic triglyceride accumulation in non-alcoholic fatty liver disease. J Gastroenterol 2013; 48(4): 434–41.
8. Bertolotti M, Lonardo A, Mussi C, Baldelli E, Pellegrini E, Ballestri S, et al. Nonalcoholic fatty liver disease and aging: epidemiology to management. World J Gastroenterol 2014; 20(39): 14185–204.

9. Jiang Y, Zhao MY, An W. Increased hepatic apoptosis in high-fat diet-induced NASH in rats may be associated with downregulation of hepatic stimulator substance. J Mol Med-Jmm 2011; 89(12): 1207–17.
10. Xiao J, Guo R, Fung ML, Liong EC, Chang RCC, Ching YP, et al. Garlic-derived S-allylmercaptocysteine ameliorates non-alcoholic fatty liver disease in a rat model through inhibition of apoptosis and enhancing autophagy. Evidence-Based Complement Alternat Med 2013; 2013: 642920.
11. Valinas MA, Lanteri ML, ten Have A, Andreu AB. Chlorogenic acid biosynthesis appears linked with suberin production in potato tuber (*Solanum tuberosum*). J Agric Food Chem 2015; 63(19): 4902–13.
12. Ambigaipalan P, Shahidi F. Antioxidant potential of date (*Phoenix dactylifera* L.) seed protein hydrolysates and carnosine in food and biological systems. J Agric Food Chem 2015; 63(3): 864–71.
13. Huang CY, Chiang WD, Pai PY, Lin WT. Potato protein hydrolysate attenuates high fat diet-induced cardiac apoptosis through SIRT1/PGC-1a/Akt signalling. J Funct Foods 2015; 12: 389–98.
14. Hu WS, Ting WJ, Chiang WD, Pai P, Yeh YL, Chang CH, et al. The heart protection effect of alcalase potato protein hydrolysate is through IGF1R-PI3K-Akt compensatory reactivation in aging rats on high fat diets. Int J Mol Sci 2015; 16(5): 10158–72.
15. Lin WT, Lee KI, Hong MC, Chiang WD. Production of potato protein hydrolysates with 2 lipolysis-stimulating activity and study of 3 their possible regulation mechanism. Taiwanese J Agric Chem Food Sci 2016; 54(2): 53–63.
16. Tsou MJ, Kao FJ, Lu HC, Kao HC, Chiang WD. Purification and identification of lipolysis-stimulating peptides derived from enzymatic hydrolysis of soy protein. Food Chem 2013; 138(2–3): 1454–60.
17. Ahima RS. Connecting obesity, aging and diabetes. Nature Med 2009; 15(9): 996–7.
18. Moore JB. Non-alcoholic fatty liver disease: the hepatic consequence of obesity and the metabolic syndrome. Proc Nutr Soc 2010; 69(2): 211–20.
19. Huang C-Y, Lee S-D. Possible pathophysiology of heart failure in obesity: cardiac apoptosis. Bio Med 2012; 2(1): 36–40.
20. Sundaram S, Johnson AR, Makowski L. Obesity, metabolism and the microenvironment: links to cancer. J Carcinog 2013; 12: 19.
21. van Koningsveld GA, Walstra P, Voragen AG, Kuijpers IJ, van Boekel MA, Gruppen H. Effects of protein composition and enzymatic activity on formation and properties of potato protein stabilized emulsions. J Agric Food Chem 2006; 54(17): 6419–27.
22. Bouziana SD, Tziomalos K. Inhibition of apoptosis in the management of nonalcoholic fatty liver disease. World J Gastrointest Pharmacol Ther 2013; 4(1): 4–8.
23. Vuppalanchi R, Chalasani N. Nonalcoholic fatty liver disease and nonalcoholic steatohepatitis: selected practical issues in their evaluation and management. Hepatology 2009; 49(1): 306–17.
24. Mazza A, Fruci B, Garinis GA, Giuliano S, Malaguarnera R, Belfiore A. The role of metformin in the management of NAFLD. Exp Diabetes Res 2012; 2012: 716404.
25. Green DR. Apoptosis – death deceiver. Nature 1998; 396(6712): 629–30.
26. Park MT, Kang JA, Choi JA, Kang CM, Kim TH, Bae S, et al. Phytosphingosine induces apoptotic cell death via caspase 8 activation and Bax translocation in human cancer cells. Clin Canc Res 2003; 9(2): 878–85.
27. Matsuda S, Kobayashi M, Kitagishi Y. Roles for PI3K/AKT/PTEN Pathway in cell signaling of nonalcoholic fatty liver disease. ISRN Endocrinol 2013; 2013: 472432.
28. Ou HC, Tzang BS, Chang MH, Liu CT, Liu HW, Lii CK, et al. Cardiac contractile dysfunction and apoptosis in streptozotocin-induced diabetic rats are ameliorated by garlic oil supplementation. J Agric Food Chem 2010; 58(19): 10347–55.
29. Goto M, Iwase A, Harata T, Takigawa S, Suzuki K, Manabe S, et al. IGF1-induced AKT phosphorylation and cell proliferation are suppressed with the increase in PTEN during luteinization in human granulosa cells. Reproduction 2009; 137(5): 835–42.
30. Chakraborty JB, Oakley F, Walsh MJ. Mechanisms and biomarkers of apoptosis in liver disease and fibrosis. Int J Hepatol 2012; 2012: 648915.
31. Tawara K, Tomikawa M, Abiko Y. Mode of action of probucol in reducing serum cholesterol in mice. Jpn J Pharmacol 1986; 40(1): 123–33.
32. Merat S, Malekzadeh R, Sohrabi MR, Hormazdi M, Naserimoghadam S, Mikaeli J, et al. Probucol in the treatment of nonalcoholic steatohepatitis: an open-labeled study. J Clin Gastroenterol 2003; 36(3): 266–8.
33. Tokushige K, Hashimoto E, Yatsuji S, Taniai M, Shiratori K. Combined pantethine and probucol therapy for Japanese patients with non-alcoholic steatohepatitis. Hepatol Res 2007; 37(10): 872–7.
34. Yamashita S, Masuda D, Matsuzawa Y. Did we abandon probucol too soon? Curr Opin Lipidol 2015; 26(4): 304–16.

*Wan-Teng Lin
Department of Hospitality Management
College of Agriculture
Tunghai University
No.1727, Sec.4, Taiwan Boulevard,
Situn District, Taichung City 40704, Taiwan
Email: 040770@thu.edu.tw

Diet in 1-year-old farm and control children and allergy development: results from the FARMFLORA birth cohort

Karin Jonsson[1]*, My Green[2], Malin Barman[1], Agneta Sjöberg[3], Hilde K. Brekke[4], Agnes E. Wold[5] and Ann-Sofie Sandberg[1]

[1]Division of Food and Nutrition Science, Department of Biology and Biological Engineering, Chalmers University of Technology, Gothenburg, Sweden; [2]Department of Internal Medicine and Clinical Nutrition, University of Gothenburg, Gothenburg, Sweden; [3]Department of Food and Nutrition, and Sport Science, University of Gothenburg, Gothenburg, Sweden; [4]Department of Nutrition, Institute of Basic Medical Sciences, University of Oslo, Oslo, Norway; [5]Clinical Bacteriology Section, Department of Infectious Diseases, University of Gothenburg, Gothenburg, Sweden

Abstract

Background: A farming environment confers strong protection against allergy development. We have previously shown that farming mothers consume more full-fat dairy than control mothers, who instead consume more low-fat dairy, margarine, and oils; margarine and oil intake was associated with increased risk of allergy development in their children.

Objectives: The aims of this study were to investigate the differences in diet between children in farming and control families at 1 year of age, to investigate the relation between the diets of the mothers and their children, and to relate the children's diet to allergy development.

Design: The diet of 1-year-old children from dairy farming families ($n = 28$) and from control families in the same rural area ($n = 37$) was assessed by 24-h dietary recalls, followed by 24-h food diaries. Allergy was diagnosed by pediatricians at 3 years of age using strict predefined criteria.

Results: Farm children had a higher intake of farm milk, whole cream, cholesterol, saturated fat, and fat in total and tended to eat more butter, while controls consumed more carbohydrates and poultry and tended to eat more margarine. Farm children also had higher intakes of homemade porridge/gruel, oily fish, and iodine. The intake of butter and whole milk in children and mothers correlated significantly in farm families but not in controls. A weak negative association was found between seafood intake and allergy development, while allergy was positively associated with the intake of pork as well as zinc in the control group; these intakes also correlated with each other.

Conclusions: Consistent with mothers in farming families, the children consumed more full-fat dairy and saturated fat than did controls, but this could not be linked to the low risk of allergy in the farming group. Seafood intake might protect against allergy development, in accordance with earlier findings.

Keywords: *atopy*; *dairy farm*; *fatty acids*; *dietary patterns*; *infants*

The incidence of allergy has increased during the last decades in countries with a Western lifestyle. A reduced exposure to microbes has been proposed to explain the increase (1, 2), but changes in diet may also contribute. For example, an increased consumption of omega-6 fatty acids has paralleled the increase in allergy development, (3) and consumption of margarine has been associated with an increased allergy prevalence (4, 5) Another common finding is that the consumption of fish by the mother and the early introduction of fish in the diet of the child is associated with protection from the development of allergy (6, 7).

Children who grow up on farms have considerably fewer allergies than those who grow up in the countryside, but not on a farm (8). Contact with livestock (9, 10), cattle feed (11), and the consumption of unpasteurized farm milk (9, 12) have been identified as independent protective factors. We have previously shown in the FARMFLORA birth cohort that farm mothers consume more full-fat milk and butter than do non-farm mothers living in rural areas, who instead consume more margarine and oils (13). Accordingly, the breast milk of farm mothers is richer in saturated fats and poorer in unsaturated fats (13). Furthermore, the consumption of margarine and oils by the mother was associated with an increased risk of allergy development in the offspring (13). Although fish consumption did not differ notably between the farm and control mothers in our cohort (13), we found that the proportions of the long-chain omega-3 (n-3) polyunsaturated fatty acid (PUFA) eicosapentaenoic acid (EPA) in serum phospholipids in 4-month-old infants were associated with less allergy development; serum EPA correlated with the breast milk proportions of EPA, which in turn correlated with the maternal consumption of oily fish during lactation (unpublished observations).

The aim of this study was to investigate whether the diet at 1 year of age differed between children raised on small dairy farms and control children in rural non-farming families, and whether the children's diet resembled those of their mothers. A second aim was to examine the relation between the diet at 1 year of age and subsequent allergy development.

Methods

Subjects

The FARMFLORA birth cohort includes 65 children from the Skaraborg County in the Southwestern part of Sweden, 28 of whom are being raised on small family-owned dairy farms, while 37 are controls living in the same rural area but not on farms, all included in this study. The recruitment of the pregnant women took place at maternity clinics between September 2005 and May 2008. Children who were born within the span of gestational weeks 36–42 were included in the study. Written consent was obtained from both parents and the study was approved by the Regional Ethics Committee in Gothenburg (No. 363-05).

Assessment of diet in 1-year-old children

At the age of 1 year (10–14 months), the parents of the children were asked to complete a 24-h dietary recall followed by a 24-h food diary of their children's diet. The 24-h recalls were performed unannounced and followed a pre-decided interview protocol based on the five-step multiple-pass method developed by the United States Department of Agriculture (14). The protocol included questions about 1) all foods and beverages consumed during the last 24 h, 2) foods that are often forgotten, 3) when and where the foods and/or beverages were consumed, and 4) additional information, such as the amounts and brands, for all the reported foods and beverages. To shorten the interview, the fifth step of the original protocol was omitted, that is, the reproduction by the interviewer of all recorded food items, giving the interviewee a chance to remember any forgotten foods consumed by the child. The parents were instructed to initiate the 24-h food diary immediately after the interview was made, including registration of the amount and brand of the foods, at what time the foods were consumed, and how the foods were prepared. Weights were recorded aided by household scales or estimated by volume with household measures.

The collected dietary information was registered and calculated based on the food composition database of the Swedish National Food Agency using the software Dietist Net Pro (Kost och Näringsdata, version 15.11.02, Stockholm, Sweden).

No data of the children's weights were collected at 1 year of age. Instead, a reference weight of Swedish 1-year-old children (10.25 kg) (15) was used to obtain a reference value of the recommended energy intake, based on current nutrient recommendations (0.33 MJ/kg, mean for boys and girls) (16).

Clinical examination

At the ages of 1.5 and 3 years, the children were examined by pediatricians to diagnose allergic rhinoconjuctivitis, asthma, and/or food allergies according to predefined protocols (17). Allergic rhinoconjuctivitis was defined as nose or eye symptoms after exposure to pollen or animal dander in combination with an allergen-specific IgE test to the correspondent inhalant allergen (Phadiatope, Phadia, Uppsala, Sweden). Asthma was diagnosed based on either persistent wheezing for ≥ 4 weeks, or ≥ 3 wheezing episodes combined with either: 1) eczema, allergic rhinoconjuctivitis, or food allergy; or 2) a response to leukotriene antagonists or inhaled glucocorticoids. For asthma diagnosis at 3 years of age, at least one wheezing episode had to have occurred after 2 years of age. Food allergy and sensitization against common food and inhalant allergens were assessed by blood tests (Phadiatope, Phadia, Uppsala, Sweden). Food allergy was defined based on immediate or late-onset reactions that rapidly improved after allergen elimination. The diagnosis was affirmed by a positive six-mix food test and/or an open-food challenge test. This was then followed by an Immunocap test (Phadia) for the identification of the relevant allergen. Atopic eczema was diagnosed according to the criteria by Williams (18) or Hanifin and Rajka (19). For the diagnosis of atopic eczema at the age of 3 years, symptoms had to be present after 2 years of age.

Statistics

Multivariate analysis

Orthogonal Projections to Latent Structures with Discriminant Analysis (OPLS-DA) (20) was used to visualize the differences in the dietary patterns of farm and control children. Data were scaled using UV-scaling, and model validation was performed by cross-validation. Error bars denote the 95% confidence level, which was computed by jackknifing (the estimation of bias and variance based on subsets of the available data).

Univariable analysis

Due to a non-normal distribution of variables, a non-parametric Mann–Whitney U test was used for the evaluation of differences in dietary intake between farmers and controls and healthy and allergic children. For categorical variables, a χ^2-test or Fishers' exact test was used. Correlations were made using Spearman's *rho*. Two-tailed P-values <0.05 were used as the limit of significance. The univariable analyses were performed using SPSS (version 22, IBM Corporation New York, USA).

Multivariable analysis

Logistic regression was used for multivariable analysis (SPSS, version 22). Variables were included as covariates in adjusted models if $P \leq 0.2$ in a univariable analysis of healthy versus allergic children.

Results

Characteristics of farm ($n=28$) and control ($n=37$) children are shown in Table 1. Farm and control children differed according to gender, with more male infants being born in the control group while farm fathers were less often allergic and had less education than control fathers.

At 3 years of age, 10 children in the control group and one in the farming group were allergic. In the allergic group, cesarean section tended to be more prevalent and male gender tended to be higher compared to the healthy group.

Energy intake

All 65 children had either the 24-h dietary recall and/or the 24-h food diary completed; 74% completed both the recall and diary, 14% completed only the dietary recall and 12% only the food diary, with no difference between farming and control families or between families with healthy or allergic children. The median energy intake of all children was 4,202 kJ from foods, excluding breast milk, and did not differ significantly between farm and control children or healthy and subsequently allergic children. The children had a median energy intake per body weight of 0.41 MJ/kg, which exceeded the current recommendations of 0.33 MJ/kg (16). Five farm children

Table 1. Characteristics of farm versus control children and healthy versus subsequent allergic children

Variables	Farmers ($n=28$)	Controls ($n=37$)	P^a	Healthy ($n=44$)	Allergic ($n=11$)	P^a
Antenatal characteristics						
Heredity[b]						
Mothers	7 (25%)	11 (30%)	0.68	9 (21%)	5 (46%)	0.12
Fathers	1 (4%)	12 (32%)	0.01	7 (16%)	3 (27%)	0.40
Maternal age at delivery, year	33 (21–42)	32 (22–41)	0.46[c]	32 (21–42)	34 (22–41)	0.71[c]
Education, level[d] (1 = lowest, 5 = highest)						
Mothers	2 (1–5)	4 (1–5)	0.20[c]	4 (1–5)	3 (1–5)	0.78[c]
Fathers	2 (1–5)	2 (1–5)	0.02[c]	2 (1–5)	2 (2–4)	0.51[c]
Smoking during last month of pregnancy						
Mothers	0 (0%)	1 (3%)	1.00	1 (2%)	0 (0%)	1.00
Fathers	1 (4%)	4 (11%)	0.38	2 (5%)	2 (18%)	0.18
Cats or dogs in house at recruitment	21 (75%)	19 (51%)	0.05	31 (71%)	5 (46%)	0.16
Siblings	18 (64%)	17 (46%)	0.15	23 (52%)	6 (55%)	0.89
Birth characteristics						
Gestational week[e]	40 (37–42)	39 (36–42)	0.13[c]	39 (36–42)	39 (36–41)	0.14[c]
Cesarean section	3 (11%)	7 (19%)	0.50	5 (11%)	4 (36%)	0.07
Birth weight[f], g	(2,780–4,740)	(2,440–4,830)	0.78[c]	(2,440–4,740)	(2,730–4,830)	0.14[c]
Infant characteristics						
Male gender	10 (36%)	23 (62%)	0.04	22 (50%)	9 (82%)	0.09
Maternal fish oil intake, 4 months postpartum	2 (11%)	0 (0%)	0.18	2 (7%)	0 (0%)	1.00
Intake of supplements of vitamin A+D at 1 year of age	17 (61%)	22 (60%)	0.92	30 (68%)	6 (55%)	0.49
Allergic at 3 years of age	1 (4%)	10 (32%)	0.02			

Data are presented as n (%) or medians (ranges).

[a]χ^2-test (or Fishers' exact test). [b]Doctor's diagnosed asthma, rhinitis, or atopic eczema. [c]Mann–Whitney U test. [d]1 = Elementary school, 2 = upper secondary school 2–3 years or equivalent, 3 = qualified graduate from upper secondary engineering course, 4 = university < 1 year, 5 = university > 1 year. [e]$n=27$ farmers and 36 non-farmers, and $n=43$ healthy and 10 allergic subjects, respectively. [f]$n=36$ non-farmers, and $n=10$ allergic subjects.

Table 2. Absolute and energy-adjusted intakes of food items/groups in farm and control children at 1 year of age

	Absolute values (g)			Energy-adjusted values (g/MJ)		
	Farmers	Controls		Farmers	Controls	
Food items/groups	($n=28$)	($n=37$)	p^a	($n=28$)	($n=37$)	p^a
Butter[b]	3 (0–10)	0 (0–5)	0.12	1 (0–3)	0 (0–1)	0.08
Margarine	0 (0–3)	2 (0–6)	0.07	0 (0–1)	0 (0–1)	0.06
Rapseed oil	1 (0–3)	1 (0.5–4)	0.77	0 (0–1)	0 (0–1)	0.98
Other oils	0 (0–1)	0 (0–01)	0.84	0 (0–0)	0 (0–0)	0.95
Oils total	2 (0–4)	2 (1–4)	0.90	1 (0–1)	1 (0–1)	0.82
Margarine and oil	3 (1–6)	5 (2–9)	0.10	1 (0–2)	1 (1–2)	0.19
Milk products ($\leq 1.5\%$ fat)[c]	0 (0–30)	15 (0–80)	0.10	0 (0–9)	4 (0–20)	0.13
Milk products ($> 1.5\%$ fat)[c,d]	58 (9–120)	25 (0–75)	0.17	15 (3–26)	7 (0–19)	0.12
Farm milk[e]	0 (0–75)	0 (0–0)	0.00	0 (0–21)	0 (0–0)	0.00
Milk total	77 (30–160)	100 (4–180)	0.93	20 (9–34)	27 (1–39)	1.00
Cream (27–41% fat)	1 (0–6)	0 (0–1)	0.02	0 (0–1)	0 (0–0)	0.02
Cheese	7 (0–19)	3 (0–12)	0.46	2 (0–4)	1 (0–3)	0.28
Oily fish	0 (0–12)	0 (0–0)	0.02	0 (0–4)	0 (0–0)	0.02
Seafood total	0 (0–12)	0 (0–3)	0.08	0 (0–4)	0 (0–1)	0.07
Pork[f]	8 (1–20)	10 (6–14)	0.83	2 (0–5)	2 (0–3)	0.68
Beef[f]	9 (3–22)	10 (6–15)	0.94	3 (1–6)	3 (1–4)	0.53
Processed meat	4 (0–25)	0 (0–18)	0.44	1 (0–6)	0 (0–4)	0.36
Poultry	0 (0–0)	0 (0–5)	0.03	0 (0–0)	0 (0–1)	0.03
Eggs	0 (0–9)	0 (0–1)	0.74	0 (0–2)	0 (0–0)	0.71
Porridge/gruel, homemade[g]	0 (0–43)	0 (0–0)	0.06	0 (0–8)	0 (0–0)	0.05
Porridge/gruel, from store[g]	76 (15–190)	110 (55–200)	0.36	22 (10–48)	30 (13–51)	0.50
Bread/rice/pasta/couscous	41 (15–58)	46 (15–77)	0.40	10 (5–18)	12 (4–16)	0.80
Crackers (non-sweetened)	0 (0–3)	0 (0–4)	0.66	0 (0–1)	0 (0–0)	0.71
Whole grain[h]	0 (0–0)	0 (0–0)	0.51	0 (0–3)	0 (0–0)	0.56
Grain foods, total[i]	46 (26–77)	60 (29–98)	0.47	13 (7–20)	13 (7–20)	0.88
Potatoes	38 (3–51)	30 (8–64)	0.99	9 (1–16)	9 (2–14)	0.76
Mashed potatoes	38 (7–51)	35 (8–65)	0.96	9 (3–16)	9 (2–16)	0.73
Root vegetables[j]	10 (0–22)	10 (0–30)	0.40	2 (0–6)	2 (0–6)	0.61
Vegetables[k]	30 (15–57)	42 (12–69)	0.40	6 (3–14)	10 (4–17)	0.55
Fruits/berries	68 (46–150)	84 (53–130)	0.67	17 (11–29)	21 (12–28)	0.90
Fruits and vegetables, sum[l]	150 (77–200)	18 (90–240)	0.22	33 (19–44)	37 (21–50)	0.46
Fruit juice	0 (0–25)	3 (0–25)	0.81	0 (0–8)	1 (0–7)	0.91
Sugar-rich foods[m]	31 (0–140)	44 (6–130)	0.82	10 (0–30)	16 (1–27)	0.99

Data are presented as medians (interquartile ranges).
[a]Mann–Whitney *U* test. [b]Includes butter-based spreads. [c]Includes sour milk products. [d]Includes farm milk. [e]Incudes both pasteurized and unpateurized farm milk. [f]Includes processed meat. [g]Wet weight. [h]For bread: $>5\%$ fiber, for pasta: $>50\%$ whole grain. [i]Bread, rice, pasta, crackers, cereals/granola, including whole grain. [j]Excludes potatoes. [k]Includes green peas, no other legumes. [l]Root vegetables, vegetables, fruits and berries. [m]Pastry, cake, candy, ice cream, fruit yoghurt, fool, and so on.

and four control children were partially breastfed at 1 year of age ($P=0.10$). Of these, one child (in the farm group) received substantial amounts of breast milk at this age and consumed only 712 kJ per day from foods other than breast milk. The duration of exclusive breastfeeding tended to be longer in farm children compared to control children (4 vs. 3.5 months, $P=0.11$), although the duration of any breastfeeding did not differ (8 months in both groups, $P=0.74$).

Diet in farm and control children

A broad variety of foods in the children's diets were reported. Food items consumed by less than 25% of the children were not included in the tables and figures; such items were olive oil, low-fat cream, lean fish, shellfish, game/lamb, nuts/seeds, peanuts, soft drinks, mashed potatoes from powder, muesli/granola, coconut milk, vegetable based milk, mushrooms, ketchup/chili sauce, whey cheese, and mayonnaise dressing.

Differences between farm and control children in the intake of food groups or food items, macronutrients and fatty acids, and micronutrients were analyzed as both absolute and energy-adjusted values (Tables 2–4). In Table 2, the median intakes of different food items and food groups are displayed. Farm children consumed more farm milk ($P < 0.001$), whole cream ($P = 0.02$), oily fish ($P = 0.02$), and homemade porridge/gruel ($P = 0.05$) than did controls, while the latter group consumed more poultry ($P = 0.03$; Table 2). Children in farming families tended to eat more butter ($P = 0.08$), while controls tended to consume more margarine ($P = 0.06$; Table 2). Significances were similar for energy-adjusted values (Table 2).

To visualize the differences in the intake of macronutrients and fatty acids between farm and control children, OPLS-DA was performed on the absolute and energy-adjusted variables (Fig. 1a and b). The absolute and energy-adjusted intakes of macronutrients and fatty acids in farm and control children are also shown in Table 3, which displays the median intakes and interquartile ranges. The differences between farm and control children were more pronounced if their diets were calculated as energy-adjusted values rather than absolute values. Farm children consumed significantly more fat ($P = 0.01$), cholesterol ($P = 0.02$), the fatty acids 4:0–10:0 ($P = 0.01$), 14:0 ($P = 0.02$), 18:0 ($P = 0.02$), saturated fatty acids in total ($P = 0.02$), as well as the fatty acids 16:1 ($P = 0.01$) and arachidonic acid ($P = 0.04$) compared to controls, who instead consumed more carbohydrates ($P = 0.02$; Table 3, energy-adjusted values).

The absolute and energy-adjusted intakes of micronutrients in farm and control children are shown in Table 4. No significant differences were found between the farm

Table 3. Absolute and energy-adjusted intakes of macro nutrients and fatty acids in farm and control children at 1 year of age

	Absolute values (g)			Energy-adjusted values (g/MJ)		
	Farmers	Controls		Farmers	Controls	
Energy and nutrients	($n = 28$)	($n = 37$)	p^a	($n = 28$)	($n = 37$)	p^a
Energy and macronutrients						
Energy, kJ	4,009 (3,383–5,093)	4,247 (3,755–4,833)	0.62			
Energy, kcal	958 (809–1,217)	1,011 (897–1,154)	0.62			
Protein, g	35 (26–43)	34 (30–43)	0.69	8.2 (7.6–9.2)	8.6 (7.7–9.2)	0.54
Carbohydrates, g	130 (110–140)	135 (124–151)	0.11	31 (29–32)	32 (30–34)	0.02
Fiber, g	11 (9–13)	11 (8–13)	0.93	2.6 (2–3.1)	2.5 (2.2–2.9)	0.60
Fat, g	33 (26–49)	32 (27–41)	0.70	8.6 (7.8–9.7)	7.6 (7–8.7)	0.01
Cholesterol, mg	85 (57–118)	60 (35–96)	0.07	22 (15–30)	17 (10–22)	0.02
Fatty acids						
Saturated fatty acids, g	14 (9–21)	13 (10–17)	0.47	3.6 (3–4.3)	3 (2.5–3.9)	0.02
4:0–10:0, g	1.0 (0.7–1.8)	0.6 (0.4–1.3)	0.06	0.26 (0.20–0.40)	0.15 (0.10–0.28)	0.01
12:0, g	0.6 (0.3–1.0)	0.5 (0.3–0.8)	0.54	0.16 (0.1–0.19)	0.12 (0.09–0.17)	0.28
14:0, g	1.4 (1.0–2.0)	1.0 (0.7–1.6)	0.06	0.39 (0.31–0.52)	0.25 (0.18–0.37)	0.002
16:0, g	7.8 (5.0–11)	7.6 (5.0–9.0)	0.42	2 (1.6–2.3)	1.8 (1.6–2)	0.07
18:0, g	2.3 (1.6–3.4)	2.0 (1.4–2.6)	0.25	0.6 (0.5–0.7)	0.5 (0.3–0.6)	0.02
20:0, g	0.08 (0.05–0.1)	0.07 (0.04–0.1)	0.80	0.02 (0.01–0.02)	0.02 (0.01–0.02)	0.37
Monounsaturated fatty acids, g	12 (9–17)	12 (9–14)	0.90	3 (2.6–3.4)	2.8 (2.5–3.1)	0.16
16:1, g	0.5 (0.3–0.6)	0.3 (0.2–0.4)	0.08	0.11 (0.07–0.16)	0.07 (0.05–0.11)	0.01
18:1, g	10 (9.0–16)	11 (9.0–13)	0.91	2.8 (2.4–3.2)	2.6 (2.3–2.9)	0.27
Poly unsaturated fatty acids, g	5 (4–6)	5 (4–7)	0.42	1.3 (1.2–1.5)	1.3 (1.1–1.5)	0.91
18:2, n-6, g	4.2 (3.3–4.6)	4.8 (3.4–5.4)	0.20	1 (0.89–1.15)	1 (0.91–1.20)	0.20
18:3, n-3, g	0.7 (0.5–0.9)	0.7 (0.5–1)	0.74	0.17 (0.13–0.22)	0.17 (0.11–0.23)	0.99
20:4, n-6, g	0.05 (0.02–0.07)	0.03 (0.02–0.05)	0.13	0.01 (0.01–0.02)	0.01 (0–0.01)	0.04
20:5, n-3 (EPA), g	0.01 (0.00–0.13)	0.01 (0.00–0.01)	0.19	0 (0–0.03)	0 (0–0)	0.24
22:5, n-3 (DPA), g	0.02 (0.00–0.07)	0.01 (0.01–0.03)	0.46	0 (0–0.02)	0 (0–0.01)	0.52
22:6, n-3 (DHA), g	0.04 (0.01–0.25)	0.02 (0.01–0.06)	0.34	0.01 (0–0.07)	0.01 (0–0.01)	0.35

EPA, eicosapentaenoic acid; DPA, docosapentaenoic acid; DHA, docosahexaenoic acid.
Data are presented as medians (interquartile ranges).
[a]Mann–Whitney *U* test.

Table 4. Intake of micronutrients in 1-year-old farm and control children

	Absolute values (weight)			Energy-adjusted values (weight/MJ)		
	Farmers	Controls		Farmers	Controls	
Nutrients	($n=28$)	($n=37$)	P^a	($n=28$)	($n=37$)	P^a
Vitamin A, RE	400 (250–660)	370 (280–600)	0.77	140 (100–180)	140 (99–200)	0.86
Vitamin B6, mg	1.0 (0.90–1.33)	1.1 (0.97–1.5)	0.18	0.27 (0.20–0.30)	0.26 (0.23–0.32)	0.31
Vitamin B12, μg	2.3 (1.8–3.8)	2.1 (1.5–2.8)	0.19	0.60 (0.40–0.80)	0.50 (0.40–0.70)	0.09
Vitamin C, mg	69 (54–87)	66 (48–95)	0.99	17 (14–20)	16 (12–22)	0.70
Vitamin D, μg	5.4 (3.7–7.4)	5.7 (3.2–7.7)	0.87	1.4 (0.90–2.0)	1.4 (0.70–2.0)	0.78
Vitamin E, mg	8.5 (6.3–11)	10 (6.9–16)	0.4	2.1 (1.7–2.8)	2.3 (1.6–3.0)	0.60
Calcium, mg	620 (460–790)	620 (480–770)	0.81	140 (110–180)	150 (110–180)	0.68
Folate, μg	120 (110–150)	130 (95–150)	0.58	32 (24–37)	29 (26–33)	0.24
Iodine, μg	38 (25–66)	33 (18–50)	0.18	10 (7.0–14)	7.0 (4.0–10)	0.03
Iron, mg	8.2 (6.7–9.5)	8.9 (5.8–11)	0.62	2.0 (1.6–2.5)	2.0 (1.5–2.9)	0.48
Magnesium, g	147 (132–171)	160 (130–170)	0.58	35 (30–40)	36 (32–39)	0.68
Niacin, NE	8.1 (6.0–9.1)	8.4 (7.0–9.5)	0.36	3.5 (3.1–3.7)	3.5 (3.0–4.0)	0.68
Phosphorus, mg	750 (540–920)	710 (580–860)	0.97	170 (150–190)	170 (150–190)	0.93
Potassium, g	1.5 (1.3–1.7)	1.5 (1.4–1.9)	0.55	0.37 (0.31–0.43)	0.36 (0.33–0.43)	0.64
Riboflavin, mg	1.0 (0.71–1.3)	0.95 (0.77–1.1)	0.68	0.24 (0.20–0.25)	0.23 (0.20–0.24)	0.75
Selenium, μg	13 (10–18)	13 (9.0–15)	0.45	3.0 (2.5–4.4)	2.9 (2.5–3.5)	0.25
Thiamine, mg	0.80 (0.68–0.95)	0.83 (0.69–1.1)	0.53	0.20 (0.16–0.23)	0.20 (0.17–0.24)	0.47
Zinc, mg	4.7 (3.8–6.1)	4.8 (3.9–5.6)	0.91	1.1 (1.0–1.3)	1.2 (1.0–1.2)	0.73

Data are presented as medians (interquartile ranges).
[a]Mann–Whitney *U* test.

and control children, except for iodine, of which farm children had a higher intake ($P=0.03$; Table 4).

Correlations between selected nutrients and food items in the children's diet

To examine the origin of the fatty acids that were consumed in different amounts of farm and control children, we correlated the absolute intakes of fatty acids and food items (Table 5). Butter, milk, cream, cheese, and pork were the main contributors of the dietary fatty acids 4:0–10:0, 14:0, 18:0, and 16:1, while oily fish was the main contributor of arachidonic acid (Table 5).

Further, the correlations between the absolute intake of iron and different foods in the children's diet were analyzed to evaluate the main contributors of iron to their diet. The children's intake of bought porridge was the only food item or food group that correlated positively with the children's iron intake ($rho=0.63$, $P \leq 0.001$, Fig. 2). Negative correlations to iron were found for grain foods ($rho=-0.32$, $P=0.01$), seafood ($rho=-0.30$, $P=0.02$), legumes ($rho=-0.29$, $P=0.02$), and charcuteries ($rho=-0.26$, $P=0.04$). When energy-adjusted intakes were analyzed, negative correlations were found also for butter ($rho=-0.37$, $P=0.01$), cheese ($rho=-0.40$, $P=0.001$), milk ($rho=-0.27$, $P=0.03$), pork ($rho=-0.42$, $P=0.001$), vegetables ($rho=-0.34$, $P=0.01$), and fruit ($rho=-0.28$, $P=0.03$).

Correlations between the diets of mothers and children

Our hypothesis was that the diets of the pregnant and lactating mother and child living on a farm resemble each other and differ from those of non-farming families. Correlations were made between the maternal and child intake of foods that differed significantly between farm and control families, either in the children's or the mothers' diets. Absolute intakes of the children's diet were used for correlations to the maternal intakes, as they were previously reported as absolute values (13). The farm children's intake of butter correlated with their mothers' intake of butter both during pregnancy ($rho=0.57$, $P=0.012$) and lactation ($rho=0.59$, $P=0.01$; Fig. 3a), and the intake of whole milk correlated with maternal intake of whole milk during pregnancy ($rho=0.51$, $P=0.03$) and tended to correlate with the intake also during lactation ($rho=0.38$, $P=0.09$; Fig. 3b). The intake or whole cream in the farm children correlated with the mothers' intake of whole milk ($rho=0.47$, $P=0.04$), but not whole cream, during pregnancy and tended to correlate with the maternal intake of whole cream during lactation ($rho=0.40$, $P=0.08$). The farm children's intake of margarine correlated with their mothers' intake of margarine during lactation ($rho=0.47$, $P=0.03$); the intakes of oily fish did not correlate at all. In the control group, no significant correlations were found between the children's

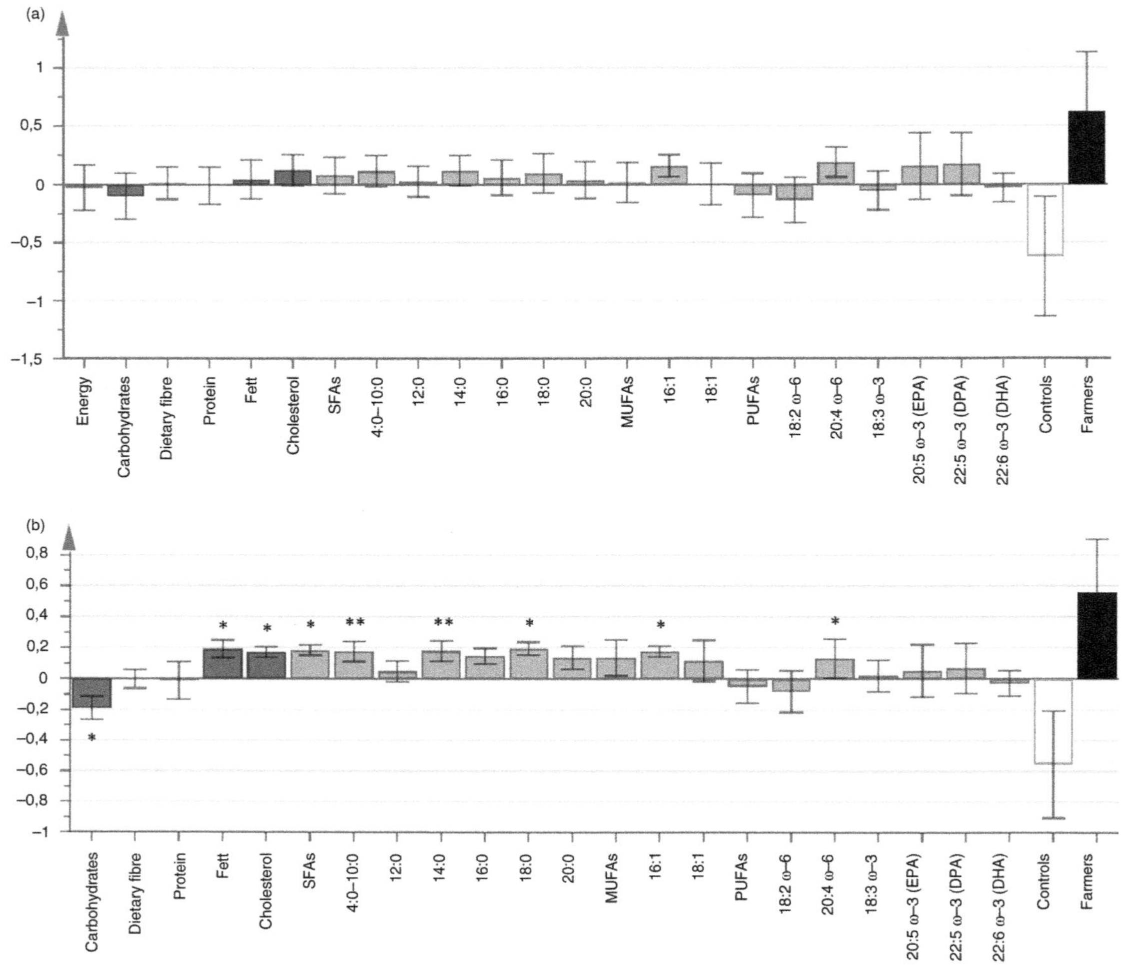

Fig. 1. Loadings plot of OPLS-DA displaying differences in absolute (a) and energy-adjusted (b) intakes of energy, macronutrients, and fatty acids in farm and control children at 1 year of age. Variables pointing in the same direction as farm children are higher in farm children and vice versa. Error bars denote the 95% confidence level, calculated using jackknifing during cross-validation. The models contain two components; $R^2X = 0.13$ (a) and 0.37 (b), and $Q^2 = 0.06$ (a) and 0.08 (b). Information about univariable significances has been added to the figure in retrospect, analyzed by univariable Mann–Whitney *U* test (*$P \leq 0.05$; **$P \leq 0.01$). $n = 28$ farm children and 37 controls. *Abbreviations:* DHA, docosahexaeonic acid; DPA, docosapentaeonic acid; EPA, eicosapentaenoic acid; MUFAs, monounsaturated fatty acids; PUFAs, polyunsaturated fatty acid; ω, omega; SFAs, saturated fatty acids.

Table 5. Correlations between the intakes of fatty acids[a] and food items in farm and control children at 1 year of age

	Fatty acids									
	4:0–10:0		14:0		18:0		16:1		20:4[b]	
Foods	*rho*[c]	*P*	*rho*[c]	*P*	*rho*[c]	*P*	*rho*[c]	*P*	*rho*[c]	*P*
Butter	0.67	<0.001	0.69	<0.001	0.56	<0.001	0.56	<0.001	0.29	0.02
Milk	0.32	0.01	0.31	0.01	0.35	0.01	0.27	0.03	0.08	0.52
Cream	0.31	0.01	0.34	0.01	0.28	0.03	0.32	0.01	0.30	0.02
Cheese	0.58	<0.001	0.54	<0.001	0.46	<0.001	0.50	<0.001	0.38	0.01
Pork	0.46	<0.001	0.42	0.001	0.58	<0.001	0.56	<0.001	0.38	0.01
Beef	0.10	0.42	0.16	0.21	0.29	0.02	0.35	0.01	0.32	0.01
Oily fish	0.06	0.65	0.05	0.72	–0.8	0.55	0.23	0.08	0.43	<0.001

[a]Fatty acids, of which the intake differ significantly between farm and control children (absolute intakes were analyzed). [b]Arachionic acid. [c]Spearman's *rho*.

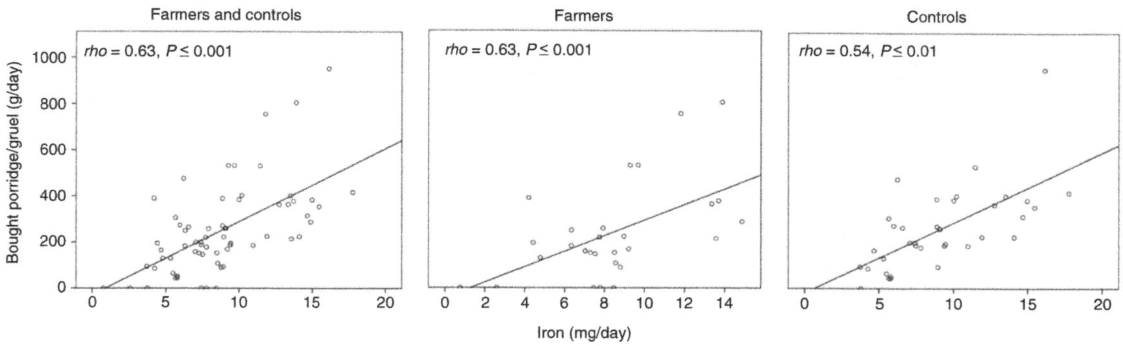

Fig. 2. Correlations between the absolute intakes of iron and commercial porridge/gruel in 1-year-old farm and control children. Spearman's *rho* with two-sided significances of $P \leq 0.05$ was used for the correlations.

intake of full-fat milk and cream, butter, margarine, and oily fish and their mothers' intake of these foods. Thus, the farming families were characterized by a common diet rich in full-fat dairy products, while no 'family pattern' could be detected in the control families.

Diet in healthy and allergic children

One farm child (4%) and 10 control children (32%) were diagnosed as allergic by the age of 3 years (Table 1). The allergic farm child had eczema, along with six children from the control group (11% in total of the 11 allergic children). Of the eczematous control children, one had a concomitant food allergy and another had asthma. In total, four children (6%) had asthma, two (3%) had food allergy, and one (2%) allergic rhinitis. A shorter duration of any (6 vs. 8 months, $P = 0.02$) and exclusive (0.5 vs. 4 months, $P = 0.01$) breastfeeding was observed in the allergic group compared to the healthy

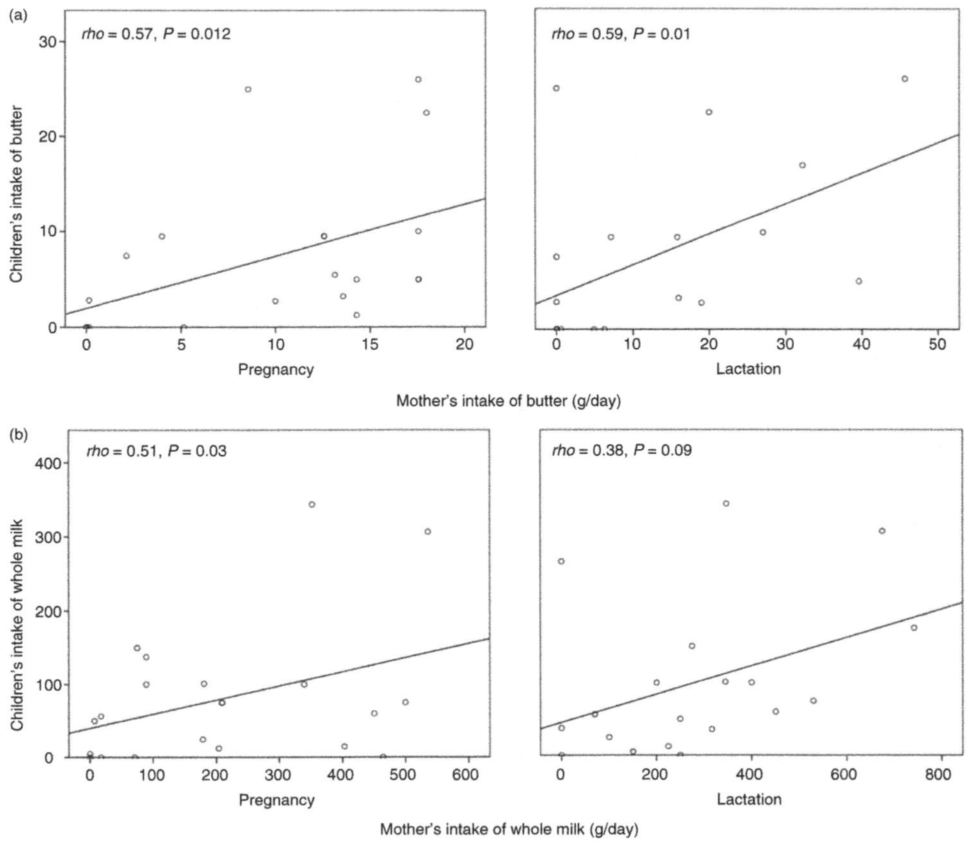

Fig. 3. Correlations between butter (a) and whole milk (b) intake in children at 1 year of age and their mothers during pregnancy and lactation. The correlations were analyzed with Spearman's *rho* and two-sided significances of $P \leq 0.05$. The children's diet and maternal diet during lactation (4 months postpartum) was assessed using 24-h dietary recalls followed by 24-h food diaries. The maternal diet during pregnancy was assessed using a semi-quantitative food frequency questionnaire.

Table 6. Food items/groups of which the intake differs between healthy and subsequent allergic children; in the entire cohort and controls only

	Absolute values (g)			Energy-adjusted values (g/MJ)		
Foods and nutrients	Healthy ($n = 44$)	Allergic ($n = 11$)	P^a	Healthy ($n = 44$)	Allergic ($n = 11$)	P^a
Farmers and controls						
Seafood, g	0 (0–10)	0 (0–0)	0.02	0 (0–3)	0 (0–0)	0.02
Pork, g	7 (0–15)	10 (7–30)	0.08	2 (0–4)	2 (2–7)	0.052
Zinc, mg	5.0 (4.0–6.0)	5.0 (4.0–7.0)	0.11	1.1 (1.0–1.2)	1.3 (1.1–1.4)	0.73
	Healthy ($n = 21$)	Allergic ($n = 10$)	P	Healthy ($n = 21$)	Allergic ($n = 10$)	P
Controls						
Seafood, g	0 (0–9)	0 (0–0)	0.14	0 (0–3)	0 (0–0)	0.14
Pork, g	4 (0–12)	12 (7–30)	0.053	1 (0–3)	3 (2–7)	0.02
Zinc, mg	5.0 (4.0–5.0)	5.0 (5.0–7.0)	0.08	1.2 (1.1–1.2)	1.3 (1.1–1.4)	0.04

Data are presented as medians (interquartile ranges).
Allergy was diagnosed at 3 years of age.
[a]Mann–Whitney U test.

group, although no significant differences were found for the rate of breastfeeding at 1 year of age (9% vs. 18%, $P = 0.13$). Significant differences in the diets of healthy and allergic children are displayed in Table 6. Healthy children consumed more seafood ($P = 0.02$) and tended to eat less pork ($P = 0.052$; Table 6). Since only one farm child developed allergy, analyses were made also in control children only; the higher intake of seafood in healthy infants became a trend ($P = 0.14$), while the lower intake of pork became significant ($P = 0.02$; Table 6). Additionally, a higher intake of zinc was observed in allergic control children ($P = 0.04$; Table 6). Crude and adjusted odds ratios for seafood and pork are displayed in Tables 7 and 8, respectively. We have observed that the proportions of the long-chain n-3 PUFA EPA in children's sera at 4 months of age were associated with protection from allergy (unpublished observations), while the maternal intake of margarine and oils during pregnancy and lactation were positively associated with allergy development (13). Therefore, we investigated whether the children's intake of pork or seafood correlated with serum EPA proportions and the maternal intake of margarine and oils. The intake of seafood at 1 year of age was found to correlate with EPA in infant sera at 4 months ($rho = 0.35$, $P = 0.01$). Similar results were obtained when energy-adjusted values were used in the calculation ($rho = 0.34$, $P = 0.02$); no correlation was found between seafood and the maternal intake of margarine and oils. Also, no correlations were found between pork and serum EPA or margarine and oil intake.

Discussion

We have previously shown that farm mothers in the FARMFLORA birth cohort consume more saturated fat and full-fat dairy products during pregnancy and lactation, while control mothers consume more margarine and oils (13). In this study, we show that similar differences between the diet of farm and non-farm families occur among 1-year-old children. Thus, children living on a dairy farm consumed significantly more full-fat cream and saturated fat and tended to consume more butter, whereas control children tended to consume more margarine. These results are in line with a cross-sectional study of 6–13-year-old Finnish farm children, who had a higher intake of farm milk, whole milk, and butter but less margarine (21). In our study, the farm children's intake of butter correlated with the mothers' butter intake, and the children's intake of whole milk correlated with maternal whole milk intake, although less pronounced. No correlations of these foods between mother and child were observed in controls, probably resulting from their less frequent consumption of full-fat dairy products.

Despite the farm mothers' higher intake of full-fat milk during lactation observed in our previous study (13), we could not find any significant differences in the consumption of full-fat or low-fat milk between the 1-year-old farm and control children (except for higher intakes of farm milk in farm children). This might be explained by national guidelines that advocate the restriction of milk consumption up to 1 year of age, which are based on concerns regarding the low iron content in milk. In accordance, the children's energy-adjusted milk intake correlated negatively with the energy-adjusted iron intake. Commercially bought porridge or gruel was the only food group or item for which the intake correlated positively with the intake of iron. In addition to milk, the intake of several other food groups correlated negatively with the iron intake; a high intake of foods like

Table 7. Logistic regression models of intake of seafood at 1 year of age and allergy in the child at 3 year of age

	Farmers and controls			Controls		
	Healthy ($n = 44$)			Healthy ($n = 21$)		
	Allergic ($n = 11$)			Allergic ($n = 10$)		
Predictor variables	OR	95% CI	*P*	OR	95% CI	*P*
Seafood alone	0.41[a]	0.14–1.26	0.12[b]	0.45	0.14–1.43	0.17
Model 1						
Seafood	0.50	0.17–1.48	0.21	0.52	0.14–1.89	0.32
Length of exclusive breastfeeding, months	0.63	0.42–0.96	0.03	0.58	0.34–0.99	0.05
Model 2						
Seafood	0.43	0.14–1.33	0.14	0.39	0.11–1.44	0.16
Length of partial breastfeeding, months	0.84	0.69–1.02	0.08	0.81	0.63–1.03	0.08
Model 3						
Seafood	0.35	0.11–1.12	0.08	0.31	0.08–1.30	0.11
Cesarean section	8.43	1.2–59.2	0.03	11.7	0.89–1.54	0.06
Model 4						
Seafood	0.43	0.14–1.29	0.13	0.42	0.12–1.45	0.17
Female gender	0.21	0.04–1.16	0.07	0.15	0.02–1.50	0.11
Model 5						
Seafood	0.47	0.26–0.83	0.01	0.47	0.14–1.52	0.20
Maternal heredity	3.14	0.71–13.9	0.13	3.43	0.61–19.2	0.16
Model 6						
Seafood	0.41	0.13–1.29	0.13	0.48	0.14–1.66	0.25
Gestational week[c]	3.14	0.71–13.9	0.13	0.74	0.46–1.21	0.23
Model 7						
Seafood	0.44	0.15–1.33	0.15	0.46	0.14–1.54	0.21
Birth weight[d], g	1.00	0.99–1.00	0.58	1.0	0.99–1.00	0.85
Model 8						
Seafood	0.39	0.12–1.27	0.18	0.44	0.14–1.38	0.16
Cats or dogs in house at recruitment	0.34	0.08–1.43	0.14	0.37	0.07–1.92	0.24
Model 9						
Seafood	0.44	0.15–1.31	0.14	0.46	0.14–1.48	0.19
Paternal smoking last month of pregnancy	2.68	0.32–22.2	0.36	1.47	0.17–12.9	0.73

Odds ratios (ORs) and confidence intervals (CIs) for every g/MJ/d of seafood intake at 1 year of age and allergy at 3 years of age.
Variables with $p \leq 0.2$ in univariable analysis are included as covariates in separate models.
[a]OR = 0.03 for every 5 g/MJ/d. [b]$P = 0.01$ in likelihood ratio testing (χ^2). [c]One healthy farmer and one allergic control child missing. [d]One allergic control child missing.

vegetables, grains, dairy, fish, and pork is likely to be an indicator of a lower intake of porridge/gruel, which is fortified with iron when bought commercially. Accordingly, negative correlations were found between the intake of bought porridge/gruel and the intake of most of the foods that correlated negatively with iron intake. However, restricting the intake of several food groups in favor of bought porridge/gruel might counteract the acceptance of a broad range of foods, which in turn may influence the future diversity of a child's diet negatively.

The children's intake of nutrients did not differ substantially between farm and control children. The majority of the children had intakes of vitamin D, iodine, and selenium that were considerably lower than current recommendations (10, 70, and 20 µg, respectively) (16). Although only significant for iodine, the children of farmers less often had a diet deficient in the above-mentioned micronutrients, vitamin D, iodine, and selenium, which is most likely explained by their significantly higher intake of oily fish; fish is a good source of all these three micronutrients. Ten farm children (36%) and four control children (11%) had fish during any of the 2 days of registration. However, the true intake of fish is difficult to capture using a dietary assessment of only 2 days, since fish is generally consumed at irregular intervals (22). For just above half of all the farm and control children,

Table 8. Logistic regression models of intake of pork at 1 year of age and allergy in the child at 3 years of age

	Farmers and controls			Controls		
	Healthy ($n=44$)			Healthy ($n=21$)		
	Allergic ($n=11$)			Allergic ($n=10$)		
Predictor variables	OR	95% CI	*P*	OR	95% CI	*P*
Pork alone	1.28	1.02–1.6	0.03	1.37[a]	1.01–1.84	0.04
Model 1						
Pork	1.39	1.01–1.92	0.04	1.70	1.03–2.81	0.04
Length of exclusive breast feeding, months	0.53	0.34–0.84	0.01	0.43	0.21–0.86	0.02
Model 2						
Pork	1.39	1.03–1.87	0.03	1.56	1.06–2.30	0.03
Length of partial breast feeding, months	0.77	0.62–0.97	0.03	0.74	0.54–0.99	0.05
Model 3						
Pork	1.25	0.98–1.59	0.07	1.33	0.98–1.80	0.07
Cesarean section	3.28	0.62–17.5	0.16	2.18	0.3–15.9	0.44
Model 4						
Pork	1.34	1.03–1.76	0.03	1.53	1.04–2.25	0.03
Female gender	0.17	0.03–1.04	0.06	0.07	0.00–1.55	0.09
Model 5						
Pork	1.28	1.02–1.6	0.03	1.40	1.01–1.94	0.04
Maternal heredity	3.33	0.76–14.7	0.11	5.67	0.85–37.6	0.07
Model 6						
Pork	1.20	0.93–1.58	0.16	1.36	0.98–1.88	0.06
Gestational week[b]	0.70	0.45–1.09	0.11	0.70	0.42–1.14	0.15
Model 7						
Pork	1.26	0.97–1.63	0.09	1.36	0.99–1.88	0.06
Birth weight[c], g	1.00	1.00–1.00	0.29	0.99	0.99–1.00	0.50
Model 8						
Pork	1.25	0.98–1.58	0.07	1.35	0.99–1.82	0.06
Cats or dogs in house at recruitment	0.54	0.12–2.35	0.41	0.67	0.12–3.75	0.65
Model 9						
Pork	1.30	1.03–1.60	0.03	1.38	1.02–1.87	0.04
Paternal smoking last month of pregnancy	6.40	0.67–61.9	0.11	3.31	0.31–35.4	0.32

Odds ratios (ORs) and confidence intervals (CIs) for every g/MJ/d of pork intake at 1 year of age and allergy at 3 years of age.
Variables with $P \leq 0.2$ in univariable analysis are included as covariates in separate models.
[a]OR = 4.8 for every 5 g/MJ/d. [b]One healthy farmer and one allergic control child missing. [c]One allergic control child missing.

respectively, the intake of supplements of vitamin A+D was reported; hence, the true vitamin D intake was larger in both groups. No correlations were found between the intake of vitamin D supplementation and fish intake (data not shown). A higher intake of oily fish was not observed among the Finnish farm children compared to controls (21). Instead, the controls consumed more fish in total; hence our findings of a higher oily fish intake in farm children may not characterize farm children's diet in general.

The intake of seafood at 1 year of age was negatively associated with being allergic at 3 years of age. The early intake of fish has previously been associated with protection against allergy development (6, 7, 23, 24). Accordingly, we have previously shown that high proportions of the long-chain n-3 PUFA EPA in sera at 4 months of age were associated with a lower risk of developing allergy in the FARMFLORA cohort, although not related to farm residence (unpublished observations). The intake of seafood in the 1-year-olds correlated with the proportions of EPA in the sera at 4 months of age, which in turn was related to EPA in breast milk and maternal intake of oily fish during pregnancy. Also, the breast milk proportions of EPA correlated with maternal fish intake during lactation. Thus, the intake of fish in the mothers and the 1-year-old children were associated. Whether it is the maternal or infant fish intake that confers protection against allergy cannot thereby be determined. Unfortunately, no serum samples were obtained at 1 year of age; hence, we did not analyze EPA or other long-chain PUFAs in sera from the 1-year-olds.

In contrast to seafood, the intake of pork was positively associated with allergy development. No substantial decrease in the odds ratio for pork and allergy was observed when adjusted for potential covariates in logistic regression. One could suspect that the consumption of more pork may result in the consumption of less fish, but no correlations were found between the children's pork and fish intakes. However, the odds ratio for the association of pork intake and allergy was moderate (1.37), and there are no previous reports of pork consumption as a risk factor for allergy development; hence, the finding should be interpreted with caution. Further, the intake of zinc was higher in children who later developed allergy than in healthy children. Correlations were made in retrospect between pork intake and dietary zinc content, and we found that these were positively correlated. Hence, the association between pork and allergy may be mediated by zinc. However, although zinc has immunomodulatory properties and could play a role in allergy development, there are no previous reports of positive associations between zinc and allergy, to the best of our knowledge.

The dietary pattern of a higher intake of full-fat dairy, including farm milk, which characterized the farm children in our study, was not related to allergy protection. However, unpasteurized milk has been associated with a lower risk of allergy in a number of studies (9, 12). In our study, the intake of farm milk was reported for 13 farm children, six of whom consumed unpasteurized milk. No control family reported the consumption of unpasteurized milk in the children. As all allergy cases except one occurred in the control group, we cannot determine whether the consumption of unpasteurized milk contributed to the pronounced protection from allergy development in the farm children.

Conclusions

We could show a similar dietary pattern in farm children and their mothers, including more full-fat dairy, fat in total, and saturated fatty acids compared to control infants, who instead tended to consume more margarine; this pattern was, however, not linked to the protective effect on allergy development of growing up on a farm. However, the farm children consumed more oily fish, and a weak negative association between seafood intake and allergy development was found; the pork intake and zinc content of the diet were instead correlated with one another and were positively associated with the risk of allergy development in the control infants.

Acknowledgements

Great thanks to the study nurses Helen Andersson and Anders Nordberg for their comprehensive work of coordinating sampling and questionnaires in this cohort. Also, the authors acknowledge the pediatricians Bill Hesselmar, Susanne Johansen, Margareta Ceder, Gunhild Lindhagen, Stefan Stentoft, and Carl-Johan Törnhage for skillful clinical diagnoses of the children, as well as all the families for their participation in this study.

Conflict of interest and funding

No conflict of interest to declare. The FARMFLORA birth cohort was supported by grants from the Swedish Research Council for Environmental, Agricultural Sciences and Spatial Planning (Formas, No. 222-2004-1958), Livsmedelsacceleratorn, SP Food and Biosciences (Former Food and Health Concept Centre), Gothenburg Sweden, West Gothia Region (VGR), Torsten and Ragnar Söderberg Foundation, the Medical Faculty of the University of Gothenburg under the LUA agreement, the Swedish Research Council (VR, No. 521-2013-3154). Funds have been received from the OA-fund, Chalmers Publication Library, to cover costs for open access.

References

1. Strachan DP. Hay fever, hygiene, and household size. BMJ 1989; 299(6710): 1259–60.
2. Wold AE. The hygiene hypothesis revised: is the rising frequency of allergy due to changes in the intestinal flora? Allergy 1998; 53(46 Suppl): 20–5.
3. Black PN, Sharpe S. Dietary fat and asthma: is there a connection? Eur Respir J 1997; 10(1): 6–12.
4. Lumia M, Luukkainen P, Kaila M, Tapanainen H, Takkinen HM, Prasad M, et al. Maternal dietary fat and fatty acid intake during lactation and the risk of asthma in the offspring. Acta Paediatr 2012; 101(8): e337–43.
5. Sausenthaler S, Kompauer I, Borte M, Herbarth O, Schaaf B, Berg A, et al. Margarine and butter consumption, eczema and allergic sensitization in children. The LISA birth cohort study. Pediatr Allergy Immunol 2006; 17(2): 85–93.
6. Nafstad P, Nystad W, Magnus P, Jaakkola JJ. Asthma and allergic rhinitis at 4 years of age in relation to fish consumption in infancy. J Asthma 2003; 40(4): 343–8.
7. Sausenthaler S, Koletzko S, Schaaf B, Lehmann I, Borte M, Herbarth O, et al. Maternal diet during pregnancy in relation to eczema and allergic sensitization in the offspring at 2 y of age. Am J Clin Nutr 2007; 85(2): 530–7.
8. Braun-Fahrlander C, Gassner M, Grize L, Neu U, Sennhauser FH, Varonier HS, et al. Prevalence of hay fever and allergic sensitization in farmer's children and their peers living in the same rural community. SCARPOL team. Swiss study on childhood allergy and respiratory symptoms with respect to air pollution. Clin Exp Allergy 1999; 29(1): 28–34.
9. Riedler J, Braun-Fahrlander C, Eder W, Schreuer M, Waser M, Maisch S, et al. Exposure to farming in early life and development of asthma and allergy: a cross-sectional survey. Lancet 2001; 358(9288): 1129–33.
10. Von Ehrenstein OS, Von Mutius E, Illi S, Baumann L, Bohm O, von Kries R. Reduced risk of hay fever and asthma among children of farmers. Clin Exp Allergy 2000; 30(2): 187–93.

11. Douwes J, Cheng S, Travier N, Cohet C, Niesink A, McKenzie J, et al. Farm exposure in utero may protect against asthma, hay fever and eczema. Eur Respir J 2008; 32(3): 603–11.
12. Perkin MR, Strachan DP. Which aspects of the farming lifestyle explain the inverse association with childhood allergy? J Allergy Clin Immunol 2006; 117(6): 1374–81.
13. Jonsson K, Barman M, Moberg S, Sjoberg A, Brekke HK, Hesselmar B, et al. Fat intake and breast milk fatty acid composition in farming and nonfarming women and allergy development in the offspring. Pediatr Res 2016; 79(1–1): 114–23.
14. Conway JM, Ingwersen LA, Vinyard BT, Moshfegh AJ. Effectiveness of the US Department of Agriculture 5-step multiple-pass method in assessing food intake in obese and nonobese women. Am J Clin Nutr 2003; 77(5): 1171–8.
15. Wikland KA, Luo ZC, Niklasson A, Karlberg J. Swedish population-based longitudinal reference values from birth to 18 years of age for height, weight and head circumference. Acta Paediatr 2002; 91(7): 739–54.
16. Nordic Nutrition Recommendations 2012: integrating nutrition and physical activity 2014. 5th ed. Copenhagen: Nordic Council of Ministers. Available from: http://www.norden.org/en/theme/nordic-nutrition-recommendation/nordic-nutrition-recommendations-2012; 2012. [cited 5 Nov 2015].
17. Hesselmar B, Sjöberg F, Saalman R, Åberg N, Adlerberth I, Wold AE. Pacifier cleaning practices and risk of allergy development. Pediatrics 2013; 131(6): e1829–37.
18. Williams HC. Diagnostic criteria for atopic dermatitis [19]. Lancet 1996; 348(9038): 1391–2.
19. Hanifin J, Rajka G. Diagnostic features of atopic dermatitis. Acta Derm Venereol 1980; Suppl. 92; 60: 44–7.
20. Bylesjö M, Rantalainen M, Cloarec O, Nicholson JK, Holmes E, Trygg J. OPLS discriminant analysis: combining the strengths of PLS-DA and SIMCA classification. J Chemometr 2006; 20(8–10): 341–51.
21. Remes ST, Iivanainen K, Koskela H, Pekkanen J. Which factors explain the lower prevalence of atopy amongst farmers' children? Clin Exp Allergy 2003; 33(4): 427–34.
22. Barbieri Enghardt H, Pearson M, Becker W. Riksmaten – barn 2003. Uppsala: The Swedish National Food Agency; 2006.
23. Dotterud CK, Storrø O, Simpson MR, Johnsen R, Øien T. The impact of pre- and post-natal exposures on allergy related diseases in childhood: a controlled multicentre intervention study in primary health care. BMC Public Health 2013; 13: 123.
24. Hesselmar B, Saalman R, Rudin A, Adlerberth I, Wold AE. Early fish introduction is associated with less eczema, but not sensitization, in infants. Acta Paediatr Int J Paediatr 2010; 99(12): 1861–7.

***Karin Jonsson**
Department of Food and Nutrition Science
Chalmers University of Technology
SE-412 96 Gothenburg
Sweden
Email: karin.jonsson@chalmers.se

7

Nutritional and developmental status among 6- to 8-month-old children in southwestern Uganda

Grace K. M. Muhoozi[1,2]*, Prudence Atukunda[1], Robert Mwadime[3], Per Ole Iversen[1,4] and Ane C. Westerberg[5]

[1]Department of Nutrition, Institute of Basic Medical Sciences, University of Oslo, Oslo, Norway; [2]Department of Human Nutrition and Home Economics, Kyambogo University, Kampala, Uganda; [3]School of Food Technology, Nutrition and Bioengineering, Makerere University, Kampala, Uganda; [4]Department of Hematology, Oslo University Hospital, Oslo, Norway; [5]Institute of Health Sciences, Kristiania University College, Oslo, Norway

Abstract

Background: Undernutrition continues to pose challenges to Uganda's children, but there is limited knowledge on its association with physical and intellectual development.
Objective: In this cross-sectional study, we assessed the nutritional status and milestone development of 6- to 8-month-old children and associated factors in two districts of southwestern Uganda.
Design: Five hundred and twelve households with mother–infant (6–8 months) pairs were randomly sampled. Data about background variables (e.g. household characteristics, poverty likelihood, and child dietary diversity scores (CDDS)) were collected using questionnaires. Bayley Scales of Infant and Toddler Development (BSID III) and Ages and Stages questionnaires (ASQ) were used to collect data on child development. Anthropometric measures were used to determine *z*-scores for weight-for-age (WAZ), length-for-age (LAZ), weight-for-length (WLZ), head circumference (HCZ), and mid-upper arm circumference. Chi-square tests, correlation coefficients, and linear regression analyses were used to relate background variables, nutritional status indicators, and infant development.
Results: The prevalence of underweight, stunting, and wasting was 12.1, 24.6, and 4.7%, respectively. Household head education, gender, sanitation, household size, maternal age and education, birth order, poverty likelihood, and CDDS were associated ($p < 0.05$) with WAZ, LAZ, and WLZ. Regression analysis showed that gender, sanitation, CDDS, and likelihood to be below the poverty line were predictors ($p < 0.05$) of undernutrition. BSID III indicated development delay of 1.3% in cognitive and language, and 1.6% in motor development. The ASQ indicated delayed development of 24, 9.1, 25.2, 12.2, and 15.1% in communication, fine motor, gross motor, problem solving, and personal social ability, respectively. All nutritional status indicators except HCZ were positively and significantly associated with development domains. WAZ was the main predictor for all development domains.
Conclusion: Undernutrition among infants living in impoverished rural Uganda was associated with household sanitation, poverty, and low dietary diversity. Development domains were positively and significantly associated with nutritional status. Nutritional interventions might add value to improvement of child growth and development.

Keywords: *child development*; *child growth*; *Uganda*; *undernutrition*

Undernutrition continues to pose challenges to Uganda's children (1). Inadequate dietary intake of nutritious food and infections including diarrheal diseases are major causes of growth faltering among infants (2–4). Undernutrition may start as early as during foetal life as a consequence of inadequate food intake of the mother as well as strenuous work during pregnancy (5–9). This causes growth faltering among the infants, which is often accelerated when complementary feeding starts and low-nutrient-density foods are used to replace breast milk (10). Inadequate food intake also results from low meal frequency. In western Uganda, 34% of children aged 6–23 months are fed only twice or less in a day (11) instead of the recommended three to four times a day (12).

Stunting in Uganda has been linked with low socio-economic status and associated factors such as poor health, sanitation and lack of appropriate knowledge on health and nutrition, gender disparities, low or no education of mothers, and suboptimal infant feeding practices (13, 14). Poor sanitary conditions often lead to infections that increase children's risk of entering a vicious cycle of infection, undernutrition, and impaired linear growth as a result of lack of appetite, increased nutrient needs, and malabsorption (11).

Stunting in early life (0–2 years) has been linked to impaired cognitive, language, and motor development (15–17). However, improved nutrition and catch-up growth have been shown to improve or normalize development after stunting (15, 16, 18). Significant growth and development of the brain occur in the last trimester of pregnancy until two years of age (19, 20). Adequate macro- and micronutrient supply is essential for the growth and maintenance of brain tissue to support cognitive and social development (21, 22). Thus, nutrition indirectly affects children's behaviour and experiences (23). Impaired cognitive function consequently affects the individual's ability to live a productive life and educational attainment (24).

In Uganda, few studies have addressed nutrition, growth, and cognitive development. In the Ugandan Nutrition and Early Child Development Project, communities received media messages on child stimulation, positive parenting, health, hygiene, and nutrition (25). The results indicated improvement in breastfeeding practices, growth rates in the youngest children, and parental attitudes and behaviour supporting early child development, but little effect on the cognitive development of children aged 3.5–6 years (25). An intervention study in rural northern Uganda addressing maternal psychological well-being, child growth, and development, with a nutrition component (dietary diversity and demonstrations of food quantities), showed improvement in cognitive and language scores using the Bayley Scales of Infant and Toddler Development (BSID III). However, there was no improvement in length-for-age *z*-scores (LAZ) (26).

The southwestern part of Uganda, including the Kabale and Kisoro districts, has been known to be nutritionally insecure (11), and the levels of stunting, underweight, and wasting were 41.7, 15.5, and 4.9% respectively, in 2011 (1). In this study, two questions were thus addressed: 1) what factors are associated with nutritional status among 6- to 8-month-old infants in Kabale and Kisoro; and 2) what is the relation between their nutritional status, cognitive, language, and motor development? This study focused on 6- to 8- month-old infants because complementary feeding is recommended to start at 6 months (12, 27), a critical time period when adequate nutrition is key in supporting cognitive and social development (21, 22).

Subjects and methods

Study area

The study was conducted in Kabale and Kisoro because of the high levels of stunting. Town centres were excluded to minimize differences in socio-economic status and feeding practices. Inhabitants were predominantly small-scale farmers cultivating small plots of land. Both districts were densely populated with populations of 534,160 (28) and 287,179 (29), respectively.

Study design and participants

The cross-sectional study was conducted between October 2013 and February 2014. The sampling unit was a household with a lead caregiver as the respondent and an infant aged 6–8 months. Households were excluded if the child had 1) congenital malformation(s), 2) a physical handicap that would influence growth or preclude anthropometric measurements, or influence nutrient intake, or 3) been diagnosed with mental or brain illness as evidenced by the child's mother or a health worker.

Sample size determination and sampling strategy

Sample size calculations were based on a prevalence of 35% for stunting among 6- to 8-month-old children in southwestern Uganda (1). Power was set at 0.8 with a significance level of 5%. To allow for a precision of ±5% and a 30% dropout rate, 500 households were required for the study.

Basing on the 2002 housing and population census, an average of six households per 150 in every village was assumed to have an infant between 6 and 8 months old. Furthermore, the included households were stratified according to the districts. Proportionate simple random sampling was used to select sub-counties to participate in the study (six sub-counties in Kabale and four in Kisoro). Using the list of all villages, nine villages were randomly selected in each of the participating sub-counties. Finally, all consenting households with children aged 6–8 months within a participating village were recruited. If a household had more than one eligible child, the youngest was selected to participate, and in the case of twins, we randomly selected one of them. All tools and questionnaires were pretested in the area and adjusted before use.

Data collection of household characteristics and anthropometry

Data were collected during home visits using a semi-structured questionnaire with both open- and close-ended questions. The questionnaire was based on previously validated questionnaires (30), with minor language modifications to make it appropriate for the study participants. It was administered to the lead caregiver through interview and included 1) socio-demographic characteristics; 2) morbidity, if their infants had any illness in the previous 2 weeks or if the infants were sick at the time of data collection; and 3) child feeding practices. Field assistants (with minimum qualification of 'Advanced level of education') had 5 days of intensive training in data collection instruments and the collection of anthropometric data using digital scales, tapes, length boards, and measurement techniques as per standardized World Health Organization (WHO) guidelines (31). A different team, composed of nutritionists (bachelors' degree holders) led by a clinical psychologist (the second author), was trained in administering the child development tools and scoring the performance of the children.

Sanitation was evaluated by observation and recording the presence or absence of stagnant water in the compound, human faeces around the house/veranda, animal droppings, and litter in the compound. If any of these were present, the score would be 0; if none was found, the score would be 1. The presence or absence and the condition of the plate stand (drying rack), bath shelter, and latrine were also obtained by observation. These were scored as good = 3, fair = 2, poor = 1, and none = 0. The scores were then combined to make the composite variable (household sanitation) with scores ranging from 0 to 12.

Nutritional status was evaluated using weight, length, head circumference (HC), and mid-upper arm circumference (MUAC), which were measured using standard procedures and calibrations recommended by WHO (31, 32). Anthropometric measurements were performed by a pair of trained field workers. Weight (to the nearest 0.1 kg) was measured with a Seca-scale (model 881, Hamburg, Germany); recumbent length was measured (to the nearest cm) with a length board (SO114530) (33); HC was measured with a non-stretchable tape; MUAC was measured with a non-stretchable tape at the midpoint between the acromion and the olecranon. The child's date of birth was obtained from child health cards. For those who did not have child health cards (8.3%), a record of events was used to determine the approximate date of birth. The anthropometric data including age in months were calculated and converted to *z*-scores (LAZ, weight-for-age *z*-scores (WAZ), weight-for-length *z*-scores (WLZ), mid-upper arm circumference *z*-scores (MUACZ), and head circumference *z*-scores (HCZ) by use of the software Anthro package (version 3.2.2), a nutritional assessment tool using the WHO standards (31, 34). Undernutrition (stunting, underweight, and wasting: LAZ, WAZ, and WLZ, respectively) was defined as a *z*-score less than two SD below the mean on the WHO reference standards (31, 35, 36). A score of less than three SD below the mean on the WHO reference standards of either LAZ, WAZ, or WLZ was defined as severe stunting, underweight, and wasting, respectively.

The socio-economic status of the households was obtained by the 'Simple Poverty Scorecard for Uganda' (37), which has 10 indicators that are strongly associated with poverty, and is sensitive to changes in poverty status. The scores were summed up and associated with poverty likelihoods via the 'National 100% look up table', a scale that ranges from 0 to 100 (least to most likely to be below the poverty line) (37). The households were then categorized as extreme (47.9–100%), moderate (2.9–47.8%), or least (0–2.8%) likelihood to be below the poverty line.

Infant feeding practices were determined by asking mothers about the first food/drink that was given to the infant, the number of times the infant was fed, the person that normally fed the infant, and the combination of foods normally given. The child dietary diversity scores (CDDS), adapted from the Household Diversity Score tool (38), were used to determine the quality of the individual child's diet (39–43). The tool has a range of 0–8 food groups: 1) grains, roots, or tubers; 2) vitamin A-rich plant foods; 3) other fruits or vegetables; 4) meat, poultry, fish, and seafood; 5) eggs; 6) pulses, legumes, and nuts; 7) milk and milk products; 8) foods cooked in oil or fat. If the child consumed any of the foods the previous 24 h that belonged to any of the group, it would be scored 1, and these were summed up to give the CDDS. The CDDS was then categorized as 0–3 low or $\geq$ 4 high (39). Previous studies showed that CDDS has a good sensitivity and specificity (40) and correlated significantly with WAZ and LAZ (42).

The Household Food Insecurity Access Scale (HFIAS), without any modifications, was used to determine household food insecurity including all nine generic questions that require a recall about the worry of food availability and accessibility in the previous 4 weeks (44, 45). If the respondent answered 'yes' to an occurrence question, a follow-up question was asked to determine whether the condition occurred rarely (once or twice), sometimes (3 to 10 times) or often (more than 10 times). The responses determined the Household Food Insecurity Access Prevalence (HFIAP) status indicator as a proxy of household food insecurity prevalence (44). Each household was then classified into either food secure, or mildly, moderately, and severely food insecure, based on FANTA's recommended cut-offs.

Cognitive, language, and motor development assessments

Infant development was determined by the BSID III (46) on three sub-scales of cognitive, language, and motor functions. The Bayley scales are known to be the most comprehensive development measures for children up to 42 months (46–48). The BSID III scales were translated to the local language and back translated to English. Furthermore, some pictures in the stimulus and picture booklets were replaced by familiar similar objects in the local setting, for example, apples for tomatoes. The raw scores were converted to composite scores according to the reference material. The mean score is 100 with an SD of 15. Scores below 70 (i.e. <2 SD below the mean for a US reference population) indicate developmental delay.

The infant development was also assessed using the Ages and Stages questionnaires (ASQ) (46, 49–51). The scores obtained from each developmental domain were calculated according to a scale from 0 (worst) to 60 (best), and each child was classified into 'normal', 'delayed', or 'needs attention' based on cut-off values for each of the five domains (48, 52). Both tools were used because ASQ is a caregiver report that captures and establishes a wide range of adaptive behaviours (53) that are not achieved using the BSID III. A 6-day intensive training session was conducted by three research assistants (bachelor's degree holders) and a nutritionist (first author) on the use of the BSID III and ASQ. Data quality assurance was done by the clinical psychologist, who supervised the administration of tests and checked on interview styles and data records throughout the study.

The administration of the tests was done by personnel fluent in English and local language to enhance adequate communication with the children and the caregivers. Administration instructions of time, reversal, and discontinuation rules were strictly followed. Feedback on administration styles and data records were reviewed at the end of each assessment day. Social-emotional and adaptive behaviour subtests of the BSID III were not used due to time constraint and some of these aspects were covered by the ASQ. Inter-rater results showed good correlation ($r=0.71$–0.87) for both scales.

Statistics

Chi-square and Pearson's correlation tests were used to determine associations of independent variables and nutritional status and the interrelations of other variables, as well as associations between nutritional status with milestone development (aspects of cognitive, language, and motor development). All putative determinants from bivariate analysis were simultaneously included in the various models. In order to identify the most significant determinants, a linear regression analysis was performed using the enter procedures, retaining only the strongest determinants. The variables that did not explain additional variance were not included in the final regression models; all necessary assumptions were met. Variables that showed a significant ($p<0.05$) association in bivariate analyses were included in linear regression models for the different nutritional status indicators to determine the predictors of the dependent variables (Supplementary Table 1). Linear regression was used to examine the relationship between nutritional status and composite scores of cognitive, language, and motor development in children taking into account other factors. The statistical analyses were performed using SPSS version 22 (54) and the level of significance was set at $p<0.05$.

Approvals

The study was reviewed by the Makerere University School of Public Health, Higher Degrees Research and Ethics Committee (no. IRB000353) and approved by the Uganda National Council for Science and Technology. It was also approved by the Norwegian Regional Committee for Medical and Health Research Ethics (no. 2013/1833). All respondents gave informed consent by reading and signing a consent form to participate in the study and allowing publication of the findings. The consent form was designed and translated into local language for the participants.

Results

Socio-demographic characteristics

All 536 households that were identified consented to participate. Then, 24 households were excluded, mainly due to incorrect reporting of children's ages, leaving a total of 512 households. Table 1 summarizes the household characteristics. The mean ($\pm$ SD) household size was 5.5 ± 2.1 and most (97%) of the households were reported to be headed by males. The mean age of household heads was 32.3 ± 9.7 years, and they had on average spent 6.2 ± 3.7 years in school. The majority (70%) were peasant farmers. General sanitation in households was fair although a substantial proportion (10.4%) lacked basic sanitary facilities such as latrines, bath shelter, and a plate stand. In some places, these amenities were present, but in poor condition. Most households suffered from moderate to severe food insecurity (43.2 and 34%, respectively). Furthermore, the mean poverty score for all households was 47.7 ± 11.9. Most households (77.9%) had a moderate likelihood of being below the poverty line.

Maternal and child characteristics

The mean ($\pm$ SD) number of years a mother had spent in school was 4.9 ± 3.4, and most of the mothers were peasant farmers. Mean age of mothers was 26.6 ± 6.5 years, and the mean age at first birth was 19.6 ± 2.8 years. The mean number of children per mother was 3.4 ± 2.3, and 3.4% of the mothers had more than eight biological children (Table 1). The proportions of boys and girls were about equal (50.8%) and (49.2%), respectively, and their mean age was 7.3 ± 0.9 months.

Child morbidity

During the last 2 weeks prior to the survey, 65.0% of the children had suffered various illnesses, and 32.4% were still sick at the time of survey. The most common illnesses were cough and flu (56.9%), diarrhoea (26.6%), and fever (sometimes referred to as malaria; 10.3%). Other illnesses reported were skin rash, sore throat, nose bleeding, and eye infections (data not shown). There were no significant differences in gender morbidity (Supplementary Table 1).

Table 1. Household socio-demographic and maternal characteristics ($n = 512$)

Characteristics			
HH size (mean [SD])	5.5 (2.1)	Household food insecurity	
3–5	289 (56.4)	Food secure	76 (14.8)
6–13	223 (43.6)	Mild food insecurity	41 (8.0)
HH head age (years) (mean [SD])	32.3 (9.7)	Moderate food insecurity	221 (43.2)
19–29	217 (42.4)	Severe food insecurity	174 (34.0)
30–40	169 (33)	Maternal characteristics	
≥41	99 (19.6)	Maternal age (years) (mean [SD])	26.6 (6.3)
HH head education (years) (mean [SD])	6.2 (3.7)	Maternal education (years) (mean [SD])	4.9 (3.4)
None	58 (12)	None	98 (19.6)
1–6	190 (39.2)	7–10	126 (25.2)
7–10	159 (32.9)	1–6	242 (48.4)
≥11	77 (15.9)	≥11	35 (7.0)
HH head occupation		Maternal occupation	
Peasant farmers	359 (70.1)	Peasant farmers	401 (78.3)
Casual labourers	70 (13.9)	Housewife	86 (16.8)
Business	29 (5.8)	Salary employed	10 (2.0)
Salary employed	27 (5.4)	Others (e.g. business and students)	15 (3.0)
Sanitation in HH		Maternal age at first child (years) (mean [SD])	19.6 (2.8)
Poor sanitation	53 (10.4)	<18	95 (18.9)
Fair sanitation	270 (52.7)	≥18	404 (81.6)
Good sanitation	189 (36.9)	Number of children per mother (mean [SD])	3.4 (2.3)
Likelihood to below poverty line		1–4	371 (72.4)
Extreme likelihood (47.9 to 100.0%)	37 (7.2)	5–8	124 (24.2)
Moderate likelihood (2.9 to 38.1%)	398 (77.9)	9–11	17 (3.4)
Least likelihood (0.0 to 0.8)	77 (15.9)	Mean child age (months) (mean [SD])	7.3 (0.9)

Values are n (%) unless otherwise stated. HH, household.

Infant feeding

Most of the index children (97%) were still breastfeeding, and many of them (96%) had started complementary feeding. About 70% of the mothers reported having given only breast milk to their babies up to 6 months, although some of them continued beyond that point, while others had not started complementary feeding at the time of survey (Table 2). Moreover, about two-thirds of the children were reported to be breastfed on demand. There was limited use of infant formula (0.6%) and sources of animal protein.

A majority of the children were first introduced to porridge alone. The combination of foods commonly given to children was beans and a carbohydrate source (e.g. potato, green banana, rice, yam, or maize meal), or a carbohydrate source alone, as reported by approximately one-third of the respondents in each case. The mean ($\pm$ SD) CDDS was 3.1 ± 1.7 (range 0–8). Few children (4.5%) were fed foods of animal origin (Table 2).

Growth and cognitive function

The means (SD) of WAZ, LAZ, and WLZ were -0.67 (1.1), -1.14 (1.2), and 0.13 (1.2), respectively. The prevalence of underweight, stunting, and wasting in all children were 12.1, 24.6, and 4.7%, respectively (Table 3). Undernutrition was significantly higher in boys than girls as shown by stunting (30.2% vs. 18.8%), underweight (15.3% vs. 8.8%), and wasting (6.5% vs. 2.8%) (Supplementary Table 1).

The mean ($\pm$ SD) composite scores for cognitive, language, and motor development based on the BSID III were 102.6 ± 13.7; 101.8 ± 14.8, and 104.4 ± 15.2, respectively. There were no severely cognitively impaired children, but the language and motor scores indicated that one (0.2%) and four (1.1%) of the children had severe impairment in the two domains, respectively. Results from the ASQ indicated delayed development in all five domains of communication, fine motor, gross motor, problem solving, and personal social ability (Table 3). There were no significant gender differences regarding impairment in cognitive, motor, or language development.

Association between various characteristics and child nutritional status

The results of the bivariate analysis using the chi-square statistics showed that bigger households and those in extreme likelihood of being below the poverty line were likely to have more underweight children ($p < 0.05$; Supplementary Table 1). Household heads with 0–7 years of school were likely to have more stunted children compared

Table 2. Breast feeding and complementary feeding ($n = 512$)

Characteristics	*n* (%)
Exclusive breastfeeding first 6 months[a]	357 (70)
Breast feeding frequency	
Whenever the child wants (on demand)	342 (69.0)
Five to eight times per day	143 (29.0)
Two to four times per day	10 (2.0)
Age at introduction of first foods	
Between three and five months	38 (27.0)
At six months	277 (54.0)
After six months	67 (13.1)
Not yet started	19 (3.7)
Child diet diversity score	
Low CDDS (0–3 food groups)	317 (62.0)
High CDDS (4–7 food groups)	194 (38.0)
Combinations of foods commonly fed to children	
A carbohydrate source[b] and beans	144 (32.6)
Porridge alone or a carbohydrate source alone	138 (31.2)
Beans alone or beans with green vegetable	77 (17.4)
Milk, eggs, silver fish, soy	20 (4.5)
Bean soup	20 (4.5)
Beans, carbohydrate source, green vegetable	15 (3.4)
A source of animal protein[c] and carbohydrate	14 (3.2)
Green vegetable, fruit alone	6 (1.4)
A source of animal protein[c], carbohydrate source, green vegetable	5 (1.1)
Porridge with milk	3 (0.7)

[a]Mothers were asked the age at which they first gave drink or food to the infant.
[b]This is a group of staple foods including potatoes, sorghum, millet, yams, cassava, maize meal, and rice.
[c]Foods such as meat, milk, fish, and eggs.
CDDS, child dietary diversity scores.

to households whose head had more years of school ($p < 0.01$); similarly children with low CDDS were more likely to be stunted than those with higher CDDS ($p < 0.05$).

Household head education was positively and significantly associated with all the nutritional status indicators, whereas maternal education was significantly associated with only WAZ and WLZ (Supplementary Table 2). There was a negative and significant association between household size and WLZ as well as MUACZ. Child birth order was negatively and significantly associated with WAZ and WLZ. The CDDS were positively and significantly associated with WAZ and LAZ. Poverty likelihood scores were negatively and significantly associated with WAZ, WLZ, HCZ, and MUACZ. Morbidity did not show any significant association with any of the indicators of nutritional status ($p > 0.05$).

The linear multivariate regression analyses indicated that the sex of a child was a main predictor of WAZ, followed by sanitation ($R^2 = 0.068$) (Table 4). Moreover, the sex of a child and CDDS were predictors of LAZ, while WLZ was predicted by likelihood to be below the poverty line ($R^2 = 0.039$ and 0.050, respectively).

Nutritional status and child development domains

Supplementary Table 3 shows results of nutritional status indicators' bivariate correlations with the BSID III and ASQ indicators. Most of the nutritional status indicators were positively ($p < 0.05$) associated with language, cognitive, and motor domains (BSID III). However, the correlations between WLZ, HCZ, and cognitive domain were not significant. In the same way, using the ASQ, most of all the nutritional status indicators were positively ($p < 0.05$) associated with the development domains, except for LAZ with fine motor and HCZ with personal social abilities, where the associations were not significant.

Multiple regression (using BSID III) showed that the cognitive domain was predicted by WAZ, the sex of a child (boy), and household head education ($R^2 = 0.104$) (Table 5). Furthermore, the language domain was predicted by both WAZ and LAZ ($R^2 = 0.068$), whereas the motor domain was predicted by the sex of a child (boy), WAZ, LAZ, and likelihood of being below the poverty line ($R^2 = 0.086$).

Discussion

Anthropometry and nutritional status

Nutritional status indicators showed growth faltering as in many other developing countries (55). Boys were particularly more at risk of undernutrition than girls. The trend of a higher level of stunting among boys compared to girls was also observed by UDHS (41% vs. 36%) (1); however, in this study, the margin was higher (30.3% vs. 18.8%). Our findings indicated higher stunting levels (24.6%) compared to the national level (12.4%) for 6- to 8-month-old children (1). However, the levels of underweight and wasting in the current study were lower (11.9 and 4.7%, respectively) than the national level (19.1 and 13.6%, respectively) (1). This finding confirms the previously found high stunting level in southwestern Uganda (41.7%) compared to the national level (33.4%) (1, 11, 14). Evident growth restriction at a young age as 6–8 months old may indicate that growth faltering starts earlier than 6 months (6–8, 10, 11), even as intrauterine growth restriction.

We noted that complementary feeding practices were poor. Some mothers (16.8%) had not started complementary feeding, and the majority (68%) of children had their first complementary food as diluted porridge nothing added. At the time of study, the proportion of children who were being fed foods containing primarily carbohydrate sources and beans was 32.6%; for carbohydrate sources alone, it was 32.6%. The consumption of animal protein foods was limited (4.5%), as also shown in another study (14), and a good combination of sources of animal protein, carbohydrates, and green vegetables was

Table 3. Child nutrition and development status

		n (%)	*n* (%)	*n* (%)
Growth indicators	Mean (SD)	< −3.00 SD	−2.99 to −2.00 SD	< −2.00 SD
Weight-for-age *z*-score	−0.68 (1.1)	19 (3.7)	42 (8.2)	61 (11.9)
Length-for-age *z*-score	−1.14 (1.2)	50 (9.8)	76 (14.8)	126 (24.6)
Weight-for-length *z*-score	0.13 (1.2)	8 (1.6)	16 (3.1)	24 (4.7)
MUAC *z*-score	0.28 (1.0)	1(0.2)	10 (2.1)	11 (2.3)
Head circumference *z*-score	0.63 (1.1)	1(0.2)	13 (2.5)	14 (2.7)
Child development scores[a]	Mean (SD)			
BSID II		< −3.00 SD	−2.99 to −2.00 SD	< −2.00 SD
Cognitive scores	102.65 (13.4)	0 (0.0)	6 (1.3)	6 (1.3)
Language composite scores	101.85 (14.7)	1 (0.2)	5 (1.1)	6 (1.3)
Motor composite scores	104.38 (14.7)	4 (1.1)	3 (0.7)	7 (1.8)
Ages and Stages Questionnaire	Mean (SD)	Needs attention	Delayed	
Communication ability	47.31 (12.0)	75 (16.6)	34 (7.5)	
Fine motor ability	53.39 (10.2)	21 (4.7)	20 (4.4)	
Gross motor ability	47.17 (12.8)	82 (18.1)	32 (7.1)	
Problem solving	52.20 (12.2)	31 (7.0)	26 (5.8)	
Personal social ability	50.40 (12.5)	36 (8.0)	32 (1.7)	

A *z*-score of < −3.00 SD indicates severe undernutrition, whereas *z*-scores between −2.99 and −2.00 SD indicate moderate undernutrition.
BSID III, Bayley Scales of Infant and Toddler Development third edition.
A score of < −3.00 SD indicates severe development delay, whereas a score between −2.99 and −2.00 SD indicates moderate development delay.
[a]*n* = 456, that is, less than the 512 enrolled children. As a result, some mothers could not be traced for the children to do tests. In some cases, the children would become irritable and testing had to be discontinued.
MUAC, mid-upper arm circumference.

rare (1.1%). There was no mention of the consumption of fat or even the use of fat in cooking. These kinds of diets do not adequately satisfy the nutrient needs (both macro- and micronutrients) of the growing infant, as required by complementary feeding guidelines (12). This was supported by a mean CDDS of 3.1, which is lower than that recommended (11, 14, 39, 56). Indeed, low CDDS was significantly associated with stunting and underweight in bivariate analyses and was also a predictor for stunting (42).

Low CDDS could be attributed to high levels of poverty, as shown in one study in southwestern Uganda (14), but also to food insecurity, as shown in this study. It was observed that mothers spent most of the day in the field cultivating and only packed leftover food or porridges for the children who had to come along. The heavy workloads of women and the poverty of Sub-Saharan Africa undermine the nutritional status of mothers, which eventually affects the nutritional status of their children (57).

Table 4. Multivariate linear regression analyses of nutritional status and putative predictors

	WAZ	LAZ	WLZ
R^2	0.068	0.039	0.052
Sex (1 = boy)	−0.26* (−0.46 to −0.062)	−0.25* (−0.47 to −0.036)	−0.14 (−0.35 to 0.071)
Household size	–	0.027 (−0.030 to 0.084)	–
Household head education	0.020 (−0.017 to 0.057)	0.018 (−0.023 to 0.058)	–
Maternal education	0.023 (−0.020 to 0.065)	0.016 (−0.029 to 0.062)	–
No. of children	−0.018 (−0.068 to 0.032)	–	−0.047 (−0.099 to 0.005)
Sanitation	0.064* (0.009 to 0.119)	0.039 (−0.021 to 0.099)	0.057 (−0.002 to 0.116)
Poverty likelihood	−0.005 (−0.013 to 0.002)	0.003 (−0.005 to 0.011)	−0.011* (−0.019 to −0.003)
CDDS	0.039 (−0.022 to 0.099)	0.086* (0.020 to 0.151)	−0.036 (−0.100 to 0.028)

Values are B unstandardized regression coefficients (95% CI).
Sex (categorical variable) was converted to a dummy variable (0 = girl; 1 = boy). The rest of the variables were continuous.
R^2, *R*-squared/coefficient of determination; CDDS, individual dietary diversity scores.
*$p < 0.05$.

Table 5. Nutritional status and independent variables with BSIDIII developmental domains

	Cognitive scores $n = 456$	Language scores $n = 456$	Motor scores $n = 456$
R^2	0.104	0.068	0.086
Sex (1 = boy)	3.62* (1.07 to 6.17)	1.69 (−1.02 to 4.40)	3.34* (0.60 to 6.07)
Household head education	0.54* (0.077 to 0.99)	0.18 (−0.27 to 0.63)	–
WAZ scores	3.44** (1.62 to 5.26)	1.75* (0.26 to 3.25)	2.45* (0.48 to 4.41)
LAZ scores	0.29 (−1.00 to 1.59)	1.49* (0.10 to 2.88)	1.46* (0.062 to 2.89)
Sanitation	0.38 (−0.30 to 1.07)	–	–
Maternal age	0.091 (−0.16 to 0.34)	–	−0.11 (−0.32 to 0.11)
CDDS	–	0.46 (−0.35–1.27)	–
MUAZ *z*-score	−0.61 (−2.04 to 0.81)	–	−0.72 (−2.25 to 0.82)
Poverty likelihood	0.032 (−0.016 to 0.13)	–	−0.098* (−0.18 to −0.013)
Maternal education	−0.36 (−0.89 to 0.17)	–	–
Birth order	−0.48 (−1.25 to 0.30)	−0.30 (−0.92 to 0.33)	–

Values are B unstandardized regression coefficients (95% CI).
$n = 456$ less than 512 enrolled children. Some mothers could not be traced for the children to do tests and some children would become irritable and tests had to be discontinued.
Sex (categorical variable) was converted to a dummy variable (0 = girl; 1 = boy). The rest of the variables were continuous.
R^2, *R*-squared/coefficient of determination; CDDS, child dietary diversity score.
$^*p < 0.05$; $^{**}p < 0.01$.

The significant association between the nutritional status of children and household characteristics related to sanitation, poverty, size, and maternal and household head education children are consistent with UNICEF's conceptual framework of the underlying causes of under nutrition (11, 14). Furthermore, in multivariate linear regression, gender and sanitation were predictors of WAZ. The observed predictors of nutritional status in the various models (sanitation, CDDS, and the likelihood of being below the poverty line) impact nutrition through their interaction with disease, the lack of purchasing power for nutritious foods that cannot be locally obtained, and the lack of knowledge about nutritious foods to give children.

Maternal age at the first child and number of children did not show significant associations with child nutritional status. It is, however, worth noting that some of the mothers were very young (11–16 years) at their first child and that 18.9% were younger than 18 years old and 3.4% had more than eight children. The negative and significant association between household size with WLZ and MUACZ probably indicates inadequate food supply for the larger households and possibly the lack of time to prepare food for infants. Collectively, these factors may have an effect on the health of the mothers, both physically and/or psychologically, that could interfere with child care, including feeding (57, 58).

Cognitive, language, and motor development versus nutritional status

Cognitive and other development domains correlated positively and significantly with almost all the nutritional status indicators. This is in line with the fact that adequate nutrition is paramount to the development of the brain directly for structural and functional development, and indirectly for children's behaviour and experience (20, 23). Good nutrition is also required for normal physical development of the body. Though both length-for-age and weight-for-age contributed to the model predicting cognitive function, length-for-age did not show significant contribution. Previous studies (15, 16, 59) have shown length-for-age as a strong predictor for cognitive function. We noticed that the boy gender made significant positive contribution in the models predicting cognitive and motor domains.

The findings of this study indicate that the infants' HCs were adequate and only 2.7% of the infants had HCZ < -2 SD. Studies have shown that HC < -2 SD may be an indicator of severe undernutrition in the first year of life that may eventually affect brain development (60) and hence cognitive function (60–62). Despite the high levels of undernutrition observed in this study, the HCs were within normal ranges, probably because the infants were young (6–8 months). The adequate HCZ could possibly explain the observed good cognitive composite scores (only 1.3% had < -2 SD on the BSID III cognitive scale). However, many of the infants scored below the cut-off values given in the ASQ tool. These scores may be the result of undernutrition as well as lack of time for play, interaction with other children, and stimulation by the mothers. This concurs with the available evidence on the effect of stimulation on child development (17, 18, 63). An early child development intervention of play and communication among caregivers was found to improve mother–child interaction, caregiving environment, and practices that improved feeding and development in children (26, 63).

The two scales (BSID III and ASQ) showed differences in detecting developmental delay evaluated as proportions of low scores. ASQ is a caregiver report that captures a wide range of adaptive behaviours (53) that BSID III does not measure. Still, the two scales showed a low, albeit significant overall agreement (Pearson correlation coefficient = 0.37). This finding is similar to a previous study that compared the validity of the two scales and found modest agreement (Pearson correlation coefficient = 0.56) (64). Moreover, the observed low values of R^2 in linear regression models suggest that several variables, though not statistically significant, each had a small impact on our outcomes. It is also possible that other variables, not included in the regression model or study, had significant impact on the outcomes.

Strengths and limitations

This study has several strengths. It was the first of its kind to use both the BSID III scales and ASQ on children of 6–8 months in the Ugandan setting, and to explore the possibility of correlating these findings to various indicators of nutritional status. We were also able to recruit a large number of children. The main limitation of this study was the cross-sectional design, precluding any conclusion about possible cause and effect. Moreover, neither BSID III nor ASQ has been validated for use in the Ugandan setting. Some of the BSID III tool kit materials were novel to the children and could have intimidated them. Also it was difficult to fit good models that could explain the outcomes in our study population, probably indicating a complex network of variables affecting the outcomes. These findings indicate a need for multi-intervention programmes.

Conclusion

Undernutrition and growth faltering had already set in as early as 6–8 months among children living in impoverished rural Uganda. Poor household sanitation, poverty, and low dietary diversity, among other factors, were associated with undernutrition in complex interrelationships. Development domains (cognitive, language, and motor) were positively and significantly predicted by the nutritional status of the children confirming previous studies. There is a need for multi-intervention programmes addressing dietary diversity, with food hygiene, infant feeding, and care practices to improve infant and child growth as well as development.

Authors' contribution

GM contributed to all aspects of the study including conceptualization of the protocol, data collection, analysis, and drafting the manuscript; PA contributed to data collection and specifically administration of BSIID and ASQ tests, data analysis, and review of the manuscript; RM, POI, and AW contributed to the conceptualization of the protocol, the supervision of all field activities, and the analysis and critical review of the manuscript. All authors approved the final manuscript.

Acknowledgements

The authors thank the local council leaders and the leaders of Kabale and Kisoro districts as well as the study participants who, despite their busy schedules, willingly gave their time. They are also grateful to the field and research assistants for their participation in data collection and entry.

Conflict of interest and funding

The authors declare that they have no conflicts of interest. Financial support was obtained from the University of Oslo.

References

1. UBOS (2012). Uganda Demographic and Health Survey 2011. Kampala, Uganda: UBOS.
2. Black RE, Allen LH, Bhutta ZA, Caulfield LE, de Onis M, Ezzati M, et al. Maternal and child undernutrition: global and regional exposures and health consequences. Lancet 2008; 371: 243–60.
3. Fishman SM, de Onis M, Blossner M, Hyder AA, Mullany L, Camu IEM, et al., editors. Comparative quantification of health risks: global and regional burden of disease attributable to selected major risk factors. Geneva, Switzerland: World Health Organization; 2004, pp. 39–161.
4. UNICEF (1991). A UNICEF policy review. Strategy for improved nutrition of children and women in developing countries. ISSN: 1013-3194. New York, USA: UNICEF.
5. Abu-Saad K, Fraser D. Maternal nutrition and birth outcomes. Epidemiol Rev 2010; 32: 5–25.
6. Salam RA, Das JK, Bhutta ZA. Multiple micronutrient supplementation during pregnancy and lactation in low-to-middle-income developing country settings: impact on pregnancy outcomes. Ann Nutr Metabol 2014; 65: 4–12.
7. Kusin JA, Kardjati S, Houtkooper JM, Renqvist UH. Energy supplementation during pregnancy and postnatal growth. Lancet 1992; 340: 623–6.
8. Kramer MS. Effects of energy and protein intake on pregnancy outcome: an overview of the research evidence from controlled clinical trials. Am J Clin Nutr 1993; 58: 627–35.
9. Kramer MS. Determinants of low birth weight methodological assessment and meta-analysis. Bull WHO 1987; 65: 663–737.
10. Shrimpton R, Victora CG, de Onis M, Lima RC, Blossner M, Clugston G. Worldwide timing of growth faltering: implications for nutritional interventions. Pediatrics 2001; 107: E75.
11. FANTA-2. The analysis of the nutrition situation in Uganda. Food and nutrition technical assistance II Project. Washington, DC: AED; 2010.
12. PAHO/WHO. Guiding priciples for complementary feeding of the breastfed child. Washington, DC: Division of Health Promotion and Protection; 2003.
13. Wamani H, Nordrehaug A, Strøm Å, Peterson S, James T, Tylleskar T. Predictors of poor anthropometric status among children under 2 years of age in rural Uganda. Public Health Nutr 2005; 9: 320–6.
14. Kikafunda JK, Agaba E, Bambona A. Malnutrition amidst plenty: an assessment of factors responsible for persistent high

levels of childhood stunting in food secure Western Uganda. AFJAND 2014; 14: 9288–313.
15. Crookston BT, Penny ME, Alder SC, Dickerson TT, Merrill RM, Stanford JB, et al. Children who recover from early stunting and children who are not stunted demonstrate similar levels of cognition. J Nutr 2010; 140: 1996–2001.
16. Mendez MA, Adair LS. Severity and timing of stunting in the first two years of life affect performance on cognitive tests in late childhood. J Nutr 1999; 129: 1555–62.
17. Sudfeld CR, McCoy DC, Danaei G, Fink G, Ezzati M, Andrews KG, et al. Linear growth and child development in low- and middle-income countries: a meta-analysis. Pediatrics 2015; 135: e1266–75.
18. Yousafzai AK, Rasheed MA, Rizvi A, Armstrong R, Bhutta ZA. Effect of integrated responsive stimulation and nutrition interventions in the Lady Health Worker programme in Pakistan on child development, growth, and health outcomes: a cluster-randomised factorial effectiveness trial. Lancet 2014; 384: 1282–93.
19. Prado EL, Dewey KG. Nutrition and brain development in early life. Nutr Rev 2014; 72: 267–84.
20. Uauy R, Dangour AD. Nutrition in brain development and aging: role of essential fatty acids. Nutr Rev 2006; 64: S24–33.
21. Innis SM. Dietary (n-3) fatty acids and brain development. J Nutr 2007; 137: 855–9.
22. Georgieff MK. Nutrition and the developing brain: nutrient priorities and measurement. Am J Clin Nutr 2007; 85: 614S–20S.
23. Prado E, Dewey K. Nutrition and brain development in early life. Washington, DC: Alive and Thrive, FHI360, 2012.
24. Kitsao-Wekulo P, Holding P, Taylor HG, Abubakar A, Kvalsvig J, Connolly K. Nutrition as an important mediator of the impact of background variables on outcome in middle childhood. Front Hum Neurosci 2013; 7: 713.
25. Engle PL, Black MM, Behrman JR, Cabral de Mello M, Gertler PJ, Kapiriri L, et al. Strategies to avoid the loss of developmental potential in more than 200 million children in the developing world. Lancet 2007; 369: 229–42.
26. Singla DR, Kumbakumba E, Aboud FE. Effects of a parenting intervention to address both maternal psychological wellbeing and child development and growth in rural Uganda: a community-based, cluster randomised trial. Lancet Global Health 2015; 3: e458–69.
27. Imdad A, Yakoob MY, Bhutta ZA. Impact of maternal education about complementary feeding and provision of complementary foods on child growth in developing countries. BMC Public Health 2011; 11(Suppl 3): S25.
28. UBOS (2014). National Population and Housing Census 2014 (Provisional results). Kampala: Uganda Bureau of Statistics (UBOS).
29. Community Connector, Gulu University (GU), Mbarara University of Science and Technology (MUST), Community Connector (CC). Kamapala, Uganda: FHI360, 2012.
30. PAHO (2004). ProPAN: process for the promotion of child feeding. cataloguing-in-publication PHL. Washington, DC: PAHO.
31. WHO (2006). Child growth standards: length/height-for-age, weight-for-age, weight-for-length, weight-for-height and body mass index for-age: methods and development. Available from: http://www.who.int/childgrowth/standards/Technical_report.pdf [cited 3 November 2015].
32. WHO (2005). Child growth standards. World Health Organization. Available from: http://www.who.int/childgrowth/training/jobaid_weighing_measuring.pdf [cited 2 November 2015].
33. UNICEF. Technical bulletin no. 18. Available from: http://www.unicef.org/supply/files/Height_Length_Measuring_Boards.pdf [cited 18 February 2016].
34. WHO. WHO Anthro. 3.2.2 Jan 2011 ed2005. Geneva: World Health organization Geneva.
35. de Onis M, Blössner M. WHO global database on child growth and malnutrition. Geneva: World health Organization (WHO). 1997.
36. WHO (2005). Global database on child growth and malnutrition, cut-off points and summary statistics. Available from: http://www.who.int/nutgrowthdb/about/introduction/en/index5.html [cited 2 November 2016].
37. Schreiner M. A simple poverty scorecard for Uganda. Available from: http://www.microfinance.com/English/Papers/Scoring_Poverty_Uganda_2009_EN.pdf; 2011.
38. Swindale A, Bilinsky P. Household Dietary Diversity Score (HDDS) for Measurement of Household Food Access: Indicator Guide (v.2). Washington, DC: Food and Nutrition Technical Assistance Project, Academy for Educational Development; 2006.
39. WHO/UNICEF (2008). Indicators for assessing infant and young child feeding practices Part 1 Definitions. Washington, DC: World Heath Organization (WHO).
40. Moursi MM, Arimond M, Dewey KG, Tréche S, Ruel MT, Delpeuch F. Dietary diversity is a good predictor of the micronutrient density of the diet of 6- to 23-month-old children in Madagascar. J Nutr 2008; 138: 2448–53.
41. Kennedy GL, Pedro MR, Seghieri C, Nantel GA, Brouwer I. Dietary diversity score is a useful indicator of micronutrient intake in non-breast-feeding Filipino children. J Nutr 2007; 137: 472–7.
42. Steyn NP, Nel JH, Nantel G, Kennedy G, Labadarios D. Food variety and dietary diversity scores in children: are they good indicators of dietary adequacy? Public Health Nutr 2005; 9: 644–50.
43. Savy M, Martin-Prével Y, Sawadogo P, Kameli Y, Delpeuch F. Use of variety/diversity scores for diet quality measurement: relation with nutritional status of women in a rural area in Burkina Faso. Eur J Clin Nutr 2005; 59: 703–16.
44. Coates J, Swindale A, Bilinsky P. Household Food Insecurity Access Scale (HFIAS) for Measurement of Household Food Access: Indicator Guide (v. 3). Washington, DC: Food and Nutrition Technical Assistance Project, Academy for Educational Development; 2007.
45. Webb P, Coates J, Frongillo EA, Rogers BL, Swindale A, Bilinsky P. Measuring household food insecurity: why it's so important and yet so difficult to do. J Nutr 2006; 136: 1404S–8S.
46. Lia CHF, Patricia K, Patrice E, Abbie R. Examining early child development in Low-Income countries: a toolkit for the assessment of children in the first five years of life. Washington, DC: The World Bank; 2009, pp. 68–9.
47. Bayley N. Bayley scales of infant and toddler development, 3rd ed. San Antonio, TX: Psychological Corporation; 2006.
48. Juneja M, Mohanty M, Jain R, Ramji S. Ages and Stages Questionnaire as a screening tool for developmental delay in Indian children. Indian Pediatr 2012; 49(6): 457–61.
49. Kerstjens JM, Bos AF, ten Vergert EM, de Meer G, Butcher PR, Reijneveld SA. Support for the global feasibility of the Ages and Stages Questionnaire as developmental screener. Early Hum Dev 2009; 85: 443–7.
50. Squires J, Twombly E, Bricker D, LaWanda P. ASQ-3 User's guide. Baltimore: Brookes; 2009.
51. Twombly E, Fink G. ASQ-3 Learning activities. Baltimore: Paul H. Brookes; 2013.

52. Gollenberg AL, Lynch CD, Jackson LW, McGuinness BM, Msall ME. Concurrent validity of the parent-completed Ages and Stages Questionnaires, 2nd ed. with the Bayley Scales of Infant Development II in a low-risk sample. Child Care Health Dev 2010; 36: 485–90.
53. Hornman J, Kerstjens JM, de Winter AF, Bos AF, Reijneveld SA. Validity and internal consistency of the Ages and Stages Questionnaire 60-month version and the effect of three scoring methods. Early Hum Dev 2013; 89: 1011–15.
54. IBM. IBM SPSS Statistics. 22nd ed. New York: IBM Corporation; 1989, 2013.
55. Victora CG, de Onis M, Hallal PC, Blossner M, Shrimpton R. Worldwide timing of growth faltering: revisiting implications for interventions. Pediatrics 2010; 125: e473–80.
56. Lutter CK, Daelmans BM, de Onis M, Kothari MT, Ruel MT, Arimond M, et al. Undernutrition, poor feeding practices, and low coverage of key nutrition interventions. Pediatrics 2011; 128: e1418–27.
57. Lartey A. Maternal and child nutrition in Sub-Saharan Africa: challenges and interventions. Proc Nutr Soc 2008; 67: 105–8.
58. Rahman A, Iqbal Z, Bunn J, Lovel H, Harrington R. Impact of maternal depression on infant nutritional status and illness: a cohort study. Arch Gen Psych 2004; 61: 946–52.
59. Berkman DS, Lescano AG, Gilman RH, Lopez SL, Black MM. Effects of stunting, diarrhoeal disease, and parasitic infection during infancy on cognition in late childhood: a follow-up study. Lancet 2002; 359: 564–71.
60. Ivanovic DM, Leiva BP, Perez HT, Olivares MG, Diaz NS, Urrutia MS, et al. Head size and intelligence, learning, nutritional status and brain development. Head, IQ, learning, nutrition and brain. Neuropsychologia 2004; 42: 1118–31.
61. Tramo MJ, Loftus WC, Stukel TA, Green RL, Weaver JB, Gazzaniga MS. Brain size, head size, and intelligence quotient in monozygotic twins. Neurology 1998; 50: 1246–52.
62. McDaniel MA. Big-brained people are smarter: a meta-analysis of the relationship between in vivo brain volume and intelligence. Intelligence 2005; 33: 337–46.
63. Yousafzai AK, Rasheed MA, Rizvi A, Armstrong R, Bhutta ZA. Parenting skills and emotional availability: an RCT. Pediatrics 2015; 135: e1247–57.
64. Schonhaut L, Armijo I, Schonstedt M, Alvarez J, Cordero M. Validity of the ages and stages questionnaires in term and preterm infants. Pediatrics 2013; 131: e1468–74.

*Grace K. M. Muhoozi
Department of Nutrition
Institute of Basic Medical Sciences
University of Oslo
P.O. Box 1046 Blindern
NO-0317 Oslo, Norway
Email: g.k.m.muhoozi@studmed.uio.no

8

Iodine status in the Nordic countries – past and present

Helena Filipsson Nyström[1,2]*, Anne Lise Brantsæter[3], Iris Erlund[4], Ingibjörg Gunnarsdottir[5], Lena Hulthén[6], Peter Laurberg[7,8], Irene Mattisson[9], Lone Banke Rasmussen[10], Suvi Virtanen[4,11] and Helle Margrete Meltzer[3]

[1]Institute of Medicine, Sahlgrenska Academy, University of Gothenburg, Gothenburg, Sweden; [2]Department of Endocrinology, Sahlgrenska University Hospital, Gothenburg, Sweden; [3]Norwegian Institute of Public Health, Oslo, Norway; [4]National Institute for Health and Welfare, Helsinki, Finland; [5]Unit for Nutrition Research, University of Iceland and Landspitali National University Hospital, Reykjavik, Iceland; [6]Department of Clinical Nutrition, Sahlgrenska Academy, University of Gothenburg, Gothenburg, Sweden; [7]Department of Endocrinology, Aalborg University Hospital, Aalborg, Denmark; [8]Department of Clinical Medicine, Aalborg University, Aalborg, Denmark; [9]National Food Agency, Uppsala, Sweden; [10]Department of Endocrinology, Bispebjerg University Hospital, Copenhagen, Denmark; [11]School of Health Sciences, University of Tampere, Finland

Abstract

Background: Adequate iodine nutrition is dependent on ground water content, seafood, and, as many countries use iodized cow fodder, dairy products. In most countries, salt fortification programs are needed to assure adequate iodine intake.
Objectives: The objectives are threefold: 1) to describe the past and present iodine situation in the Nordic countries, 2) to identify important gaps of knowledge, and 3) to highlight differences among the Nordic countries' iodine biomonitoring and fortification policies.
Design: Historical data are compared with the current situation. The Nordic countries' strategies to achieve recommended intake and urine iodine levels and their respective success rates are evaluated.
Results: In the past, the iodine situation ranged from excellent in Iceland to widespread goiter and cretinism in large areas of Sweden. The situation was less severe in Norway and Finland. According to a 1960 World Health Organization (WHO) report, there were then no observations of iodine deficiency in Denmark. In Sweden and Finland, the fortification of table salt was introduced 50–75 years ago, and in Norway and Finland, the fortification of cow fodder starting in the 1950s helped improve the population's iodine status due to the high intake of milk. In Denmark, iodine has been added to household salt and salt in bread for the past 15 years. The Nordic countries differ with regard to regulations and degree of governmental involvement. There are indications that pregnant and lactating women, the two most vulnerable groups, are mildly deficient in iodine in several of the Nordic countries.
Conclusion: The Nordic countries employ different strategies to attain adequate iodine nutrition. The situation is not optimal and is in need of re-evaluation. Iodine researchers, Nordic national food administrations, and Nordic governmental institutions would benefit from collaboration to attain a broader approach and guarantee good iodine health for all.

Keywords: *iodine*; *goiter*; *history*; *thyroid*; *fortification*; *Iceland*; *Norway*; *Sweden*; *Denmark*; *Finland*

Adequate iodine intake is necessary for the normal production of the thyroid hormones tetraiodothyronine (T4) and triiodothyronine (T3). In 1952, the World Health Organization (WHO) stated that in order to assure normal thyroid metabolism, the average adult iodine intake should be 150 μg/day. Low iodine intake may result in hypothyroidism and goiter (1). Pregnant and lactating women have greater need of iodine and the recommended dose is 175–250 μg iodine/day to target a median urinary iodine concentration (UIC) of 150–249 μg/L during pregnancy and >100 μg/L during lactation (2–5). Thyroid hormones are especially important during fetal life and early years for the development of the brain (2, 6, 7). Severe iodine deficiency (ID) in pregnancy may result in physical and mental retardation – cretinism (8, 9). Studies also indicate that moderate to mild ID may impact neuropsychological development in school-aged children and impair growth and motor function (10, 11). A longitudinal study in the United Kingdom showed that inadequate maternal iodine status, assessed by means of UIC in early pregnancy, was associated with lower verbal IQ in their 8-year-old children (12). In a similar study in Australia, mild ID in pregnancy was associated with lower educational outcomes in children at age 9 years (13). These studies indicate that moderate to mild ID may have a long-term, adverse impact on fetal neurodevelopment, but convincing evidence is lacking. Yet, these findings, as well as reports that suboptimal iodine intake is found in countries that have for decades been considered iodine-sufficient, have raised concerns that ID is overlooked as a public health concern in developed countries, including the Nordic countries (14–19).

The balance between too little and too much iodine

The daily iodine intake is mostly a sum of the population's dietary habits of fish and other seafood, dairy products (if the cow fodder is iodized), the water iodine content, and the current iodine fortification programs.

The single most important iodine issue globally is avoiding ID and the resulting deleterious consequences for fetal and child brain development. When a population is living under conditions of mild ID, the thyroid maintains normal hormone production, but compensation mechanisms result in goiter and a higher frequency of hyperthyroidism with autonomous areas in a toxic multinodular goiter (TMNG) with secondary health consequences (2, 20, 21). When iodine intake levels are changed over time, this affects the incidence and prevalence of thyroid diseases. When a population goes from moderate or mild ID to normal iodine levels, the incidence of TMNG decreases and more young people develop Graves' disease (GD), as iodine sufficiency results in an increased incidence of autoimmune thyroid disease. The increased incidence of GD is probably temporary and the incidence of autoimmune hypothyroidism rises in line with iodine level increments (22). High iodine intake can generate both hypothyroidism and hyperthyroidism. Iodine prophylaxis is therefore a complex issue that must be handled with care and detail.

Socio- and health economic consequences of iodine deficiency

The access to iodine varies in different parts of the world because of different levels of iodine in ground water (23) and soils. The use of fish and other seafood (24) and of iodine-rich dairy products (25) varies and so does the degree of iodized salt use. In many areas with iodine-poor soils far from the sea, ID continues to be a significant health issue (26).

Goiter is the obvious and visible manifestation of ID, but severe health and socioeconomic consequences are also apparent through other expressions of ID: cretinism, neurological disability, mental retardation, hypothyroidism, and TMNG. Therefore, the term iodine deficiency disorders (IDD) was introduced in 1983 (27). There is an association between goiter prevalence and the number of cretins born. When the goiter prevalence is 30–40%, few cretins are born, but if it increases to 70–80%, 10% of all children born are cretins. On a continuum of consequences for mental development, cretinism is the most severe form. The prevalence of mental retardation in ID areas may exceed the prevalence of cretinism by 10 times (27), making combatting IDD the most cost-effective measure.

Iodine prophylaxis

From Chinese and Hindu writings, we know that the use of seaweed to combat goiter has been known for thousands of years and was still in use at the beginning of the 19th century; after iodine was found in seaweed in 1811 by Courtois, the first prophylactic attempts began in the 1820s. Iodine prophylaxis was established in 1921 after Marine and Kimball's classical experiment in which they treated schoolgirls in the United States (US) with iodine, leading to a dramatic reduction in the prevalence of goiter. After some debate, iodine prophylaxis was introduced in Switzerland in 1922. In 1923–1924, iodine fortification of table salt and tap water was tried in several communities in the Great Lakes region in the US. Over the following decades, goiter prophylaxis programs were introduced worldwide (27).

In 1986, the International Council for Control of Iodine Deficiency Disorders (ICCIDD) was founded (27). In 2014, the ICCIDD became the Iodine Global Network (IGN). The IGN has initiated and improved many iodine prophylaxis programs. The IGN also sets up monitoring guidelines and encourages national and subcontinental reporting.

The iodization of salt is the most commonly used tool for iodine prophylaxis, but the amount of iodine added to table salt varies from country to country (27). In developing countries, the use of iodized oil has been proven a safe and easy form of administering iodine to the population (28). Mandatory iodine prophylaxis programs are more likely to deliver a sustained source and, in turn, a public health benefit (29). The importance of political decisions and continuous surveillance must, however, be emphasized, all the more so due to factors such as migration and changes in food consumption over time.

The objectives of this article are 1) to describe past and present iodine status in the five Nordic countries, 2) to identify important gaps of knowledge, and 3) to highlight differences between the Nordic countries' iodine fortification policies that need to be adapted to ensure adequate iodine status in the general population and in groups at risk of ID.

Present investigation

The five Nordic countries

Geological and climatic conditions of importance for intake levels

There is a cycle of iodine in nature. Most iodine resides in the world's oceans. Large amounts of iodine were leached from surface soil by glaciations, snow, and rain and carried by rivers and floods into the sea. Therefore, many mountainous areas, but also lowlands far from the oceans, are depleted of iodine (30).

During the last Ice Age, the Nordic countries, Iceland, Norway, Denmark, Sweden, and Finland, were covered with ice. Iceland is located in the sea on the transatlantic rift with continuous volcanic activity. Norway and Sweden are on the same peninsula, with mountain areas in Norway and the northwestern parts of Sweden. The south of Sweden is lowland and was partly covered by the sea when the ice receded. Finland and Denmark are separated from the peninsula by the Baltic Sea and have no mountain areas; Denmark and parts of Finland were seabed long ago.

After the last Ice Age, approximately 14,000 years ago, Denmark was the first of today's Nordic countries to be populated. People later migrated across the narrow sound to southern Sweden and over the North Sea to southern Norway. During the Viking age, in the ninth and tenth centuries AD, Norwegians (and Irish) inhabited Iceland. Icelandic, Danish, Norwegian, and Swedish people share a common genetic heritage, while Finland was populated from the east, a heritage that is evident today through the Finnish language, which is quite different from that of the other Nordic countries. However, Finland's major genetic influence is from Europe. The Swedish influence in Finland has been significant, both genetically and culturally.

Geographical and climatic conditions favored animal herding; in addition, the gene for lactase was preserved over multiple generations. Milk and dairy products thus became staple foods in all the Nordic countries. Coastal areas had more favorable conditions and were therefore more densely populated; inland or mountain areas were more sparsely populated. Fish intake was high in coastal areas and areas to which fish was transported, but in inland areas, saltwater fish, which has higher iodine content, was rarely consumed.

The five Nordic neighbors employ different strategies to ensure adequate iodine intake (Table 1).

Iceland

Iceland has been known for its population's good iodine status. In 1939, Sigurjonsson reported findings that the thyroid gland in the Icelandic population was smaller than was generally accepted in other countries at the time (31). This was attributed to the uniquely high consumption of fish, on average 200 g/day (32), but also to high iodine levels in haddock and cod, the most commonly consumed species (33, 34). Dairy products are another important source of iodine for the Icelandic people (32–36), as dairy products have high iodine content because fish meal is used in cow fodder (37). In 1939, the average milk intake was 1 liter/person/day, resulting in an iodine contribution from fish and dairy products of 570 μg iodine/person/day (32).

In 1978–1979, the average iodine intake in Iceland was estimated to be 336 μg/person/day. In a follow-up study, urinary iodine excretion (UIE) was 395 μg/day in men and 270 μg/day in women (38). In 1990, the Icelandic Nutrition Council reported an average iodine intake of 299 μg/person/day (32). In that survey, for the first time, a subgroup that was potentially at risk of ID was identified: young women with a low intake of fish and dairy products and with an iodine intake in the range of 86–130 μg/day (32).

In many countries, iodized salt is the primary source of iodine because the intake of fish and seafood is low, but in Iceland, iodized salt is not commonly used and the iodine content in water is low (ISGEM the Icelandic Food Composition www1.matis.is/ISGEM/details1.aspx?FAEDA=0290 030116) (Table 1). Also, combined with a decline in the intake of products containing iodine, the iodine content in milk has almost halved since 1962 (38, 39). This is attributable to the reduced use of fishmeal in cow fodder. More iodine is now added to cow fodder, and the added iodine contributes more to the total iodine content of milk today. The fish meal content of cow fodder varies between 4.4 and 19.4% (40).

Young women and their risk of ID were further highlighted in the Public Health Institute of Iceland's survey in 2002. The fish intake in this group had decreased to 40 g/day and milk consumption had also declined. In a 1990 survey, young women only obtained two-thirds of the recommended iodine intake from their diet (32). Similar trends have been observed in children and adolescents (41), also in the last national survey from year 2010–2011 (36). Hence, the diet of young Icelanders has come to more closely resemble the diet of the other Nordic countries. Iceland exemplifies the fragility of iodine sufficiency at the national level and that there is a need to carefully monitor trends in iodine status. It is especially important to monitor women of child-bearing age to secure healthy brain development in their children.

Norway

Prior to 1950, there were several areas where goiter was endemic in Norway. In 1917, Dr Carl Schiøtz described his findings of goiter among 10,000 schoolchildren in the inland district of Hedmark (42) (Fig. 1). At the age of 14, the prevalence was 24% among girls and 10% among boys (Fig. 2). He gave a detailed account of cretins.

Table 1. Comparisons of the Nordic countries regarding geological conditions, iodine levels in water, and historical data on iodine intake levels

	Iceland	Norway	Denmark	Sweden	Finland
Covered by ice during Ice Age	Yes	Yes	Yes	Yes	Yes
Marine sediments	No	No	Yes	South Eastern parts	Southern parts
Water iodine level (median)	0.12 μg/L	<2 μg/L	12.2±8.3 μg/L (mean)	3.7 μg/L	Dug wells: 2.12 (range <0.2–761) mean 10.7±26.8 μg (L Drilled wells 3.04 (range <0.2–232) mean 6.78±35.1 μg(L
Iodine status before iodination	Sufficient	Severe to moderately deficient	Moderate to mildly deficient	Severely deficient	Moderately deficient
Degree of sea fish intake during 1900–1950	High	High in the coastline low in the inland	High in the coastline low in the inland	High in the coastline low in the inland	High in the coastline low in the inland
Fortification of cow fodder historically (starting point)	Fish meal used in cow fodder voluntary	Mandatory from 1950, level: 2 μg/g salt.	Voluntary	Voluntary	Voluntary
Start of iodination to the population		Late 1930s	2000	1936	1946
Type of iodination		Table salt for household use only	Household salt and salt for commercial bread production	Table salt	Household salt and cow fodder
Level of iodine added		5 μg/g salt	13 μg/g salt	50 μg/g salt	25 μg/g salt
Type of legislation		Voluntary	Mandatory	Voluntary	Voluntary
Monitoring by authorities	No	No	Yes	No	Some
Actual cow milk iodine concentration (μg/L)	2006: 85–283 (average 145)	Before year 2000: 150 2000–2012: 100–150 2012–2015: 190 2015: 200		2001: 160 2009: 117	2015: 150
Mean amount of fish by adults (gram per day per person)	National dietary survey in 2010–2011: fish and seafood 46	National dietary survey in 2011: fish and seafood: 67 fish: 52	National dietary survey 2011–2013: 37	National diet survey 2010–2011 fish and shellfish, women 37, men 43	National diet survey 2012 40
Major source for iodine in the population	Fish	Milk	Milk and salt	Salt	Milk
Iodine sufficiency in the adult general population	Yes	Yes/Mild ID (depending on milk intake)	Mild ID	Yes	Mild ID

The ongoing iodization program, regulations, and monitoring and the current iodine sources and iodine status in the normal population are also presented.

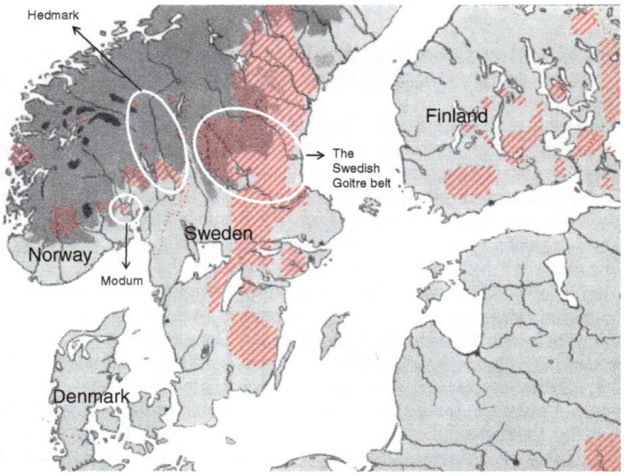

Fig. 1. Map of the Nordic countries (except Iceland) in 1960 (55). Dark gray represents mountain areas and striped areas are goiter regions. Sweden still has large areas of goiter 24 years after the start of the iodization program and the salt iodine content was increased in 1966. Goitrous areas are also seen in Norway and Finland.

The well-known goiter district of Modum was extensively studied in 1934–1935 (43) (Fig. 1). The prevalence of goiter was very high, especially among school children in the community (80%). Also, the prevalence of goiter was higher among subjects who did not consume fish than among those who ate fish (43). From 1950 onwards, the iodine fortification of cow fodder became mandatory (2 μg/g) to improve livestock reproductive performance (44), a measure that resulted in a dramatic increase in iodine concentrations in milk and dairy products in Norway. Interestingly, this was paralleled in the United Kingdom (45). In the reinvestigation of school children

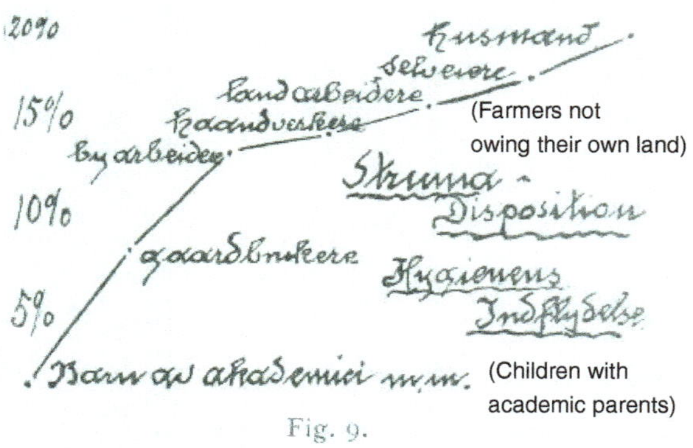

Fig. 2. Social factors that influenced the goiter frequency in Norway. This is a handwritten note by Carl Schiøtz, who investigated the prevalence of goiter in the Norwegian inland county Hedmark in 1914. In the figure, he indicates the prevalence according to social class: the lowest prevalence was among children of academics, the highest prevalence among farmers not owning their own land (a cotter) (English translation in brackets).

in Modum in 1977, the goiter rate was found to have dropped to 1.5% and goiter was no longer considered a problem among Norwegian children (46). The sufficient iodine intake was attributed to the high iodine content of milk, but also to the fact that saltwater fish was more widely consumed in the 1970s (46).

Studies carried out in men from 10 locations sampled in 1971–1972 (47, 48) and in 1985 pointed at satisfactory UIE; the dietary intake of iodine of Norwegians was suggested to be 150–250 μg iodine/person/day (44). Based on these publications, Norwegian health authorities have since 1950s considered Norwegians to be iodine-replete (Table 1).

The only study carried out so far which has calculated the iodine intake in a representative group of Norwegians was conducted in 1997, the NORKOST 2 study (49). The mean dietary intake of iodine was within the recommended dose for men (176 μg/day), while in women the intake was slightly below the recommended dose (136 μg/day). Only 7% of the adult population had a daily intake of iodine below the lowest recommended intake level of 70 μg iodine/day, which is a threshold for normal thyroid function. None exceeded 1,000 μg/day. However, vitamins and/or mineral supplements were not included in the estimations in this study.

Currently, the largest study of iodine intake in the world is the Norwegian Mother and Child Cohort Study (MoBa) (19, 50). Iodine intake from food and supplements was estimated using a food frequency questionnaire and validated by means of comparison with 24-h UIE in a subsample of 119 participants (19, 51). Of 61,904 women, 16% had an iodine intake <100 μg/day, 54% had iodine intake below the Nordic recommendation of 175 μg/day, and only 22% reached the WHO/UNICEF/ICCIDD recommendation of 250 μg/day. The insufficient iodine intake levels shown in pregnant women have set alarm bells ringing at the Norwegian Directorate of Health, and an Iodine Committee is now trying to assess the situation and has been commissioned to present proposals for the alleviation of ID in vulnerable groups.

In Norway, the fortification of salt with iodine is voluntary and very few brands contain iodine. The permitted level is 5 μg iodine/g salt, which is too low to impact the iodine intake of those who use this salt. The food industry is not allowed to use iodine-fortified salt in Norway.

The amount of iodine in drinking water is influenced by geological conditions. In samples from 12 different sites, the average water iodine content was found to be 1.7 μg/L in 2002. Samples from coastal cities had higher concentrations than samples from inland towns (range 0.6 μg/L (Rjukan) to 5.5 μg/L (Stavanger) (Table 1).

An increasing number of Norwegians take dietary supplements, and today many multivitamin-mineral supplements contain iodine. In the MoBa Study, 32% of the pregnant women took iodine-containing supplements which on average contributed 100 μg iodine/day to these women's diet (19).

Hence, in Norway, the iodine fortification of cow fodder had unintended positive effects on the human population. Milk, in combination with the intake of other dairy products, has made this food category the major source of iodine in the Norwegian diet (49, 52) However, the consumption of milk, yoghurt, and lean fish has declined over the past decades in some groups and explains why suboptimal iodine intake is becoming more prevalent in Norway (19, 51).

Denmark

Cretinism may develop when iodine intake is <25 μg/day, and goiter may appear when iodine intake is <100 μg/day. Endemic goiter is defined as either goiter found in 10% of the adult population or found in 5% among school children (53). In Denmark, neither cretinism nor endemic goiter has been reported in the population. Small local studies in the 1920s subsequently reported an incidence of goiter of 15%, but high goiter frequency was not confirmed in a national study of 350,101 Danish school children performed in 1972–1973 (54). In 1960, Denmark was among the few countries reporting no endemic goiter (55) and was not, until recently, considered to be an ID area.

However, when the focus shifted from school children to other population groups, the consequences of ID became apparent. First, the incidence rate of TMNG was high with clinical and subclinical hyperthyroidism particularly common in the elderly (22). Second, by the end of their pregnancies, pregnant women did not have sufficient iodine levels (56). In 1969, the population in Denmark had UIE levels of 64 μg/person/day, with variations within the country (57). Lower UIE was detected in Jutland, with 50 μg/person/day than in Zealand with 70–100 μg/person/day (58). Also, in a national Danish dietary survey from 1985, the average intake was calculated to be 114 μg iodine/day (59), which was below the level of 150 μg/day recommended by the WHO.

Available data in Denmark suggested that the iodine situation had been stable for 35 years until the Ministry of Health in Denmark decided to initiate a nationwide iodization program in 1997 (53). Before the iodization program, 27.8% of the population was taking multivitamins containing iodine (53). Iodized salt had been on the Danish market for a long time (kelp salt tablets containing 10–20 μg iodine/g salt) and, in the 1970s, at least three table salts containing iodine were supplied to the market (iodine content 10–40 μg/g), but they only covered a few per cent points of the market. Also, from 1974 until June 1998, the sale of iodized salt and other iodized products was illegal in Denmark, similar to the ban on other fortified food products with no proven health benefits.

Before the iodization of salt began, a monitoring program, the Danish Investigation of Iodine Intake and Thyroid Diseases (DanThyr), was initiated. The aim was to investigate iodine intake, the prevalence of goiter, and the incidence of thyroid diseases in Aalborg, with moderate ID, and Copenhagen, with mild ID. The main reason for the difference in iodine status in these cities was differences in the water iodine content (60, 61). In Copenhagen, the iodine concentration in tap water is 19 μg/L, and in Aalborg, it is 5 μg/L (61). In general, western Denmark has lower water iodine concentrations than those in eastern Denmark (Table 1). The intake of milk represented 44% of the total iodine intake; the intake of fish accounted for 15% of the iodine intake in the Danish population (62). The most prominent determinants for high iodine intake were the use of multivitamins containing iodine, eating at least 200 g fish/week, and having a milk intake of more than 0.5 liter/day (62). The results showed that individuals in Aalborg did not reach the recommended intake levels even if they followed the advice regarding intake of fish and milk. This finding highlighted that dietary changes could not redress the ID problems in Denmark and that an iodization program was needed (62).

First, the Danish Veterinary and Food Administration introduced a voluntary program of universal salt iodization. As this turned out to be ineffective, it was replaced in 2000–2001 by a mandatory program of iodine fortification of household salt and salt in bread produced in Denmark (13 μg iodine/g salt) (21) (Table 1). Even though the iodine program was cautious and increased the iodine intake with 50 μg/day, the DanThyr monitoring program has observed effects on prevalence of goiter, nodules, and thyroid dysfunctionality. The incidence of overt hypothyroidism increased more in those areas that had previously had mild ID than in areas with moderate ID; there was a 53% higher incidence of spontaneous (presumably autoimmune) hypothyroidism. On the other hand, in previously moderate ID areas, there were initially 49% more cases of overt hyperthyroidism; however, this proved a temporary phenomenon, and the incidence of hyperthyroidism is now considerably below the periodization level. One phenomenon under surveillance is whether GD is becoming more common in young people (21, 63). Denmark has demonstrated that small changes in iodine intake can have dramatic effects on the spectra of thyroid diseases.

In the last DanThyr monitoring study in 2008–2010, the UIC levels were again found to have decreased (64). The exact reason for this is unknown; there was no reduction in the use of multivitamin supplements containing iodine, fish intake, fluid intake, egg consumption, or milk intake; however, the content of iodine in milk had decreased.

Sweden

In Sweden, goiter was first described by Carl von Linné in 1746–1747 (65) (Fig. 3) and by the end of the 19th century, goiter was observed among 20–30% of the children in Gästrikland and Dalarna counties (66). Twenty years later, the prevalence of goiter had increased to 60–65% in these areas (67–70). A national investigation was undertaken in 1929 that confirmed endemic goiter and cretinism in Dalarna, Gästrikland, mid-Norrland, and in Småland (25, 71, 72) (Fig. 1), areas at a distance from the western seas' salty winds (25) and thus far from the principal product contributing to iodine intake: herring. As herring was transported to the larger cities (73, 74), urban populations and those living along the roads were well supported (75). During the 19th century, several factors contributed to a higher frequency of goiter. 1) The introduction of potatoes to the popular diet not only saved many from starvation but also led to a less iodine-rich diet. 2) The herring disappeared for long periods. 3) The rise in population meant that new areas were being cultivated, areas that were less fertile compared with the land that had once been the seabed. The areas with a high incidence of goiter were known as the goiter belt (Fig. 1), inside of which, the ground water iodine content may have been lower than in outside areas (unpublished observation).

The iodization of table salt was introduced in Sweden in 1936. Initially, 10 μg iodine was added per gram of salt (76), but in 1966 the amount was increased to 50 μg iodine per gram of salt (77), as goiter continued to be prevalent in some areas (78–81) (Table 1). Today, WHO considers the Swedish population to be iodine-sufficient because the population has been subject to almost lifelong iodization (26, 82, 83). Smaller studies support this assumption (79, 84, 85), and it was confirmed in a national study in 2006–2007, in which 889 Swedish school children aged 6–12 years from 30 schools participated (73, 74). Median UIC was 125 μg/L with a low proportion of children with UIC < 100 μg/L and > 200 μg/l, indicating an optimal intake of iodine (73). Also, the old goiter belt had disappeared (74).

Hypo- and hyperthyroidism are the most widespread forms of thyroid diseases in Sweden. Autoimmune hypothyroidism is common, but the incidence of hyperthyroidism in Sweden is lower than the ranges indicated in international reports. Seventy-five percent of patients

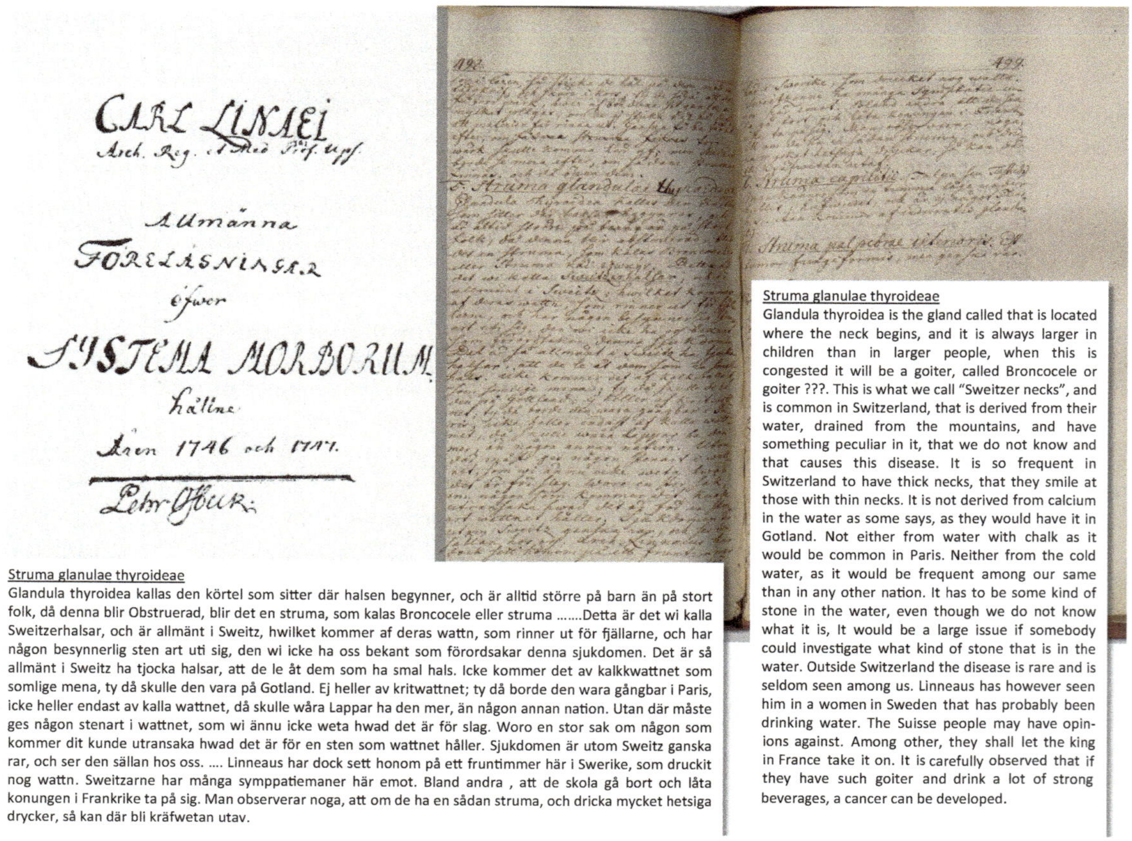

Fig. 3. Goiter as it was first described in Sweden; lecture notes by Per Osbeck that attended one of Carl von Linné's classes, 1746–1747's copy from the Hagströmer Library; Stockholm, Sweden.

with hyperthyroidism had GD and the intensity of the disease decreased by age (86, 87). Sweden is a country in which severe ID avoidance relies heavily on an adequate iodization program which, in turn, requires a satisfactory long-term monitoring strategy. However, the milk iodine concentration has decreased lately (88) and salt consumption is switching from iodized salt to salt with no added iodine, highlighting the need for future monitoring, especially of vulnerable groups.

Finland

The first known observations of goiter in Finland were made 180 years ago in some communities in the eastern parts of the country (89). In 1928, Adlercreutz reported that the water iodine content was low in Finland. The levels were lower in eastern Finland than in the west, and there was an inverse association between goiter and water iodine content (90). In 1938, Finland was classified as a country with endemic goiter, with most of the disease burden being found in eastern Finland (91) (Fig. 1). In reports from 1928–1929, the goiter frequency in school children from some areas was 10–15%, but in 1953–1954, it was 30–40% in others. The mean incidence in all elementary Finnish school children was, however, 4.4%. As late as in the 1950s, the entire country was moderately iodine-deficient, also now with endemic goiter being observed mainly in eastern Finland. However, there was considerable discussion about whether other goitrogenic factors might have additional effects on the ID population in the east, as iodine intake levels were not, in fact, very different. The goitrogenic effects of 5-vinyl-2-thiooxazoliodone (VTO, goitrin), a thionamid that blocks the intrathyroidal hormonal synthesis in milk, was much discussed (27). No distinct consensus was reached, but goitrogenic plants were eradicated from the pastures.

Iodized salt was available as early as 1949, but the use of salt with iodine was very low and the iodine content in salt was insufficient. Only 20% (or 15 μg) of the iodine intake came from iodized salt (89, 92).

The first attempts to interest the medical authorities in an iodine prophylaxis program were made in the 1930s and 1940s but was met with little response. In the late 1950s, a voluntary salt iodization program was initiated. In response to the initiative of A.I. Virtanen, the State Commission of Nutrition agreed with Finnish packing and importing firms that only import of salt containing 25 μg KI/g would be permitted. The use of iodized salt steadily increased and, in 1969, it was used in 75% of households, reaching 95% of households in 1979. However, the overall use of salt has decreased (89) and, in the 1980s, the fortification of table salt represented only one-third of the total iodine intake, while the intake of dairy products provided two-thirds of the Finns' iodine intake, thanks to the active iodization of livestock fodder (92).

In areas with endemic goiter, domestic animals also suffered from goiter and ID. After the decision to iodize table salt and cow fodder in Finland in the 1950s (Table 1), milk production increased (27), along with an increase of the iodine content in milk, from 30 μg/L in 1950 to 180 μg/L in the 1970s (89, 93, 94). Dairy products became the main iodine source (50%) as early as the 1950s. In the 1980s, when the iodine intake in Finland was 300 μg/d, 60 μg was derived from table salt and 200 μg from dairy products and eggs (27, 93). In the 1980s, the iodine intake in Finland was the highest in Europe (89) and, in 1986, it was stated that the use of iodized salt was no longer necessary because of the very active iodization strategy in household animals (89).

After the iodine prophylaxis program in humans and animals, the frequency of goiter declined. In 1965–1966, the mean prevalence was 0.25% and in the areas that had previously had the highest prevalence, it was 0.7% (89). Over the course of 15–20 years, the proportion of TMNG among patients with hyperthyroidism decreased from 80 to 10% (95) and, in the mid-1980s, GD dominated (89). For decades, Finland had a very effective iodization strategy, which rested heavily on the iodine content in dairy products and iodized salt, and on unchanged consumption patterns.

In the last decade or so, iodine levels have decreased in the general population to the extent that it has resulted in mild ID (96). Similarly, a decrease in milk and iodized salt consumption is noted. Therefore, a working group was initiated with representatives from the Ministry of Health and Social Affairs, the Ministry of Agriculture, the Finnish Food and Drink Industries' Federation, the National Institute for Health and Welfare, and the National Nutrition Council to do the necessary groundwork for new iodine recommendations and find practical new solutions that could be implemented especially by the food industry and mass catering services. A new recommendation was launched by the National Nutrition Council in 2015 (96). Finland is an example of a country with a very effective iodization strategy that relied heavily on the iodine content of dairy products and on unchanged consumption patterns.

Iodine status in populations at risk of ID in the Nordic countries

Pregnant women

As already mentioned, in Iceland, fish and milk intake has recently decreased among younger women (32). It is well known that the intake of fish and dairy products is linked to iodine status (25–27), but the recommendation to the population to consume fish at least twice a week and at least two portions of dairy products daily is based on concern for bone health and cardiovascular risk (21); iodine status was not an issue when the advice was issued. However, this recommendation also serves to promote adequate iodine intake. In Iceland, pregnant women in the second and third trimesters had UIC 180 µg/L (97), which is within the levels recommended during pregnancy by the WHO (Table 2). However, also the women that consumed fish and dairy products below the recommended levels had sufficient UIC levels at 160 µg/L, even if this value may be questioned because of the small size of the sample (97). Half of the women in this investigation took multivitamins, possibly containing iodine during pregnancy. Multivitamins with or without iodine can be bought, but giving information about iodine is not prioritized by health care workers at the Icelandic maternal health centers.

As already mentioned, a large percentage of the pregnant women in the Norwegian MoBa study had insufficient iodine intake, and only 21.7% reached the WHO/UNICEF/ICCIDD iodine intake recommendation of 250 µg/day (19, 51). The use of supplements containing iodine was reported by 31.6% of mothers-to-be (Table 2). The primary source of iodine from food was dairy products, contributing 67% of daily iodine intake in non-supplement and 43% in iodine-supplement users. The median intake of iodine from food was 141 µg/day and the additional contribution from supplements in iodine-supplement users was 107 µg/day. Dietary behaviors associated with the risk of low and suboptimal iodine intake were no use of iodine-containing supplements and low intake of milk/yoghurt, seafood, and eggs (19).

After the introduction of an iodine fortification program, the situation for Danish women has improved, but mild to moderate ID continues among pregnant women, especially for the women who are among the 12.7% that do not take multivitamin tablets also containing iodine (98) (Table 2).

In Sweden, no specific attention is given to the iodine question during pre-natal care, as the pregnant population in Sweden has appeared to be iodine-sufficient (99, 100). However, recently concerns have arisen regarding the truth of these assumptions, due to the following trends in Swedish society, which are 1) changes in food consumption patterns tending to a lower dairy product intake; 2) reduced iodine content in dairy products (88, 101); 3) a rise in the use of non-iodized salts, such as flake and gourmet salt; 4) low use of iodized salt in processed foods, promoting a lower iodine intake in the population; and 5) the salt reduction program launched by the National Food Agency (NFA) to lower the incidence of hypertension. This will affect pregnant and lactating women in particular. Retrospective local data have recently been published from Uppsala and Karlstad showing a median UIC of 99 µg/L in the third trimester in 469 women (102), further underlining these assumptions. Young women in Sweden have an intake of fish of 30 g/day, milk 230 g/day, and cheese 25 g/day (103); this may not be enough to cover the increased need of iodine. Hence, ID in pregnancy in Sweden may be imminent and there is an urgent need for monitoring studies to enable decision-making on future strategies to ensure adequate iodine nutrition (Table 2).

In Finland, there are no data on women during pregnancy, but studies are ongoing (Table 2).

Lactation

There is a large knowledge gap regarding the iodine situation for mothers and children during lactation in most Nordic countries (Table 2). The only country with available data is Denmark. Here, the use of multivitamins containing iodine during the lactation period drops to almost half compared to the use of such supplements during pregnancy, falling from 83 to 47%. Regardless of whether women take supplements containing iodine or not, Danish women do not attain the WHO target levels during breastfeeding (104). The situation is further aggravated for smokers, as smoking halves the milk iodine

Table 2. Comparison of risk populations in the Nordic countries according to available data

Success in risk groups	Iceland	Norway	Denmark	Sweden	Finland
Pregnant women	Sufficient	Mild ID	Mild ID	Mild ID	Unknown To be analyzed
Percentage of pregnant women using iodine-containing multivitamins	Unknown	32%	87%	Unknown To be analyzed	Unknown
Lactating women	Unknown	Unknown	Mild ID	Unknown To be analyzed	Unknown To be analyzed
Percentage of lactating women using iodine-containing multivitamins	Unknown	Unknown	47%	Unknown	Unknown
Children < I year	To be analyzed	Unknown	Unknown	Unknown	To be analyzed
Adolescents	Sufficient	To be analyzed	Unknown	Unknown study planned	Unknown

This table also illustrates the lack of data (unknown) in several areas in all the countries, but also that several ongoing studies will address some of the lack of knowledge (to be analyzed). The situation during pregnancy is unsatisfactory and none of the countries are aware of an optimal situation during lactation. Data are lacking in small children, and Iceland is the only country with known sufficient levels in adolescents. ID = iodine deficiency.

concentration (105). Trials are ongoing in Sweden and Finland, and new results on iodine during lactation are expected; however, no data are underway from Iceland or Norway (Table 2).

Children and adolescents

Two periods should be given special attention during childhood, which are the first year of life and adolescence. The first year of life is crucial for brain development; during adolescence many teenagers drastically reduce their milk consumption. In Denmark, however, the milk intake continues to be quite high during adolescence. In 2015, school children in eastern Denmark had iodine excretion within the recommended levels (median UIC; boys 146 μg/L, girls 128 μg/L) (106), underscoring that school children appear not to be at risk in Denmark or in the other Nordic countries for which there is data (73, 74, 98). Data are currently being collected on children <1 year in Iceland and in Finland, but there is no overall information on this risk group in the Nordic countries. The urinary iodine levels have been measured in adolescent girls on Iceland. In this age group, dairy products were the primary contributor to the girls' total iodine intake (43%), with only 24% coming from fish. The majority had a lower-than-recommended intake from fish (65%) and/or dairy products/day (40%), but the UIC was within the normal range defined by the WHO –200 μg/L (107). The dietary habits of young Icelandic girls have become more similar to the Western European diet, that is, like the diets in the United Kingdom, Denmark, and Norway (51, 62, 108). Studies are in progress to measure UICs in children and adolescents in Norway, Sweden, and Finland, but the study populations are not nationally representative samples (Table 2). Hence, there is a large knowledge gap on iodine status among small children and adolescents in the Nordic countries.

Regulations relating to iodine intake and authorities engagement with iodine-related issues in the Nordic countries

The iodine situation on Iceland is not regulated by law and there are no strategies for iodine intake, as this is not an issue of concern. Hence, there is no regular monitoring. In Norway, iodine fortification is prohibited beyond the 5 μg iodine/g salt. In Sweden and Finland, iodine fortification is regulated under European Union law, but it is voluntary, giving both the population and the food industry great freedom and responsibility for maintaining adequate iodine levels. Also, in Denmark, a voluntary approach was tried in 1998 that was not a success, and Denmark has thus ended up with a mandatory fortification of salt for commercial bread production (109) (Table 1).

The Nordic countries also differ in terms of which authorities are in charge of iodine intake. In Iceland, the responsible authority for nutritional status of the population remains to be determined. In Norway, the Ministry of Health and Care Services, working through the Directorate of Health, has the responsibility for nutritional advice and the population's health situation. In Denmark, it is the responsibility of the Danish Veterinary and Food Administration under the Ministry of Environment and Food. The NFA in Sweden is responsible for food safety and public health nutrition. However, the NFA is organized under the Ministry of Enterprise, which primarily focuses on the development of agriculture and the countryside. The responsible minister is the Minister of Agriculture, not the Minister of Health Care and Public Health. Issues related to iodine nutrition need to be coordinated between the two ministries. In Finland, the National Nutrition Council, which is under the Ministry of Agriculture and Forestry, issues nutrition-related recommendations. The new iodine recommendation launched in 2015 seems to have had some effect already, because several food and mass catering companies have recently announced that they intend to switch to iodized salt in food production. No monitoring studies have been performed subsequent to this very recent development.

Discussion

The historical perspective of present risk situation in the Nordic countries

Despite the many similarities, there were, historically, considerable differences in the access to foods with high iodine content among the Nordic populations, and they continue to vary in their intake of fish and dairy products. These factors, combined with different levels of iodine content in water, have resulted in disparate situations. Before iodization, the whole range was in evidence, from adequate iodine levels on Iceland to severe ID with cretinism in Sweden. It needs to be emphasized that, without iodization and appropriate action and monitoring measures, this may become the case again. In countries where the situation has been satisfactory for many years, government involvement and the responsibility taken by the authorities in connection with monitoring the situation and legislation seem to be substantially less than in Denmark, which is the country with the mildest ID and a short history of mandatory iodine fortification. It is not the degree of the ID, but rather the length of the period during which governments have taken action, that determines the level of responsibility assumed by government administrations. In Norway, Sweden, and Finland, a picture of apparently sufficient iodine levels and the fact that fortification measures were initiated almost a lifetime ago have resulted in the iodine situation being given little priority; modern surveillance has never been introduced. However, iodine levels are dynamic and affected by changes in society. Lying back and relaxing is not a good option.

The risk situation in the Nordic countries today

In addition to the fish intake being high in Iceland, the fish species that are consumed contain more iodine. Haddock and cod are lean fishes and contain considerably more iodine than fatty fish species. In Norway, lean fish comprise more than half of all fish consumed; but the consumption of fatty fish, such as herring, mackerel, and farmed salmon is on the rise. Herring was traditionally a common source of protein in the Norwegian and Swedish diets. Swedish and Finnish consumption patterns are, however, dominated by fatty fish, mainly farmed salmon and trout containing low amounts of iodine compared to wild salmon. Saltwater fish generally has higher iodine content. It is not only the amount of fish, but also the sort of fish that make a difference.

In all Nordic countries, except for Denmark (110), the food habits in the populations have changed during the past decades (36). In Norway, data from the national nutrition survey in 2010–2011 show that less than 25% of the adult population complied with the fish intake recommendation, which advises a weekly intake of 300–450 g fish (111). The proportion of pregnant women in MoBa whose intake matched this recommendation was $<10\%$ (112).

It is only in Iceland, with fish as the dominant source of iodine, that the population at large and pregnant women reach targeted levels. Subgroups with a low intake of fish, such as young girls, may, however, be at risk in the future if the ongoing decline in iodine intake continues, further pointing to the need for regular monitoring. There are also risk groups on Iceland that have never been investigated.

Another food which is being consumed less in the Nordic counties is milk. As Norway and Finland rely heavily on dairy product consumption as a source of iodine, these nations are at greater risk than the others from a decline in milk intake. In Norway, there has been a steady decline in milk consumption over the past decades, and Finland has recently developed mild ID after years of iodine sufficiency. Again, it needs to be emphasized that risk groups have not been properly investigated in these countries and the situation may in fact be much more serious than is apparent.

The iodization of cow fodder is critical for milk iodine concentration and the iodized feeding to domestic animals started long before iodization to people. The aim was to improve the health of the dairy cow and increase milk production, but eventually this measure also had a positive health impact on populations with a large dairy product intake. In Norway, the iodization of cow fodder is mandatory, but in Denmark, Sweden, and Finland, cow fodder iodization is voluntary. This means that changes in cow fodder content may in turn influence the concentration of iodine in milk. As rape seed contains substances that inhibit iodine secretion into cows' milk, the addition of rape seed cakes to soya protein in the fodder lowers the concentration of iodine in milk (113). Also, iodine levels in cow fodder may fall without considering the medical consequences for humans. In Sweden, milk iodine content has fallen (101), but resources are lacking for further investigations. Recently, the European Food Safety Authority (EFSA) advocated a reduction of the maximum iodine content allowed in cow fodder to minimize the risk of excessive iodine levels in small children, but this seems not to have materialized. A reduction of iodine content in milk will have sizable effects in the countries where milk is a main iodine source. A country must be aware of the risks connected to having a single primary iodine source and consider a change in strategy to broaden iodine nutrition to several sources to minimize the effects from societal changes that are beyond control from the medical or nutritional authorities.

Although the WHO, in their 2014 report, 'Guideline: fortification of food-grade salt with iodine for the prevention and control of iodine', recommends the mandatory legislation for salt iodization in all countries (114), the authorities in the Nordic countries advocate that salt consumption needs to be lowered due to the risk of hypertension. In Norway, this will do little to impact on iodine nutrition, but in Finland and Sweden, with a higher iodine fortification levels in salt, a reduction may influence the total iodine intake. This may be one reason for the reoccurrence of ID in the general population in Finland and the possible reoccurrence of ID in pregnant women in Sweden (102). Not only the amount of salt ingested but also the prevalence of the use of non-iodized salt plays an important role in iodine nutrition. Trends in society, such as the use of gourmet salt and flake salt that contain no iodine, make people in Sweden especially vulnerable, as the contribution from household salt to iodine intake is large. It is safe to lower the salt intake, but the salt ingested needs to be iodized.

More risk groups need to be evaluated in the Nordic countries; the number of unknown variables listed in Table 2 is unacceptable. However, pregnant women have been consistently evaluated in most of the Nordic countries. Despite the fact that each country has different practices in order to bring iodine levels within the targeted range, the situation seems unsatisfactory for women expecting children in the Nordic countries (102), except for the Icelandic population. Finnish data on pregnant women is still lacking, but as ID has reoccurred in the general population, it is unlikely that the condition is better in Finnish pregnant women.

Ways to target adequate iodine nutrition

It is also important to consider not only that the median iodine intake is sufficient, but also to consider the total iodine exposition in the population. In Denmark, the intake of bread is normally distributed in the population, compared with milk consumption or fish intake, for which distribution in the population is skewed. Iodization of salt in bread will result in a more uniform iodine level to people when the basic iodine intake is more dependent on dairy products, as in Norway. Presenting data in Finland about mild ID has also resulted in a successful implementation strategy and raised awareness of the need to use forms of iodized salt among the general population and among food industry representatives.

Other ways to increase the iodine intake may be strategies such as stating the iodine content for dairy products, raising awareness in the population, regulating iodine content in cow feed, making iodization mandatory, changing or adding sources of iodization, and introducing systematic monitoring, with the latter being the responsibility of the authorities. An increased awareness of the IDD should be also achieved in the personnel of national health systems, especially gynecologists, obstetricians, and pediatricians, who should regularly monitor iodine intake and thyroid status in women approaching pregnancy, in pregnant and lactating women, and adolescents. European Union (EU) law allows only nutrients >15% of the daily reference intake to be declared (Regulation (EU) no 1169/2011). For iodine, this means that only iodine levels >22 μg/100 g in foods is declared. Hence, regulations may hamper such strategies.

Conclusion

Current activities in the Nordic countries to increase iodine nutrition

In Norway, studies from the MoBa cohort have raised concerns over the iodine situation in the country and official awareness is on the rise. There is an urgent need for public health strategies to monitor and secure adequate iodine status in Norway. In Finland, actions are already ongoing to ensure satisfactory conditions. A new recommendation, issued in February 2015, states that all salt should contain 25 μg iodine per gram, and that only iodized salt should be used in mass catering and in homes. Also, the food industry, including bakeries, is urged to use iodized salt in all products. The new recommendation was widely covered by the Finnish media, which seems to have created a public demand for favoring iodized salt. The Finnish population is relatively health conscious, a factor that may have been crucial for the success of this measure, and hopefully the Finnish authorities will take responsibility for regular monitoring going forward. The reoccurrence of mild ID in the general population in Denmark and Finland is similar to what has happened in other countries, like in the United Kingdom (115), Australia (116), Germany (117), and New Zealand, where iodization programs recently have been initiated (118). In Denmark, where monitoring efforts are ongoing, the authorities are now collecting expert opinions and the advice is to increase the iodine content in salt from 13 μg/g to 20–22 μg/g. Hence, in Norway, Finland, and Denmark, authorities have started to take joint action based on new data.

The trend is for dietary habits in the Nordic countries to become more alike and, thus, the Nordic countries face similar iodine challenges. Health strategies would, therefore, benefit from coordination, and joint Nordic strategies should be designed. There are many lessons to be learned from neighboring countries in combatting ID and guaranteeing adequate iodine nutrition to all inhabitants. The systematic monitoring of iodine status in different groups is important to follow trends in iodine status; this should be a major task for the health authorities.

Acknowledgements

The authors are obliged to the Nordic Council of Ministers, Nordic Working Group for Diet, Food and Toxicology (NKMT) that made this article possible financially.

Conflict of interest and funding

The authors declare they have no conflicts of interest. This project has received grants from the Nordic Council of Ministers and receives financial support from the Swedish central government under the LUA/ALF agreement.

References

1. Hetzel BS. Iodine deficiency disorders (IDD) and their eradication. Lancet 1983; 2(8359): 1126–9.
2. Zimmermann MB. The adverse effects of mild-to-moderate iodine deficiency during pregnancy and childhood: a review. Thyroid 2007; 17(9): 829–35.
3. Velasco I, Carreira M, Santiago P, Muela JA, Garcia-Fuentes E, Sanchez-Munoz B, et al. Effect of iodine prophylaxis during pregnancy on neurocognitive development of children during the first two years of life. J Clin Endocrinol Metab 2009; 94(9): 3234–41.
4. Agostoni C, Berni Canani R, Fairweather-Tait S, Heinonen M, Korhonen H, La Vieille S, et al. Scientific opinion on dietary reference values for iodine. EFSA J 2014; 12(5): 3660.
5. Nordic Nutrition recommendations 2012. 5th ed. Copenhagen: Nordic Council of Ministers; 2014.
6. Glinoer D. The importance of iodine nutrition during pregnancy. Public Health Nutr 2007; 10(12A): 1542–6.
7. Morreale de Escobar M, Obregón MJ, Escobar del Rey F. Iodine deficiency and brain development in the first half of pregnancy. Public Health Nutr 2007; 10(12A): 1554–70.
8. Stanbury JB, Ermans AM, Hetzel BS, Pretell EA, Querido A. Endemic goitre and cretinism: public health significance and prevention. WHO Chron 1974; 28(5): 220–8.
9. Walker SP, Wachs TD, Gardner JM, Lozoff B, Wasserman GA, Pollitt E, et al. Child development: risk factors for adverse outcomes in developing countries. Lancet 2007; 369(9556): 145–57.
10. Zimmermann MB, Connolly K, Bozo M, Bridson J, Rohner F, Grimci L. Iodine supplementation improves cognition in iodine-deficient schoolchildren in Albania: a randomized, controlled, double-blind study. Am J Clin Nutr 2006; 83(1): 108–14.
11. Zimmermann MB, Jooste PL, Mabapa NS, Mbhenyane X, Schoeman S, Biebinger R, et al. Treatment of iodine deficiency

in school-age children increases insulin-like growth factor (IGF)-I and IGF binding protein-3 concentrations and improves somatic growth. J Clin Endocrinol Metab 2007; 92(2): 437–42.
12. Bath SC, Steer CD, Golding J, Emmett P, Rayman MP. Effect of inadequate iodine status in UK pregnant women on cognitive outcomes in their children: results from the A von Longitudinal Study of Parents and Children (ALSPAC). Lancet 2013; 382(9889): 331–7.
13. Hynes KL, Otahal P, Hay I, Burgess JR. Mild iodine deficiency during pregnancy is associated with reduced educational outcomes in the offspring: 9-year follow-up of the gestational iodine cohort. J Clin Endocrinol Metab 2013; 98(5): 1954–62.
14. Bath SC, Rayman MP. Iodine deficiency in the U.K: an overlooked cause of impaired neurodevelopment? Proc Nutr Soc 2013; 72(2): 226–35.
15. Zimmermann MB, Gizak M, Abbott K, Andersson M, Lazarus JH. Iodine deficiency in pregnant women in Europe. Lancet Diabetes Endocrinol 2015; 3(9): 672–4.
16. Charlton KE, Gemming L, Yeatman H, Ma G. Suboptimal iodine status of Australian pregnant women reflects poor knowledge and practices related to iodine nutrition. Nutrition 2010; 26(10): 963–8.
17. Stagnaro-Green A, Dogo-Isonaige E, Pearce EN, Spencer C, Gaba ND. Marginal iodine status and high rate of subclinical hypothyroidism in Washington DC women planning conception. Thyroid 2015; 25(10): 1151–4.
18. Andersen SL, Sorensen LK, Krejbjerg A, Moller M, Klitbo DM, Nohr SB, et al. Iodine status in Danish pregnant and breastfeeding women including studies of some challenges in urinary iodine status evaluation. J Trace Elem Med Biol 2015; 31: 285–9.
19. Brantsaeter AL, Abel MH, Haugen M, Meltzer HM. Risk of suboptimal iodine intake in pregnant Norwegian women. Nutrients 2013; 5(2): 424–40.
20. Bulow Pedersen I, Knudsen N, Jorgensen T, Perrild H, Ovesen L, Laurberg P. Large differences in incidences of overt hyper- and hypothyroidism associated with a small difference in iodine intake: a prospective comparative register-based population survey. J Clin Endocrinol Metab 2002; 87(10): 4462–9.
21. Laurberg P, Jorgensen T, Perrild H, Ovesen L, Knudsen N, Pedersen IB, et al. The Danish investigation on iodine intake and thyroid disease, DanThyr: status and perspectives. Eur J Endocrinol 2006; 155(2): 219–28.
22. Laurberg P, Cerqueira C, Ovesen L, Rasmussen LB, Perrild H, Andersen S, et al. Iodine intake as a determinant of thyroid disorders in populations. Best Pract Res Clin Endocrinol Metab 2010; 24(1): 13–27.
23. Fordyce FM, Johnson CC, Navaratna UR, Appleton JD, Dissanayake CB. Selenium and iodine in soil, rice and drinking water in relation to endemic goitre in Sri Lanka. Sci Total Environ 2000; 263(1–3): 127–41.
24. Bourre JM, Paquotte P. Seafood (Wild and Farmed) for the elderly: contribution to the dietary intakes of iodine, selenium, DHA and vitamins B12 and D. J Nutr Health Aging 2008; 12(3): 186–92.
25. Sjöberg K. Strumasjukdomarnas profylax och behandling. Thesis at Uppsala University, Sweden, 1972, pp. 5–50.
26. Andersson M, Takkouche B, Egli I, Allen HE, de Benoist B. Current global iodine status and progress over the last decade towards the elimination of iodine deficiency. Bull World Health Organ 2005; 83(7): 518–25.
27. Lamberg BA. Iodine deficiency disorders and endemic goitre. Eur J Clin Nutr 1993; 47(1): 1–8.
28. Delange F. Administration of iodized oil during pregnancy: a summary of the published evidence. Bull World Health Organ 1996; 74(1): 101–8.
29. WHO (2006). Guidelines on food fortification with micronutrients. Geneva: World Health Organization.
30. Hetzel B. The story of iodine deficiency: an international challenge in nutrition. Hetzel BS, ed. Oxford, UK: Oxford University Press; 1989.
31. Sigurjonsson J. Study on the human thyroid in Iceland. Reykjavik, Iceland: University of Iceland; 1940.
32. Gunnarsdottir I, Gustavsdottir AG, Thorsdottir I. Iodine intake and status in Iceland through a period of 60 years. Food Nutr Res 2009; 53: 1925, doi: http://dx.doi.org/10.3402/fnr.v53i0.1925
33. Steingrimsdottir L, Thorgeirsdottir H, Olafsdottir AS. The diet of Icelanders. Reykjavik, Iceland: Icelandic nutrition council; 2002.
34. Steingrimsdottir L, Thorgeirsdottir H, Aegisdottir S. The diet of the Icelander. Reykjavik, Iceland: Icelandic nutrition council; 1990.
35. Sigurjonsson J. Survey of diet and health in Iceland. Reykjavik, Iceland: University of Iceland; 1940.
36. Thorgeirsdottir H, Valgeirsdottir H, Gunnarsdottir I, Gisladottir E, Gunnarsdottir BE, Thorsdottir I. Main results. Reykjavik, Iceland: Directorate of Health, Icelandic Food and Veterinary Authority, Unit for nutrition research Landspitali – The National University Hospital of Iceland and University of Iceland; 2011.
37. Reykjdal O, Hilmarsson OTh, Audunsson GA. Iodine in agricultural produce (in Icelandic). Agr Conf 2007; 4: 516–18.
38. Sigurdsson G, Franzson L. Urinary iodine excretion in Icelandic men and women. Icelandic Med J 1988; 74: 183–7.
39. ISGEM (2008). Icelandic database for food composition. Reykjavik, Iceland: ISGEM.
40. Iodine, selenium and mercury in meat, milk and eggs. Center of Food Technology; 2008. Available from: http://www.matis.is/media/utgafa/matra/Jod_Lokaskyrsla_0804.pdf
41. Thorsdottir I, Gunnarsdottir I. The diet of Icelandic 9 and 15-year-old children and adolescents 2003–4. Reykjavik, Iceland: Unit for Nutrition Research and Icelandic Health Institute; 2006.
42. Schiøtz C. Steller norge forsvarlig med sine skolebarn og sin ungdom? Kristiania, Norway: Nei! Cappelens Forlag; 1917.
43. Devold O, Batt F, Closs K, Backer J. En strumaundersøkelse fra modum. Norsk Magazin for Lægevitenskap, 1937, pp. 899–937.
44. Frey H, Rosenlund B, Try K, Theodorsen L. Iodine deficiency in Europe. New York: Plenum press; 1993, pp. 297–300.
45. Phillips DI. Iodine, milk, and the elimination of endemic goitre in Britain: the story of an accidental public health triumph. J Epidemiol Community Health 1997; 51(4): 391–3.
46. Frey H, Tangen T, Lovik J, Thorsen RK, Sand T, Rosenlund B, et al. [Endemic goiter no longer exists in the community of Modum]. Tidsskr Nor Laegeforen 1981; 101(22): 1184–6.
47. Frey H, Rosenlund B, Storli U. [Urinary excretion of iodine in some Norwegian population groups 1971–1972]. Tidsskr Nor Laegeforen 1974; 94(15): 982–7.
48. Halvorsen AO, Muri R. [Iodine excretion in 24-hour urine]. Tidsskr Nor Laegeforen 1974; 94(15): 987–90.
49. Dahl L, Johansson L, Julshamn K, Meltzer HM. The iodine content of Norwegian foods and diets. Public Health Nutr 2004; 7(4): 569–76.
50. Magnus P, Irgens LM, Haug K, Nystad W, Skjaerven R, Stoltenberg C, et al. Cohort profile: the Norwegian mother and child cohort study (MoBa). Int J Epidemiol 2006; 35(5): 1146–50.
51. Brantsaeter AL, Haugen M, Julshamn K, Alexander J, Meltzer HM. Evaluation of urinary iodine excretion as a biomarker

for intake of milk and dairy products in pregnant women in the Norwegian Mother and Child Cohort Study (MoBa). Eur J Clin Nutr 2009; 63(3): 347–54.
52. Dahl L, Opsahl JA, Meltzer HM, Julshamn K. Iodine concentration in Norwegian milk and dairy products. Br J Nutr 2003; 90(3): 679–85.
53. Rasmussen LB, Andersson G, Haraldsdottir J, Kristiansen E, Molsted K, Laurberg P, et al. Iodine. Do we need an enrichment program in Denmark? Int J Food Sci Nutr 1996; 47(5): 377–81.
54. Laurberg P, Jørgensen T, Perrild H, Ovesen L, Knudsen N, Pedersen IB, et al. Surveillance of thyroid disorders and iodine intake in the Danish population before and after mandatory iodide fortification of salt: the DanThyr program. In: Preedy VR, Burrow GN, Watson RR, eds. Comprehensive handbook on iodine: Nutritional, Endocrine and Pathological Aspects. Oxford: Elsevier; 2009, pp. 1159–68.
55. Kelly F, Snedden WW. Endemic goitre. Geneva: World Health Organization; 1960. Contract No.: 44.
56. Pedersen KM, Borlum KG, Knudsen PR, Hansen ES, Johannesen PL, Laurberg P. Urinary iodine excretion is low and serum thyroglobulin high in pregnant women in parts of Denmark. Acta Obstet Gynecol Scand 1988; 67(5): 413–16.
57. Pedersen KM, Nöhr SB, Laurberg P. Jodindtagelse i Danmark. Ugeskrift for Laeger 1997; 159: 2201–6.
58. Munkner T. Urinary excretion of 127 Iodine in the Danish population. Scand J Clin Lab Invest 1969; 110(Suppl): 134.
59. Haraldsdottir J, Holm L, Höjmark Jensen J, Möller A. Dietary habits in Denmark 1985 1. Main results. Søborg, Denmark: Levnedsmiddelstyrelsen; 1986. Contract No.: 136.
60. Pedersen KM, Laurberg P, Nohr S, Jorgensen A, Andersen S. Iodine in drinking water varies by more than 100-fold in Denmark. Importance for iodine content of infant formulas. Eur J Endocrinol 1999; 140(5): 400–3.
61. Rasmussen LB, Larsen EH, Ovesen L. Iodine content in drinking water and other beverages in Denmark. Eur J Clin Nutr 2000; 54(1): 57–60.
62. Rasmussen LB, Ovesen L, Bulow I, Jorgensen T, Knudsen N, Laurberg P, et al. Dietary iodine intake and urinary iodine excretion in a Danish population: effect of geography, supplements and food choice. Br J Nutr 2002; 87(1): 61–9.
63. Laurberg P, Pedersen KM, Vestergaard H, Sigurdsson G. High incidence of multinodular toxic goitre in the elderly population in a low iodine intake area vs. high incidence of Graves' disease in the young in a high iodine intake area: comparative surveys of thyrotoxicosis epidemiology in East-Jutland Denmark and Iceland. J Intern Med 1991; 229(5): 415–20.
64. Rasmussen LB, Carle A, Jorgensen T, Knuthsen P, Krejbjerg A, Perrild H, et al. Iodine excretion has decreased in Denmark between 2004 and 2010 – the importance of iodine content in milk. Br J Nutr 2014; 112(12): 1993–2001.
65. Linné Cv. Carl Linaei Allmänna föeläsningar öfwer Systema Morborum hållna noted by Pehr Osbeck. 1746–47.
66. Söderbaum P. Om förekomsten av struma inom Gefleborgs och Stora Kopparbergslän på grund af undersökningar, gjorda av medlemmar af Gefleborgs-Dala Läkare-och Apoteksförening. Hygia 1893; 55(II): 416–18.
67. Fjellander G. Endemisk struma i Husby distrikt. Gefleborgs-Dala Läkare- och Apotekare-Förenings Förhandlingars häfte 1913; 26: 22–8.
68. Hollström KF. Om förekomsten av struma bland skolbarn i Falun och om profylaktisk användning av jodhaltigt matsalt. Nordisk Hygiensk Tidskrift, 1929, pp. 219–32.
69. Gibson G, BA. Till frågan Kan struma i Sverige bekämpas? Svenska Läkartidningen 1924; 21: 113–16.
70. Gibson G, BA. Till frågan Kan struma i Sverige bekämpas? Svenska Läkartidningen 1927; 24: 1317–20.
71. Höjer J. Kropfstudien Die Verbreitung des endemischen Kropfes in Schweden. Svenska Läkarsällskapets handlingar 1931; 57: 1–104.
72. Höjer J. Strumaundersökningar. Nor Hyg Tidskr 1928; IX: 61–125.
73. Andersson M, Berg G, Eggertsen R, Filipsson H, Gramatkovski E, Hansson M, et al. Adequate iodine nutrition in Sweden: a cross-sectional national study of urinary iodine concentration in school-age children. Eur J Clin Nutr 2009; 63(7): 828–34.
74. Filipsson Nystrom H, Andersson M, Berg G, Eggertsen R, Gramatkowski E, Hansson M, et al. Thyroid volume in Swedish school children: a national, stratified, population-based survey. Eur J Clin Nutr 2010; 64(11): 1289–95.
75. Sjoberg KH. [Iodine and diet]. Lakartidningen 1978; 75(25): 2477–9.
76. Medicinalstyrelsen. Förebyggande åtgärder mot endemisk struma. Cirkulär 1936; 30.
77. Medicinalstryelsen. jodering av koksalt. Cirkulär 1966; 11.
78. Johnsson S. [Endemic struma – average frequency]. Lakartidningen 1965; 62(26): 2049–56.
79. Sjoberg KH, Sundlof G. [The occurrence of struma before and after iodine prophylaxis]. Lakartidningen 1971; 68(9): 980–4.
80. Gullström A. Om strumaprofylax. Svenska Läkartidningen 1943; 40: 455–9.
81. Hollström KF. Om förekomsten av struma bland skolbarn i Falun och om profylaktisk användning av jodhaltigt matsalt. Svenska Läkartidningen 1946; 43: 163–71.
82. Vitti P, Delange F, Pinchera A, Zimmermann M, Dunn JT. Europe is iodine deficient. Lancet 2003; 361(9364): 1226.
83. Dohan O, De la Vieja A, Paroder V, Riedel C, Artani M, Reed M, et al. The sodium/iodide symporter (NIS): characterization, regulation, and medical significance. Endocr Rev 2003; 24(1): 48–77.
84. Milakovic M, Berg G, Nystrom E, Lindstedt G, Gebre-Medhin M, Eggertsen R. Urinary iodine and thyroid volume in a Swedish population. J Intern Med 2004; 255(5): 610–14.
85. Milakovic M, Berg G, Eggertsen R, Lindstedt G, Nystrom E. Screening for thyroid disease of 15–17-year-old schoolchildren in an area with normal iodine intake. J Intern Med 2001; 250(3): 208–12.
86. Abraham-Nordling M, Bystrom K, Torring O, Lantz M, Berg G, Calissendorff J, et al. Incidence of hyperthyroidism in Sweden. Eur J Endocrinol 2011; 165(6): 899–905.
87. Nystrom HF, Jansson S, Berg G. Incidence rate and clinical features of hyperthyroidism in a long-term iodine sufficient area of Sweden (Gothenburg) 2003–2005. Clin Endocrinol (Oxf) 2013; 78(5): 768–76.
88. Lindmark Månsson H. Den svenska mejerimjölkens sammansättning 2009. Stockholm, Sweden: Svensk Mjök (Swedish Milk); 2012. Report No.: Contract No.: 7094.
89. Lamberg BA. Endemic goitre in Finland and changes during 30 years of iodine prophylaxis. Endocrinol Exp 1986; 20(1): 35–47.
90. Adlercreutz E. Orientierende untersuchung uber der Verbreitung des Kropfes in Finnland and uber deren Zusammenhang mit dem Jodvorkommen im Wasser. Acta Med Scand 1928; 69: 1–45, 186–221, 325–91.
91. Wahlberg J. Die Schilddrusenkrankheiten in Finland. Acta Med Scand 1938; 94(Suppl).
92. Lindberg O, Andersson LC, Lamberg BA. The impact of 25 years of iodine prophylaxis on the adult thyroid weight in Finland. J Endocrinol Invest 1989; 12(11): 789–93.
93. Varo P, Saari E, Paaso A, Koivistoinen P. Iodine in Finnish foods. Int J Vitam Nutr Res 1982; 52(1): 80–9.

94. Vilkki P. Iodine in Finnish diet and its relation to goitre incidence. Ann Acad Fenn Ser A II Chem 1956; 71.
95. Lamberg B-A, Liewendahl K, Välimäki M. Present state of endemic goitre in Finland. Iodine deficiency in Europe, a continuous concern. New York: Plenum Press; 1993.
96. Iodine recommendation of the National Nutrition Council in Finland: the National Nutrition Council recommends the following actions to improve the iodine intake of the population. 2015. [cited 7 May 2016]. Available from: http://www.ravitsemusneuvottelukunta.fi/files/attachments/en/vrn/vrn_jodi_toimenpidesuositus_10_2.2015_english.pdf
97. Gunnarsdottir I, Gustavsdottir AG, Steingrimsdottir L, Maage A, Johannesson AJ, Thorsdottir I. Iodine status of pregnant women in a population changing from high to lower fish and milk consumption. Public Health Nutr 2013; 16(2): 325–9.
98. Andersen SL, Sorensen LK, Krejbjerg A, Moller M, Laurberg P. Challenges in the evaluation of urinary iodine status in pregnancy: the importance of iodine supplement intake and time of sampling. Eur Thyroid J 2014; 3(3): 179–88.
99. Elnagar B, Eltom A, Wide L, Gebre-Medhin M, Karlsson FA. Iodine status, thyroid function and pregnancy: study of Swedish and Sudanese women. Eur J Clin Nutr 1998; 52(5): 351–5.
100. Eltom A, Elnagar B, Elbagir M, Gebre-Medhin M. Thyroglobulin in serum as an indicator of iodine status during pregnancy. Scand J Clin Lab Invest 2000; 60(1): 1–7.
101. Lindmark Månsson H. The Swedish Milk composition. Stockholm, Sweden: Svensk Mjölk (Swedish Milk); 2010. Report No.: Contract No.: Report nr 7090–P.
102. Granfors M, Andersson M, Stinca S, Akerud H, Skalkidou A, Sundstrom Poromaa I, et al. Iodine deficiency in a study population of pregnant women in Sweden. Acta Obstet Gynecol Scand. 2015; 94(11): 1168–74.
103. Amcoff E, Edberg A, Enghardt Barbieri H, Lindroos AK, Nälsén C, Pearson M. Livsmedels- och näringsintag bland vuxna i Sverige. Uppsala: National Food Agency; 2012.
104. Andersen SL, Moller M, Laurberg P. Iodine concentrations in milk and in urine during breastfeeding are differently affected by maternal fluid intake. Thyroid 2014; 24(4): 764–72.
105. Laurberg P, Nohr SB, Pedersen KM, Fuglsang E. Iodine nutrition in breast-fed infants is impaired by maternal smoking. J Clin Endocrinol Metab 2004; 89(1): 181–7.
106. Rasmussen LB, Kirkegaard-Klitbo DM, Laurberg P, Jørgensen T, Ovesen L, Perrild H. Iodine excretion in school children in Copenhagen. Dan Med J 2016; 63(5): pii: A5223.
107. Gunnarsdottir I, Gunnarsdottir BE, Steingrimsdottir L, Maage A, Johannesson AJ, Thorsdottir I. Iodine status of adolescent girls in a population changing from high to lower fish consumption. Eur J Clin Nutr 2010; 64(9): 958–64.
108. Lightowler HJ, Davies GJ. Iodine intake and iodine deficiency in vegans as assessed by the duplicate-portion technique and urinary iodine excretion. Br J Nutr 1998; 80(6): 529–35.
109. Fødevareministeriets bekendtgørelse Last Update, 627 (2000 29 June).
110. Pedersen AN, Christensen T, Matthiessen J. Danskernes kostvaner 2011–2013. Hovedresultater. Søborg: DTU Fødevareinstituttet; 2015.
111. Norwegian Directorate of Health. Norkost 3. En landsomfattende kostholdsundersøkelse blant menn og kvinner i Norge i alderen 18–70 år. [National dietary survey, report in Norwegian]. 2015. [cited 7 May 2016]. Available from: https://helsedirektoratet.no/Lists/Publikasjoner/Attachments/301/Norkost-3-en-landsomfattende-kostholdsundersokelse-blant-menn-og-kvinner-i-norge-i-alderen-18-70-ar-2010-11-IS-2000.pdf
112. von Ruesten A, Brantsaeter AL, Haugen M, Meltzer HM, Mehlig K, Winkvist A, et al. Adherence of pregnant women to Nordic dietary guidelines in relation to postpartum weight retention: results from the Norwegian Mother and Child Cohort Study. BMC Public Health 2014; 14: 75.
113. Laurberg P, Andersen S, Knudsen N, Ovesen L, Nohr SB, Bulow Pedersen I. Thiocyanate in food and iodine in milk: from domestic animal feeding to improved understanding of cretinism. Thyroid 2002; 12(10): 897–902.
114. World Health Organization. Guideline: fortification of food-grade salt with iodine for the prevention and control of iodine deficiency disorders. Geneva: World Health Organization; 2014.
115. Vanderpump MP, Lazarus JH, Smyth PP, Laurberg P, Holder RL, Boelaert K, et al. Iodine status of UK schoolgirls: a cross-sectional survey. Lancet 2011; 377(9782): 2007–12.
116. Li M, Eastman CJ, Waite KV, Ma G, Zacharin MR, Topliss DJ, et al. Are Australian children iodine deficient? Results of the Australian National Iodine Nutrition Study. Med J Aust 2006; 184(4): 165–9.
117. Johner SA, Gunther AL, Remer T. Current trends of 24-h urinary iodine excretion in German schoolchildren and the importance of iodised salt in processed foods. Br J Nutr 2011; 106(11): 1749–56.
118. Edmonds JC, McLean RM, Williams SM, Skeaff SA. Urinary iodine concentration of New Zealand adults improves with mandatory fortification of bread with iodised salt but not to predicted levels. Eur J Nutr 2016; 55(3): 1201–12.

*Helena Filipsson Nyström
Department of Endocrinology
Sahlgrenska University Hospital
Gröna Stråket 8
SE-41345, Gothenburg, Sweden
Email: helena.filipsson@telia.com

9

Perspectives on the probiotic potential of lactic acid bacteria from African traditional fermented foods and beverages

Mduduzi Paul Mokoena*, Taurai Mutanda and Ademola O. Olaniran

Discipline of Microbiology, School of Life Sciences, College of Agriculture, Engineering and Science, University of KwaZulu-Natal (Westville Campus), Durban, South Africa

Abstract

Diverse African traditional fermented foods and beverages, produced using different types of fermentation, have been used since antiquity because of their numerous nutritional values. Lactic acid bacteria (LAB) isolated from these products have emerged as a welcome source of antimicrobials and therapeutics, and are accepted as probiotics. Probiotics are defined as live microbial food supplements which beneficially affect the host by improving the intestinal microbial balance. Currently, popular probiotics are derived from fermented milk products. However, with the growing number of consumers with lactose intolerance that are affected by dietary cholesterol from milk products, there is a growing global interest in probiotics from other food sources. The focus of this review is to provide an overview of recent developments on the applications of probiotic LAB globally, and to specifically highlight the suitability of African fermented foods and beverages as a viable source of novel probiotics.

Keywords: *antimicrobials*; *probiotics*; *lactic acid bacteria*; *fermented foods*

Traditional fermentation is a form of food processing achieved by using microorganisms, especially lactic acid bacteria (LAB), and yeast. Although it is an ancient food preservation technology, it is still part of the cultural norm usually being practiced at a local or household level among indigenous communities in Africa and most of the developing world (1–3). Unlike their unfermented counterparts, fermented foods are preferred by consumers because of their characteristic taste, texture, and color (4). Fermented traditional foods and beverages in developing countries constitute one of the main dietary components, with some being used as light meals or refreshments.

LAB isolated from various fermented foods produce organic acids and a high diversity of antimicrobial agents, which are responsible for the upkeep of quality and the palatability of fermented foods. At a local level, LAB are used in African communities to produce a variety of fermented foods which include cereal-based fermented porridges, beverages, fermented fruits and vegetables (including roots or tubers), fermented milks, and fermented meats (4, 5). Of the various types of fermentations used to obtain fermented foods and beverages, lactic acid and alcoholic fermentations are the most popular. Other types are alkaline fermentation and amino acid fermentation (5).

The role of LAB in improving the shelf life and nutritional quality of fermented foods and beverages, controlling diarrhea, as well as their antimicrobial properties have been established (6–9). However, despite an increasing interest in probiotic LAB, there is a paucity of literature regarding novel and emerging uses of LAB as probiotics, especially from the African continent. In addition, strict regulation by international bodies has resulted in limited probiotic products passing the clinical trial stage. Rural communities are known to be consuming fermented foods laden with probiotic microflora, from which they derive health benefits. This paper reviews different topical traditional fermented foods and beverages in Africa which are potential sources of novel probiotics, and explores global progress on the isolation of probiotic LAB candidates. The applications of LAB as antidiabetic agents, cholesterol-reducing agents, immune system modulation agents, and as drug-delivery vehicles, as well as their novel applications in mental and emotional well-being of humans were discussed in detail.

Food and beverage fermentation by LAB

Fermented foods have been part of the human diet since the dawn of human civilization, and have been used as a means of improving the shelf life, safety, digestibility, and nutritional value for more than 6,000 years (10–16). Lactic acid food fermentation is a process whereby microorganisms and their enzymes are used to convert fermentable sugars in the food substrate into mainly lactic acid and other limited products. Fermentation is widely used for food preservation in households and in food industries to develop a variety of food products (13). This food preservation technology is inexpensive; hence, it is of economic importance in developing countries (4). Microorganisms responsible for the fermentation can be the microflora indigenously present on substrates, or they can be added as starter cultures after cooking or preparing the food or beverage.

Fermentation of traditional foods is mainly carried out by LAB, which has earned the 'generally regarded as safe' (GRAS) status. Fermentation improves the organoleptic properties of foods and their acceptability. Popular fermented food products in Africa include fermented milks, sour porridges, and alcoholic and non-alcoholic beverages (17). Cereals are a staple diet globally and they can be processed through fermentation to acquire desirable modifications of taste, flavor, acidity, and food digestibility (4). There is a vast diversity of African traditional fermented foods and beverages distributed throughout the continent, with typical examples presented in Table 1.

In addition to the various fermented plant products, fermented meats and fish form part of the African diet and also of diet in other parts of the world (18–21), although these are arguably not yet common. Nonetheless, fermented meats can be adequate purveyors of probiotic bacteria if properly applied. Fermented meat products are defined as meat that is inoculated with a microbial starter culture during processing under controlled conditions to give desirable characteristics. Meat fermentation can also be achieved by allowing it to spontaneously ferment by natural meat microbial flora. A recent review (22) discusses the application of novel technologies and microbial cultures in the development of functional fermented meats. Zakpaa et al. (19) established that the microbial composition of Ghanaian fermented meats consists of LAB species, *Streptococcus* spp., *Staphylococcus* spp., and *Micrococcus* spp. Of these,

Table 1. Various African traditional fermented foods and beverages

Fermented product	Region	Raw substrates	Microorganisms implicated	Published references
Ogi	West Africa	Maize, sorghum, millet	*Lactobacillus plantarum* *L. fermentum, S. cerevisiae* *Candida krusei, Corynebacterium* spp., *Acetobacter* spp.	(23, 117)
Iru	West Africa	African locust bean	*Bacillus, Staphylococcus* spp.	
Gari	West Africa	Cassava	*Leuconostoc mesenteroide* *Lactobacillus plantarum* *Bacillus subtilis, Candida krusei*	
Mahewu	Southern Africa	Maize or sorghum	*Lactobacillus bulgaricus,* *L. brevis*	(7, 9, 17)
Munkoyo (chibwantu)	Southern Africa	Maize	*Weisella* and *Lactobacillus* spp.	(24, 25, 27)
Borde Shamita	North East Africa	Barley	*Lactobacillus* spp.	(118)
Togwa	East Africa	Cassava, maize, sorghum, millet	*Lactobacillus* spp., *Pediococcus pentosaceus, Weissella confusa, Issatchenkia orientalis, S. cerevisiae, Candida pelliculosa* and *C. tropicalis*	(25)
Mabisi/Amasi	Southern Africa	Milk	*Lactococcus, Lactobacillus* and *Streptococcus* spp., *Leuconostoc* spp.	(17, 119)
Amabere amaruranu	Southern Africa	Milk	*Streptococcus thermophilus, Lactobacillus plantarum,* and *Leuconostoc mesenteroides; Yeasts*	(120)
Marula/buganu	Southern Africa	Amarula fruit	Yeasts	(9)
Bushera	East Africa	Sorghum or millet	*Lactobacillus* spp., *Streptococcus* spp., *Leuconostoc* spp., *Pediococcus* spp., *Weissella* spp.	(121)
Chibuku	Southern Africa	Sorghum	*Lactobacillus* spp., *Saccharomyces cerevisiae*	(9)
Umqombothi	Southern Africa	Maize or sorghum	*Lactobacillus* spp., *S. cerevisiae*	(122)

Streptococcus and *Staphylococcus* spp. are characterized as pathogenic, and the LAB species and *Streptococcus* spp. as probiotics. These results suggest that using a robust probiotic starter culture might be useful in improving the quality of fermented meats, as it may inhibit the growth of potentially pathogenic organisms. Fermentation is one of the most important fish preservation methods in many parts of the world and particularly in the coastal regions of African countries (21). The fermentation processes applied are generally indigenous and adaptable to the culture of the people. However, lack of standardization of the processing methods and hygiene levels compromise the safety and quality of fermented fish products in Africa. Thus, more research needs to be dedicated to finding solutions to these issues.

Fermented foods are produced using different manufacturing techniques, raw materials, and microorganisms depending on available raw materials and local practices. However, the four main fermentation processes are alcoholic, lactic acid, acetic acid, and alkali fermentation. While a majority of these fermentations are carried out by bacteria, in alcohol fermentation, yeasts are the predominant microorganisms used for production of ethanol-containing beverages, such as wines and beers, where LAB play a limited role (4).

LAB are critical in the production of most fermented foods and beverages, but there is a paucity of knowledge about the specific health benefits such foods confer on consumers and the characteristics of the bacterial strains used for their production. Moreover, literature on probiotic microbes from different fermented foods from Africa that have found applications in the food and pharmaceutical industries is scarce.

Diversity of African traditional fermented foods and beverages and associated microbes

Ogi, *iru*, and *gari* (Table 1) are the Nigerian fermented foods that have been commercialized; the rest are still being produced at the household level. *Ogi* is a fermented product of maize or sorghum or millet grains. *Iru* is a fermented product of African locust bean; and *Gari* is a fermented cassava product, produced by peeling fresh roots, grating them into mash, and putting in sacks for fermentation (23). The main microorganisms used for the fermentation in these products are LAB and yeasts.

Borde and *Shamita* (Table 1) are important Ethiopian traditional fermented beverages, produced by an overnight fermentation of certain cereals predominantly by LAB (24). LAB associated with *Borde* and *Shamita* fermentation have antimicrobial properties against various food-borne pathogens; the inhibitory products are extracellular and diffusible. *Togwa* (Table 1) is a Tanzanian fermented beverage that could be prepared from cassava, maize, sorghum, and millet, or their combinations. Yeasts and LAB are the predominant microorganisms found in *togwa* (25).

Amasi or sour milk, *umqombothi* or sorghum beer, and *amahewu* (Table 1), a non-alcoholic fermented maize meal, are South African foods and beverages. *Amasi* is produced by using specific LAB such as *Lactobacillus delbrueckii* and *Streptococcus* spp. *Amahewu* is produced with LAB starter culture, whereas *umqombothi* is produced from maize or sorghum via wild yeast fermentation, and LAB from malted sorghum adjuncts play a limited role (7). Fermented beverages such as those obtained from amarula fruits using yeast and LAB are popular in parts of Limpopo and Mpumalanga Provinces in South Africa.

Sour porridge is maize or sorghum, which is fermented using mainly LAB to improve and develop palatability, flavor, and nutrition (26). *Chibuku* (Table 1) is a Zimbabwean traditional sorghum beer commercially produced by yeast fermentation of sorghum (9), whereas *mabisi*, *munkoyo*, and *chibwantu* (Table 1) are Zambian traditional food and beverages produced through yeast and lactic acid fermentations (27).

Production of these traditional fermented foods depends on the availability of infrastructure to store and transport the product. Isolation and screening of microorganisms from natural sources has been the most effective means for obtaining robust and genetically stable strains for industrially important food products (28, 29). However, the microbial diversity of the different fermented foods from different localities in Africa still needs to be characterized using more reliable tools such as next generation sequencing and other molecular techniques. This will enable the selection of more robust, probiotic microorganisms with desirable characteristics to be used as starter cultures and will ensure the safety of the foods and beverages and pharmaceutical products.

Role and importance of LAB in traditional fermented foods

General role of LAB

Fermentation may be the most simple and economical way of improving cereal nutritional value, sensory properties, and functional qualities available at the local community level (15, 30). Lactic acid fermentation of cereals has been used as a strategy to decrease the content of antinutrients, such as phytate and tannins, and for improving the bioavailability of micronutrients (31). Many bacteria associated with fermented foods produce antimicrobial bioactive molecules, such as hydrogen peroxide, organic acids, and bacteriocins, that make them effective biopreservatives (12, 32) and produce nutraceuticals to create functional foods with increased bioavailability of nutrients (33, 34). Table 2 presents an overview of some of the various applications of LAB isolates.

LAB as probiotics

LAB comprise a significant component of the human gut flora and have several beneficial roles in the

Table 2. An overview of some of the applications of selected LAB strains

LAB Strain(s)	Applications	Published References
Lactobacillus rhamnosus	Reduction of dental caries risk	(63, 123)
L. casei	Mitigation of Type II diabetes and obesity	(67, 124)
Bifidobacterium longum SPM 1207; *Lactobacillus* spp.	Lowering of cholesterol and low-density lipoproteins	(77, 80, 83)
Lactobacillus spp.	Inhibition of *Listeria monocytogenes* & *Clostridium* spp.	(20, 90)
Lactobacillus reuteri; L. plantarum	Antifungal agents	(3, 20, 92)
L. casei; L. planturum	Drug-delivery vehicles	(93, 97, 98, 101)
L. acidophilus, L. salivarius, L. rhmnosus, L. brevis, L. casei	Immune system modulation and mental health	(39, 42, 53, 115)
Lactobacillus spp.	Reduction of mycotoxins in fermented maize products	(7)

gastrointestinal tract. Thus, a better understanding of the intestinal microbial populations will contribute to the development of new strategies for the prevention and/or treatment of several diseases (35). Probiotics are live microbial food supplements which beneficially affect the host by improving the intestinal microbial balance (36–38). Probiotic LAB belong to the genera *Lactobacillus*, *Bifidobacterium*, *Enterococcus*, *Lactococcus*, *Streptococcus*, and *Leuconostoc* (39, 40). Probiotics are consumed in the form of yoghurt, fermented milks, or other fermented foods (37, 41). These products containing living microorganisms have been traditionally used to restore gut health (42). Thus, bacteria known as probiotics because of their positive impact on human health and well-being have been added to various foods for the past decades (42, 43).

Probiotic bacteria from the genus *Lactobacillus* are inherently present in fermented foods and many diseases caused by pathogens invading the gastrointestinal tract can be prevented by maintaining proper intestinal flora by consuming probiotics or fermented foods. Probiotics have a great potential for improving nutrition, soothing intestinal disorders, improving the immune system, optimizing gut ecology, and promoting overall health because of their ability to compete with pathogens for adhesion sites, to antagonize pathogens, or to modulate the host's immune response (33, 43, 44).

Bifidobacterium species are strictly anaerobic, inhabit the large intestines, and more than 30 species have been identified. These microbes are added in baby formula milk and dairy products such as yoghurt or their growth in the large intestines is stimulated by prebiotics from diet. They assist in the metabolism of lactose, generation of lactate ions from lactic acid, and vitamin synthesis (40, 45). Generally, probiotic bacteria do not colonize the human intestinal tract permanently, but some strains are able to transiently colonize and modulate the indigenous microbiota (42). LAB are highly beneficial organisms for humans and their use should be promoted for good health.

Candidate probiotic microbial strains must satisfy the criteria for safety, production or manufacturing, administration and application, and survival and colonization in the host (46). *In vitro* experiments are used to investigate whether the selected microbial strains fulfill these criteria and enable screening of microorganisms for their potential as probiotic strains (46). Potential probiotics are further subjected to *in vivo* experiments to validate their efficacy. In this regard, it has been experimentally demonstrated that feeding day-old chicks with a commercial LAB-based probiotic culture after they were challenged with *Salmonella enteritidis* or *Salmonella typhimurium* significantly reduced recovery of *Salmonella* (47). Similarly, it has been demonstrated that fish fed with probiotic-supplemented diets presented significantly higher growth rates and feeding performance than those fed with control diet (48).

Probiotic LAB isolated from fermented food samples exhibit excellent antimicrobial activity against pathogenic bacteria and fungi (3). Bacteria with such notable probiotic properties can be used as a potential source of probiotic for use in pharmaceutical preparations, and as functional foods for the betterment of public health. Developing countries in Asia and Africa have a rich diversity of fermented foods and beverages which can be exploited for isolation of such novel probiotics.

The role of LAB in immune system modulation and mental health

Most probiotic foods contain LAB belonging to the genera *Lactobacillus* but not exclusively (39). Certain strains of probiotics are able to stimulate and regulate several aspects of the natural and acquired immune response, although differences in the ability of *Bifidobacterium* and *Lactobacillus* strains to influence the functioning of the immune system have been reported (33). The interactions of these probiotics and their unique metabolic capabilities are critical to their ability to colonize the gastrointestinal tract and immune system modulation.

More than 100 species of *Lactobacillus acidophilus*, *Lactobacillus salivarius*, *Lactobacillus rhamnous*, *Lactobacillus brevis*, and *Lactobacillus casei* have been characterized and identified. They are implicated in enhancing the innate and acquired immunity as well as cause inhibition of proinflammatory mediators (49). Probiotic protective microorganisms prevent pathogens from adhering to the intestines by competing for substrates and places of adhesion, simultaneous production of antibacterial molecules, and stimulating the production of specific antibodies and mucus. Thus, early colonization of the gut with probiotic bacteria is critical for the development of the gut protection barrier.

Several studies have indicated that LAB play a positive role in modulating the host immune system and display of antimicrobial activities against common food-borne pathogens and in preventing and treating diarrhea (11, 28, 33, 34, 50, 51). The current understanding of the role of probiotic bacteria in the human and animal systems is preliminary, partly because of the complexity of the gastrointestinal ecosystem and the increasing variety of strains considered as probiotics (52). However, these mechanisms may be multifactorial and each probiotic strain may have specific functions affecting the host. Specific probiotic bacteria are known to modulate local and systemic immune responses, although the mechanisms of immune modulation are still not fully elucidated. Nevertheless, there is an understanding that bacterial components are recognized by the immune system through their interaction with specific receptors, resulting in the modulation of the immune responses (42).

Another study (53) suggests that there is a connection between microbes inhabiting the human GUT and many aspects of physiology, including brain health. The authors point out that fermentation alters dietary compounds in food and maintain that fermentation-enriched chemicals (lactoferrin, bioactive peptides) and the newly formed phytochemicals such as unique flavanoids may act upon the human intestinal microflora. They further suggest that consumption of fermented foods has a potential to positively affect human health and mental well-being by stimulating the actions of the GUT microflora, via the production of bioactive chemicals and neuropeptides that manifest behaviourally through magnified antioxidant and anti-inflamattory activity, and reduction of intestinal permeability. Other studies established that agmatine and other polyamines associated with fermented meats, fish, and certain beverages have benefits related to brain health (54, 55). All these studies highlight the great strides already made on the role of probiotic foods and beverages on human physiology.

Potential role of LAB as a remedy for lifestyle health problems

Prevention and treatment of dental caries

Evidence suggests that species of *Lactobacillus* and *Bifidobacterium* may have beneficial effects in the oral cavity by inhibiting cariogenic bacteria (54, 56, 57). However, scarcity of information on the probiotic action in the oral cavity suggests that more studies should be conducted on the colonization of mouth by probiotics and their potential effect on and within oral biofilms. With increasing antibiotic drug resistance, the concept of probiotic therapy is compelling and merits further investigation in the field of oral medicine (58–60).

The potential application of probiotic bacteria as a remedy for oral infections is of research interest, and clinical studies carried out thus far suggest that probiotics could be critical in preventing and treating dental caries, periodontal disease, and halitosis (43). *Streptococcus mutans* is regarded as the main cause of dental decay and various lactobacilli are associated with progression of the lesion (61, 62). In one study (63), *Lactobacillus rhamnosus* GG, ATTC (LGG) was demonstrated to be antagonistic to many bacteria, including *S. mutans*, which is responsible for tooth decay. This study shows that consuming milk containing *L. rhamnosus* GG significantly reduces the risk of caries. The effect of probiotics on dental caries has been reviewed elsewhere. Although these studies indicate a positive role of probiotics in oral health, more studies need to be conducted to evaluate the efficacy of several probiotics for this purpose.

A survey of novel technologies for the prevention of dental caries has been conducted, and these include the use of probiotics (64). Dental caries and their biofilms can be treated by using probiotic lactobacilli and bifidobacteria from dairy products, tablets, lozenges, and chewing gum in various dose regimens. Results from randomized clinical trials are promising although further large-scale trials with orally derived anticaries bacteria are essential for the success of bacteriotherapy (65). Most reccently, probiotics have proven to be effective in dealing with dental caries (66). However, more studies are needed to explore the use of probiotics appropriately in the field of dentistry.

Prevention of Type II diabetes and obesity

Earlier studies suggest that probiotic bacteria play an important role in management of insulin-independent diabetes, with one study particularly indicating that the oral administration of *L. casei* in mice causes a decrease in plasma glucose levels (67). Nutrients with prebiotic and probiotic properties have positive consequences for host well-being with regard to obesity and diabetes. Bacterial metabolism of nutrients in the gut is suggested to influence the release of bioactive compounds which interact with host cellular targets to control energy metabolism and immunity, resulting in less fat mass development, diabetes, and low levels of inflammation associated with obesity (68). A human randomized, double-blind, placebo-controlled trial concluded that probiotic bacteria induce beneficial changes in gut microbiota, reduce the systemic inflammatory state through altering systemic endotoxin levels, thereby reducing the systemic inflammatory response observed in type II diabetes mellitus subjects (69).

Studies with mice indicate that antidiabetic activity of probiotic LAB could emanate from continuous reduction of the blood glucose through the suppression of glucose absorption from the intestine, thus indicating that specific strains of LAB are crucial for the management of type II diabetes (70). Consumption of yoghurt, rich in probiotic bacteria, may exert antidiabetic and antioxidant properties in human subjects and human microflora and is likely to have a major role in maintaining the homeostasis of human metabolism, suggesting that probiotics intake is a useful approach for modulation of human microbiota (71). Elsewhere, it has been established that probiotic soy milk could modulate blood lipoprotein levels and thus may be considered in managing diabetes complications and atherosclerotic risks (72).

Lowering serum cholesterol levels

Cholesterol plays a significant role in human heart health. However, because the human body produces enough cholesterol, dietary cholesterol is extraneous and is a leading cause of cardiovascular diseases such as stroke and heart attack (73). Studies conducted to explore the role of probiotic bacteria in the reduction of serum cholesterol showed promising results where cholesterol precipitated out during *in vitro* studies with a possibility of the same being excreted under *in vivo* conditions (74). However, more research needs to be conducted in this regard as these studies were inconclusive. Moreover, some authors warn that overconsumption of prebiotics and probiotic bacteria could cause intestinal discomfort, and the risk of probiotics being purveyors of antibiotic resistance genes needs further investigation (75).

According to one study, there is a difference in fecal cholesterol-associated short chain fatty acids pattern in conventional rats fed with the oat-based diets with probiotic bacteria in comparison to the group fed with rice-based diet (76). Probiotic bacteria able to reduce cholesterol in blood can be obtained from carnivores because they normally eat meat containing high fat and rarely develop cardiovascular conditions. Isolation and characterization of such strains of bacteria has a potential application in controlling cholesterol levels in humans (73).

Bifidobacterium longum SPM 1207 is able to reduce serum total cholesterol and low-density lipoproteins which are associated with bad cholesterol levels, while slightly increasing serum high-density lipoproteins, which are associated with good cholesterol. This suggests that a combination of LAB from the genus *Bifidobacterium* and *Lactobacillus* could result in robust probiotics as the latter genera produce bacteriocins (77–79). A *Lactobacillus oris* HMI68 was successfully isolated from a mother's milk and this strain demonstrated cholesterol-reducing property and was regarded as a candidate probiotic (80).

Interestingly, *Lactobacillus plantarum* and *L. brevis* from pickle cabbage decreased levels of serum cholesterol, total glycerides, and low-density lipoprotein cholesterol but increased high-density lipoprotein cholesterol levels in mice treated with the probiotic bacteria (81). The study suggests that in addition to lowering blood cholesterol, the bacterial strains have the potentials to enhance the activities of antioxidant enzymes, relieve lipid-induced oxidative stress, and serve as probiotics. In addition, *Lactobacillus* spp. and *Weissella* spp. isolated from fermented Indian koozh and cucumber exhibited cholesterol-reducing potential (82).

Recently, the effect of probiotic consumption on the Iraqi human body weight and lipid profile was investigated and probiotic strains showed lowering effects on abdominal adiposity, body weight, and other measures of subjects with obese tendencies, suggesting a positive influence on metabolic disorders (83). In particular, this study showed that consumption of probiotic strains reduces total cholesterol and low-density lipoproteins while increasing levels of high-density lipoproteins. This counteracts obesity effects and regulates lipid metabolism.

LAB as a source of antimicrobial agents

Bacteriocins from LAB

Bacteriocins are a heterogeneous group of potent antimicrobial peptides primarily active against closely related organisms, mostly gram-positive bacteria (84). They are ribosomally synthesized during the primary phase of growth (85). Bacteriocins are small cationic molecules of about 30–60 amino acids, forming amphiphilic helices and stable at 100 °C for 10 min. Thus, they vary in spectrum of activity, mode of action, molecular weight (MW), genetic origin and biochemical properties (86). They are classified into three groups: lantibiotics, non-lantibiotics of low MW, and non-lantibiotics of higher MW (87). LAB strains that produce bacteriocins protect themselves from their own toxins by the expression of a specific immunity protein which is encoded in the bacteriocin operon (88).

In fermented foods, LAB display various antimicrobial activities, including bacteriocin production. Consequently, several bacteriocins with potential industrial applications have been purified and characterized. Bacteriocin-producing cultures have been applied to inhibit *Listeria monocytogenes* and *Clostridium* in various fermented meats, vacuum-packaged products, and in vegetable-based foods (20, 84). Bacteriocins can be vital when cold chain is interrupted during transportation of heat-sensitive foods. Artificial chemicals are currently widely used to limit food spoilage organisms, but their potential health risks has led researchers to seriously consider the possible use of bacteriocins or their synergistic effect with chemicals, phenolic compounds, and antimicrobial proteins (86, 89).

The spread of antibiotic resistance and demand for food products with fewer chemical preservatives necessitates the search for new alternatives to avoid the abuse of therapeutic antibiotics (87). LAB isolated from home-made fermented vegetables produce antibacterial substances against both gram-positive and gram-negative common food-borne bacterial pathogens. This broad spectrum of inhibition suggests that the LAB strains have a potential to be used as natural biopreservatives in various food products.

Bacteriocins are mainly bactericidal, with some being bacteriostatic, rendering them useful in the food and pharmaceutical sectors. Their site of action is the bacterial cytoplasmic membrane and on energized membrane vesicles to disrupt the proton motive force (84, 86). However, their drawback could lie in the fact that they inhibit mainly closely related organisms, implying that they may inhibit other desired starter cultures, and may not be active against gram-negative pathogens and food spoilers. Bacteriocins have been found to be effective against gram-positive toxigenic and pathogenic bacteria. Addition of chelating agents has been effective in rendering gram-negative bacteria susceptible to bacteriocins (86). A recent study has established that the use of heterofermentative *Lactobacillus* spp. in the production of Dutch-type cheese-like products reduces the populations of technologically harmful microorganisms that negatively affect the quality, safety, and shelf life of the end products (90).

Antifungal agents and other antimicrobial agents from LAB

As the number of antibiotic-resistant microbial species increases, fungi and yeasts are no exception, and both human fungal pathogens and spoilage molds in food and feeds are becoming resistant. Interestingly, yeasts and molds are becoming resistant also to preservatives such as sorbate and benzoate as well as chemical detergents (91). LAB produce various antimicrobial compounds such as lactic acid, propionic acid, and diacetyl, which cause pH reductions that inhibit many microorganisms, including fungi (91).

In addition to other functions, *Lactobacillus reuteri* produces reuterin, which has a broad spectrum activity against protozoa, fungi, and both gram-positive and gram-negative bacteria and reuterocyclin, which is a negatively charged, hydrophobic, broad spectrum antibiotic which is restricted only to work against gram-positive bacteria (92). Organic acids, bacteriocins, and antifungal peptides produced by microorganisms can also be isolated from grass silage. *L. plantarum* isolated from grass silage exhibit antifungal activity by producing organic acids, other molecular mass metabolites, and cyclic dipeptides (20).

LAB as drug-delivery vehicles

Because of their properties such as GRAS status, adjuvant profile, mucosal adhesion, and low intrinsic immunogenicity, LAB have been adjudged to have a potential as a carrier for oral immunization, where the adjuvant function of different *Lactobacillus* species was explored. In one such study (93), *L. casei* and *L. plantarum* consistently showed strong adjuvanticity in different experimental model systems. These results thus demonstrated that the generation of *Lactobacillus*-based live vectors as vaccines instead of pathogen-derived live vaccines is feasible (93). This represents preliminary immunological data of recombinant LAB strains expressing antigens from pathogens.

Live bacterial vaccine vectors can be applied for antigen delivery (94). However, increased stability and low production costs should be pursued in addition to the multiple advantages associated with the use of bacteria as vaccine vectors in order to reap maximum benefits. There is growing interest regarding the use of peptides from LAB in medicinal and personal care products, but there is paucity of clinical data to substantiate their efficacy.

Targeted drug delivery to the colon using probiotics, alone or in combination with prebiotics, ensures direct treatment at the disease site leading to lower dosing and fewer systemic side effects (95). As the habitat of probiotics, the colon is better placed as a portal for the entry of drugs into the circulation system (96). While it has been suggested that muco-adhesive polymers such as lectins and fibrin can be used to improve drug delivery through different routes such as gastrointestinal, nasal, ocular, buccal, vaginal, and rectal routes, LAB are more ideal candidates for drug delivery, especially in the gastrointestinal and nasal routes (97). In addition, LAB have potential as an alternative approach to the treatment of human asthma (98).

Nasal vaccination using live bacterial vectors, where attenuated respiratory pathogens are applied, is more effective than non-colonizing microbes such as LAB. However, in contrast to systemically administered vaccines, recombinant live bacteria generally induce strong mucosal immune responses in the respiratory tract and distal mucosal sites. Although many applications of LAB as host factory and delivery vehicles need further research (99, 100), the already established safety profile and efficiency of this system purports a promising future of GRAS bacteria as expression vectors that can revolutionize the field of recombinant protein expression.

The two main advantages of using probiotics as an alternative approach to health care management are their inherent diverse mechanism of action and being living organisms. The current challenges with this system are probiotic strain identification, characterization, screening, and understanding its mechanism of action for a particular disease. Several approaches including microencapsulation and use of compatible material have been studied with a view to circumvent these challenges (101).

Major factors impacting on the use of LAB as probiotics

Probiotics are living and non-pathogenic bacteria that have beneficial effects on their host's health (33, 102). The major interest in LAB is driven by the fact that upon consumption, these microorganisms are beneficial to the host by boosting the good microflora of the gastrointestinal tract (GIT), and because probiotics are normally associated with LAB, it makes sense to use traditional fermented foods as the main source of probiotics (102, 103). Probiotic bacteria are commonly marketed as fermented foods and dairy products are popular carriers of probiotics (33, 104). Fermented foods are well suited to promote the positive health image of probiotic bacteria because fermented cereals and dairy products already have a positive health image; consumers are familiar with the fact that fermented foods contain microorganisms; and probiotics used as starter cultures combine the positive images of fermentation and probiotic cultures (104).

Probiotic food products are conventionally sold in the form of fermented milk because milk has been accepted as a nutritious and healthy product, and as an important source of calcium, proteins, phosphorus, and riboflavin (39). However, with an increase of more health conscious consumers in developed countries, there is a demand for non-dairy probiotic fermented food products because some consumers are negatively affected by the lactose and cholesterol content associated with fermented dairy products (39, 105–107). The fat content, sustained viability, and numbers of probiotic bacteria are some of the factors currently affecting the use of LAB as probiotics. Several factors that are considered in the criteria for the selection of candidate probiotic LAB are briefly described below.

Bile and low pH tolerance

LAB with high tolerance for low pH and bile salts demonstrate the ability to survive in the stomach and intestine, and to successfully compete with other bacteria in this environment and to colonize the GIT of the host. The probiotic potential of six LAB strains was evaluated with respect to tolerance for acidity and to bile salts. All six strains were resistant to pH 3.0 and pH 4.0 after 24 h of incubation showing viability rates of 10^9 CFUml^{-1} and 10^{12} CFUml^{-1}, respectively. Moreover, all six strains also demonstrated a high resistance to bile salt concentration of 0.3% (w/v), giving a cell viability of 10^5–10^8 CFUml^{-1} after 24 h of treatment (38). High exopolysaccharide-producing LAB such as *Streptococcus thermophilus* strains exhibit a higher tolerance to bile salts than the *Lactobacillus delbrueckii* subsp. *bulgaricus* strains (108).

Starter culture populations

Probiotics are live microorganisms providing benefits to humans when they are consumed in adequate amounts. To effect these benefits, fermented foods must contain probiotic microorganisms in populations above 10^6 CFUml^{-1} or g throughout its shelf life. Accordingly, consumption of more than 100 g per day of a typical commercial bio-yoghurt containing more than 10^6 CFUml^{-1} is necessary to satisfy adequate numbers of viable cells (109). High population of probiotics in commercial fermented milk products is achieved by adding them during or after the fermentation process separately from the starter culture. For traditional fermented foods, this implies that they must be produced by ensuring probiotics populations of not less than 10^6 CFUml^{-1}, otherwise they might not provide maximum benefit to consumerism (110).

Adhesion to gut epithelial tissue

Candidate probiotic LAB isolates should demonstrate the ability to adhere to gut epithelial tissue and to colonize the GIT. The relative importance of these characteristics is highlighted by the fact that many of the probiotics available, except *L. rhamnosus*, do not colonize their targeted hosts and consequently do not remain in the GIT for any significant period of time (3, 111, 112).

Antimicrobial activity and safety

A typical probiotic strain should exhibit antimicrobial effects by producing some of the several compounds such as organic acids, fatty acids, hydrogen peroxide, and diacetyl (112). Probiotics should improve safety to the host by inactivating pathogens but must not demonstrate any pathogenic or toxic activities to the host. In addition, candidate probiotics must have no transferable antibiotic resistance genes and must prevent the production of biogenic amines from dietary proteins (3, 113).

Other selection criteria for probiotic LAB

Other properties an ideal probiotic LAB candidate must display include resistance to antibiotics, antimutagenicity properties, rapid production of lactic acid, viability and retention of activity in delivery vehicles, ability to stimulate the host immune response, and the ability to influence metabolic activities such as vitamin production, cholesterol assimilation, and lactose metabolism (3, 114).

Current status and future prospects of probiotic bacteria

Probiotic is the current buzz word in the human diet arena and has captured major attention from researchers across the world, including developing countries, because of its enormous health potential (115, 116). The term probiotics was first used in 1965 and defined at that time as microbially derived factors that stimulate growth of other organisms. However, in 1989 the term probiotics was modified to mean live microbes that are beneficial to the host (115). Although probiotic microorganisms have been used for centuries in food production, global research on their products and applications has recently began. There is an increasing interest in utilizing probiotic LAB for treating GIT disorders and as drug-delivery vehicles (33). Because of increase in antibiotic resistance, probiotics and their products, such as bacteriocins, promise to be good alternatives as antimicrobials. Globally, many communities recognize the importance of probiotic microorganisms as evidenced by increasing demands for dairy products, especially yoghurt. Due to increasing food prices, communities in rural and urban areas in developing countries should be encouraged to continue consuming their household fermented foods and beverages as part of normal diet to exploit the probiotic benefits of these products.

Food products that simultaneously contain probiotics and prebiotics are called synbiotics. This combination ensures the survival of probiotics through the gut and facilitates their delivery into the large intestine. Prebiotics stimulate the growth and activity of endogenic intestinal microflora (33). Most African traditional fermented foods and beverages fit the synbiotics definition perfectly, as they comprise of residual stomach-indigestible polysaccharides together with the LAB used for fermentation. Recent advancements in the science of probiotics research at a molecular level include using high throughput sequencing techniques. This will enable researchers to decipher unique probiotic gene products with novel applications. The use of probiotics offers an innovative approach for developing formulations applied as functional foods for managing diseases such as chronic inflammatory gastrointestinal disorders and many lifestyle diseases.

Concluding remarks

The value of fermented food cannot be overemphasized, as they have always played a vital role in diet and nutrition. The benefits associated with fermented foods, such as increased shelf life, palatability, and nutritional value, suggest the importance of these foods. The probiotic effects of various fermented foods and their associated microbial cultures look promising and warrant further research. Fermentation products of probiotic LAB from traditional foods can be a suitable alternative source of antimicrobial agents, incorporated in the fight against emerging antibiotic-resistant microorganisms. Food fermentation is a method of preserving food by presenting a hurdle against pathogenic bacteria, and can mitigate diarrhea in communities with inferior potable water quality. Traditional foods, appropriately produced, are safe and acceptable, and qualify as a source of probiotics with novel applications.

While the mechanisms of action of probiotic LAB and their products, including bacteriocins, warrant further experimentation (*in vitro* and *in vivo*), and controlled clinical trials to exploit the maximum value is important, current developments suggest that consumption of fermented foods and beverages should be encouraged in all communities, especially in developing countries where probiotic dairy products may come at a great price. Probiotic bacteria have a potential in solving current and emerging lifestyle diseases. Surprisingly, LAB from fermented foods were recently found to play a positive role in mental health. Most of the probiotic microbial cultures in literature and currently available in the market are from outside Africa even though this continent has such a rich diversity of fermented foods that needs to be exploited as a source of probiotics. Hence, the search for novel probiotic bacteria from African fermented foods and beverages; and from other parts of the world should be intensified. Finally, metagenomics can play a crucial role in this process by providing insights into the genes, structure, and function of products from probiotic microorganisms.

Conflict of interest and funding

The authors have not received any funding or benefits from industry or elsewhere to conduct this study. This study was supported by the University of KwaZulu-Natal, Durban, South Africa.

References

1. Aderiye B, Laleye S. Relevance of fermented food products in southwest Nigeria. Plant Foods Hum Nutr 2003; 3: 1–16.
2. Mosha T, Vincent M. Nutritional value and acceptability of homemade maize/sorgum-based waning mixtures supplemented with *rojo* bean flour, ground sardines and peanut paste. Int J Food Sci Nutr 2004; 55: 301–15.
3. Pundir RK, Rana S, Kayshap N, Kaur A. Probiotic potential of lactic acid bacteria isolated from food samples: an *in vitro* study. J Appl Pharm Sci 2013; 3: 085–93.
4. Nout MJR, Motarjemi Y. Assessment of fermentation as a household technology for improving food safety: a joint FAO/WHO workshop. Food Contr 1997; 8: 221–6.
5. Steinkraus K. Classification of fermented foods: worldwide review of household fermentation techniques. Food Contr 1997; 8: 311–17.
6. Moyane JN, Jideani AIO. The physicochemical and sensory evaluation of commercial sour milk (*amasi*) products. Afr J Food Sci 2013; 7: 56–62.
7. Chelule PK, Mokoena MP, Gqaleni N. Advantages of traditional lactic acid bacteria fermentation of food in Africa. In: Mendez-Vilas A, ed. Current research, technology and education topics in applied microbiology and microbial biotechnology. Madrid: FORMATEX; 2010.
8. Hati S, Mandal S, Prajapati JB. Novel starters for value added fermented dairy products. Current Res Nutr Food Sci 2013; 1: 83–91.

9. Gadaga TH, Mutukumira AN, Narvhus JA, Feresu SB. A review of traditional fermented foods and beverages of Zimbabwe. Int J Food Microbiol 1999; 53: 1–11.
10. Holzapfel W. Use of starter cultures in fermentation on a household scale. Food Contr 1997; 8: 241–58.
11. Lei V, Friis H, Michaelen KF. Spontaneously fermented millet product as a natural probiotic treatment for diarrhoea in young children: an intervention study in Northern Ghana. Int J Food Microbiol 2006; 110: 246–53.
12. Ananou S, Maqueda M, Martinez-Bueno M, Valdivia E. Biopreservation, an ecological approach to improve the safety and shelf-life of foods. In: Mendez-Vilas A, ed. Communicating current research and education topics and trends in applied microbiology. Madrid: FORMATEX; 2007.
13. Guarner F, Khan AG, Garisch J, Eliakim R, Gangl A, Thomson A, et al. Probiotics and prebiotics. Milwaukee, USA: World Gastroentorology Org; 2008, p. 22.
14. Scott R, Sullivan WC. Ecology of fermented foods. Human Ecol Rev 2008; 15: 25–31. Available from: http://www.humanecologyreview.org/pastissues/her151/scottandsullivan.pdf [cited 21 January 2015].
15. Borresen EC, Henderson AJ, Kumar A, Weir TL, Ryan EP. Fermented foods: approaches and formulations for nutritional supplementation and health promotion. Recent Patents on Food. Nutrition & Agriculture 2012; 4: 134–40.
16. Georgala A. The nutritional value of two fermented milk/cereal foods named 'Greek Trahanas' and 'Turkish tarhana': a review, J Nutr Disorders Ther 2013; S11: 002. doi: http://dx.doi.org/10.4172/2161-0509.S11-002
17. Oyewole OB. Lactic fermented foods in Africa and their benefits. Food Contr 1997; 8: 289–97.
18. Dirar H. The indigenous fermented foods of the Sudan: a study in African Food and Nutrition. Oxfordshire, UK: CAB International; 1993.
19. Zakpaa D, Imbeah C, Mak-Mensah E. Microbial characterization of fermented meat products on some selected markets in the Kumasi metropolis, Ghana. African J Food Sci 2009; 3: 340–6.
20. De Vuyst L, Leroy F. Bacteriocins from lactic acid bacteria: production, purification, and food applications. J Mol Microbiol Biotechnol 2007; 13: 194–9.
21. Anihouvi V, Kindossi J, Hounhouigan J. Processing and quality characteristics of some major fermented fish products from Africa: a critical review. Int Res J Biol Sci 2012; 1: 72–84.
22. Ojha K, Kerry J, Duffy G, Beresford T, Tiwari B. Technological advances for enhancing quality and safety of fermented meat products. Trends Food Sci Tech 2015; 44: 105–116.
23. Kuye A, Sanni LO. Industrialization of fermented food processes: how far in Nigeria? J Sci Ind Res 1999; 58: 837–43.
24. Girum T, Eden E, Mogessie A. Assessment of the antimicrobial activity of lactic acid bacteria isolated from *Borde* and *Shameta*, traditional Ethiopian fermented beverages, on some foodborne pathogens and effect of growth medium on inhibitory activity. Int J Food Safety 2005; 5: 13–20.
25. Mugula JK, Nnko SAM, Narvhus JA, Sorhaug T. Microbiological and fermentation characteristics of togwa, a Tanzanian fermented food. Int J Food Microbiol 2003; 80: 187–99.
26. Abdelgadir WS, Ahmed TK, Dirar HA. The traditional fermented milk products of the Sudan. Int J Food Microbiol 1998; 44: 1–13.
27. Schoustra SE, Kasase C, Toarta C, Poulain AJ. Microbial community structure of three traditional Zambian fermented products: *mabisi*, *chibwantu* and *munkoyo*. PLoS One 2013; 6: 1–12.
28. Adnan AFM, Tan IKP. Isolation of lactic acid bacteria from Malaysian foods and assessment of the isolates for industrial potential. Bioresource Tech 2007; 98: 1380–5.
29. Harlander SK. Genetic improvement of microbial starter cultures. In: Ruskin FR, ed. Applications of biotechnology to traditional fermented foods. Washington, DC: National Academy Press; 1992.
30. Blandino A, Al-Seeri ME, Pandiella SS, Cantero D, Webb C. Cereal-based fermented foods and beverages. Food Res Int 2003; 36: 527–43.
31. Hotz C, Gibson RS. Traditional food-processing and preparation practices to enhance the bioavailability of micronutrients in plant-based diets. The J Nutr 2007; 137: 1097–100.
32. O'sullivan L, Murphy B, Mcloughlin P, Duggan P, Lawlor PG, Hughes H, et al. Prebiotics from marine macroalgae for human and animal health applications. Mar Drugs 2010; 8: 2038–64.
33. Toma MM, Pokrotnieks J. Probiotics as functional food: microbiological and medical aspects. Acta Univ Latv Biol 2006; 710: 117–29.
34. Divya JB, Varsha KK, Nampoothiri MK, Ismail B, Pandey A. Probiotic fermented foods for health benefits. Eng Life Sci 2012; 12: 377–90.
35. De Almad C, De Almada C, Martinez R, Sant'ana A. Characterization of the intestinal microbiota and its interaction with probiotics and health impacts. Appl Microbial Technol 2015; 99: 4175–99.
36. Salminen S, Von Wright A, Morelli L, Marteau P, Brassart D, De Vos WM, et al. Demonstration of safety of probiotics – a review. Int J Food Microbiol 1998; 44: 93–106.
37. Parvez S, Malik KA, Kang SA, Kim H-Y. Probiotics and their fermented food products are beneficial for health. J Appl Microbiol 2006; 100: 1171–85.
38. Grosu-Tudor SS, Zamfir M. Probiotic potential of some lactic acid bacteria isolated from Romanian fermented vegetables. Ann RSCB 2012; 17: 234–9.
39. Prado FC, Parada JL, Pandey A, Soccol CR. Trends in non-dairy probiotic beverages. Food Res Int 2008; 41: 111–23.
40. Masood MI, Qadir MI, Shirazi JH, Khan IU. Beneficial effects of lactic acid bacteria on human beings. Crit Rev Microbiol 2011; 37: 91–8.
41. Kiani L. Bugs in our guts – not all bacteria are bad: how probiotics keep us healthy. Ulster, UK: CSA Discovery Guides; 2006, pp. 1–21.
42. Shinde PB. Probiotic: an overview for selection and evaluation. Int J Pharm and Pharm Sci 2012; 4: 14–21.
43. Bonifait L, Chandad F, Grenier D. Probiotics for oral health: myth or reality. JCDA 2009; 75: 585–90.
44. Kore KB, Pattanaik AK, Sharma AK, Marajkar PP. Effect of feeding traditionally prepared fermented milk *dahi* (curd) as probiotics on nutritional status, hindgut health and haematology in dogs. Indian J Trad Knowl 2012; 11: 35–9.
45. Gibson GR, Roberfroid MB. Dietary modulation of the human colonic microbiota: introducing the concept of prebiotics. J Nutr 1995; 125: 1401–12.
46. Dash SK. Selection criteria for probiotics. XXXVII Dairy Conference, Kala Academy, Panjim, Goa, 7–9 February 2009.
47. Higgins JP, Higgins SE, Vincente JL, Wolfenden AD, Tellez G, Hargis BM. Temporal effects of lactic acid bacteria probiotic culture on *Salmonella* in neonatal broilers. Poultry Sci 2007; 86: 1662–6.
48. Lara-Flores M, Olvera-Novoa MA. The use of lactic acid bacteria isolated from intestinal tract of Nile tilapia (*Oreochromis niloticus*), as growth promoters in fish fed low protein diets. Lat Am J Res 2013; 41: 490–7.
49. Grover HS, Luthra S. Probiotics- the nana soldiers of oral health. J Indian Acad Clin Med 2011; 13: 48–54.

50. Mensah P. Fermentation – the key to food safety assurance in Africa. Food Contr 1997; 5/6: 271–8.
51. Mattila-Sandholm T, Myllarinen P, Crittenden R, Mogensen G, Fonden R, Saarela M. Technological challenges for future probiotic foods. Int Dairy J 2002; 12: 173–82.
52. Mercenier A, Pavan S, Pot B. Probiotics as biotherapeutic agents: present knowledge and future prospects. Current Pharm Design 2002; 8: 99–110.
53. Selhub EM, Logan AC, Bested AC. Fermented foods, microbiota, and mental health: ancient practice meets nutritional psychiatry. J Physiol Anthropol 2014; 33: 3.
54. Galgano F, Caruso M, Condelli N, Favati F. Focused review: agmatine in fermented foods. Front Microbiol 2012; 3: 199.
55. Taksande B, Faldu D, Dixit M, Sakaria J, Aglawe M, Umekar M. Agmatine attenuates chronic unpredictable mild stress induced behavioral alteration in mice. Eur J Pharmacol 2013; 720: 115–20.
56. Meurman JH. Probiotics: do they have a role in oral medicine and dentistry? Eur J Oral Sci 2005; 113: 188–96.
57. Jain P, Sharma P. Probiotics and their efficacy in improving oral health: a review. J Appl Pharm Sci 2012; 2: 151–63.
58. Singh A. Oral probiotics: the beneficial microbes for dental & periodontal health. Int J Med Sci 2012; 3: 26–30.
59. Tellez G, Rodriguez-Fragoso L, Kuttapura G, Velasco X, Menconi A, Latorre J, et al. Probiotics for human and poultry use in the control of gastrointestinal disease: a review of real-world experiences. Alternative Integr Med 2013; 2: 1–6.
60. Barman I, Talukdar A. Probiotics: "a new horizon in oral health promotion". Int J Adv Res 2015; 3: 682–8.
61. Loesche WJ. Microbiology of dental decay and periodontal disease. In: Baron S, ed. Medical microbiology 4. Galveston, TX: University of Texas Medical Branch at Galveston; 1996, pp. 1–30.
62. Featherstone JBD. Prevention and reversal of dental caries: role of low level fluoride. Community Dent Oral Epidemiol 1999; 27: 31–40.
63. Nase L, Savilahti E, Saxelin M, Ponka T, Poussa T, Korpela R, Meurman JH. Probiotic bacterium, Lactobacillus rhamnosus GG, in milk on dental caries and caries risk in children. Caries Res 2001; 35: 412–20.
64. Barlow J. The use of probiotics for oral health. In: Barlow J, ed. The clinical use of probiotics. United Kingdom: Probiotics International Ltd; 2010, pp. 36–39.
65. Twetman S. Are we ready for caries prevention through bacteriotherapy? Braz Oral Res 2012; 26: 4–70.
66. Chen F, Wang D. Novel technologies for the prevention and treatment of dental caries: a patent survey. Expert Opin Ther Pat 2010; 20: 681–94.
67. Naidu AS, Bidlack WR, Clemens RA. Probiotic spectra of lactic acid bacteria (LAB). Crit Rev Food Sci Nutr 1999; 39: 13–126.
68. Bushan J, Chachra S. Probiotics – their role in prevention of dental caries. J Oral Heal Comm Dent 2010; 4: 78–82.
69. Alokail MS, Sabico S, Al-Saleh Y, Al-Daghri NM, Alkharfy KM, Vanhoutte PM, et al. Effects of probiotics in patients with diabetes mellitus type 2: study protocol for randomized, double-blind, placebo-controlled trial. Trials 2013; 14: 1–8.
70. Honda K, Moto M, Uchida N, He F, Hashizume N. Anti-diabetic effects of lactic acid bacteria in normal and type 2 diabetic mice. J Clin Bioch and Nutr 2012; 51: 96–101.
71. Naydenov K, Anastasov A, Avramova M, Mindov I, Tacheva T, Tolekova A, et al. Probiotics and diabetes. Trakia J Sci 2012; 10: 300–6.
72. Babashahi M, Mirlohi M, Ghiasvand R, Azadbakht L. Comparison of soymilk and probiotic soymilk effects on serum high-density lipoprotein cholesterol and low-density lipoprotein cholesterol in diabetic Wistar rats. ARYA Atheroscler 2014; 11: 1–6.
73. Ma H. Concept and protocol to isolate cholesterol-reducing bacteria from carnivores. Nat Sci 2004; 2: 11–17.
74. De Roos NM, Katan MB. Effects of probiotic bacteria on diarrhea, lipid metabolism, and carcinogenesis: a review of papers between 1988 and 1998. Am J Clin Nutr 2000; 71: 405–11.
75. Ooi L-K, Liong M-T. Cholesterol effects of probiotics and prebiotics: a review of *in vivo* and *in vitro* findings. Int J Mol Sci 2010; 11(6): 2499–522.
76. Martensson O, Maite-Duenas C, Irastorza A, Holst O, Rudling M, Norin E, et al. Effects of fermented, ropy, non-dairy, oat-based products of serum lipids and faecal excretion of cholesterol and short chain fatty acids in germfree and conventional rats. Nutr Res 2002; 22: 1461–73.
77. Kumar M, Nagpal R, Kumar R, Hemalatha R, Verma V, Kumar A, et al. Cholesterol-lowering probiotics as potential biotherapeutics for metabolic diseases. Exp Diabetes Res 2012; 2012: 902917.
78. Lee J, Heo G, Lee JW, Oh Y, Par JA, Park Y, et al. Analysis of kimchi microflora using denaturing gradient gel electrophoresis. Int J Food Microbiol 2005; 102: 143–50.
79. Lee J-H. Comparative and functional genomic analysis of Bifidobacterium longum. Minneapolis, Minnesota, USA: PhD, University of Minnesota, 2007.
80. Anandharaj M, Sivasankari B. Isolation of potential probiotic Lactobacillus oris HMI68 from mother's milk with cholesterol-reducing property. J Biosci Bioeng 2014; 118: 153–9.
81. Gao D, Zhu G, Gao Z, Liu Z, Wang L, Guo W. Antioxidative and hypolipidemic effects of lactic acid bacteria from pickled Chines cabbage. J Med Plants Res 2011; 5: 1439–46.
82. Anandharaj M, Sivasankar IB, Santhanakaruppu R, Manimaran M, Rani R, Sivakumar S. Determining the probiotic potential of cholesterol-reducing *Lactobacillus* and *Weissella* strains isolated from gherkins (fermented cucumber) and south Indian fermented koozh. Res Microbiol 2015; 166(5): 428–39.
83. Al-Ajeeli F, Flayyih M, Lkhazrajy L. Study the effect of probiotic consumption on the Iraqi human body weight and lipid profile. EurJ Biol Med Sci Res 2015; 3: 52–61.
84. Holzapfel WH, Geinsen R, Schillinger U. Biological preservation of foods with reference to protective cultures, bacteriocins and food-grade enzymes. Int J Food Microbiol 1995; 24: 343–62.
85. Zacharof MP, Lovitt RW. Bacteriocins produced by lactic acid bacteria: a review article. APCBEE Procedia 2012; 2: 50–6.
86. Abee T, Krockel L, Hill C. Bacteriocins: modes of action and potentials in food preservation and control of food poisoning. Int J Food Microbiol 1995; 28: 169–85.
87. Parada JL, Caron CR, Medeiros ABP, Soccol CR. Bacteriocins from lactic acid bacteria: purification, properties and use as biopreservatives. Braz Arch Biol Tech 2007; 50: 521–42.
88. Cintas LM, Casaus MP, Herranz C, Nes IF, Hernandez PE. Review: bacteriocins of lactic acid bacteria. Food Sci Tech Int 2001; 7: 281–305.
89. Galvez A, Abriouel H, Lopez RL, Omar NB. Bacteriocin-based strategies for food biopreservation. Int J Food Microbiol 2007; 120: 51–70.
90. Aljewicz M, Cichosz G. Protective effects of Lactobacillus cultures in Dutch-type cheese-like products. LWT – Food Sci Tech 2015; 63: 52–6.
91. Schnurer J, Magnusson J. Antifungal lactic acid bacteria as biopreservatives. Trends Food Sci Tech 2005; 16: 70–8.
92. Rattanachaikunsopon P, Phumkhachorn P. Lactic acid bacteria: their antimicrobial compounds and their uses in food production. Ann Biol Res 2010; 1: 218–28.

93. Pouwels PH, Leer RJ, Shaw M, Den Bak-Glashouwer M-JH, Tielen FD, Smit E, et al. Lactic acid bacteria as antigen delivery vehicles for oral immunization purposes. Int J Food Microbiol 1998; 41: 155–67.
94. Medina E, Guzman CA. Use of live bacterial vaccine vectors for antigen delivery: potential and limitations. Vaccine 2001; 19: 1573–80.
95. Dicks LMT, Heunis TDJ, Van Staden DA, Brand A, Sutyak Noll K, Chikindas ML. Medical and personal care applications of bacteriocins produced by lactic acid bacteria. In: Drider D, Rebuffat S, eds. Prokaryotic antimicrobial peptides: from genes to applications. Springer Science + Business Media, LLC; 2011, pp. 391–421.
96. Pooja C, Naveen M, Rathore MS, Anurekha J, Kumar JA. Probiotic assisted colon targeted drug delivery system: research scope. Asian J Pharm Clin Res 2011; 4: 12–15.
97. Saraswathi B, Balaji A, Umashankar MS. Polymers in mucoadhesive drug delivery system-latest updates. Int J Pharm Pharmaceut Sci 2013; 5: 423–30.
98. Kim H-J, Kim Y-J, Lee S-H, Kang M-J, Yu H-S, Jung Y-H, et al. Effect of Lactobacillus rhamnosus on asthma with an adoptive transfer of dendritic cells in mice. J Appl Microbiol 2013; 115: 872–9.
99. Mielcarek N, Alonso S, Locht C. Nasal vaccination using live bacterial vectors. Adv Drug Deliv Rev 2001; 51: 55–69.
100. García-Fruitós E. Lactic acid bacteria: a promising alternative for recombinant protein production. Microbial Cell Factories 2012; 11: 157.
101. Yadav NR, Bhitre MJ, Ansari IK. Probiotic delivery systems: applications, challenges and prospective. Int Res J Pharm 2013; 4: 1–9.
102. Jafari B, Rezaie A, Alizadeh S. Isolation and identification of potentially probiotic bacteria from traditional dairy products of Ardabil region in Iran. Ann Biol Res 2011; 2: 311–17.
103. Mahasneh AM, Abbas MM. Probiotics and traditional fermented foods: the eternal connection. Jordan J Biol Sci 2010; 3: 133–40.
104. Heller KJ. Probiotic bacteria in fermented foods: product characteristics and starter organisms. Am J Clin Nutr 2001; 73: 374S–9S.
105. Heenan CN, Adams MC, Hosken RW. Growth medium for culturing probiotic bacteria for applications in vegetarian food products. LWT-Food Sci Technol 2002; 35: 171–6.
106. Heenan CN, Adams MC, Hosken RW, Fleet GH. Survival and sensory acceptability of probiotic microorganisms in a nonfermented frozen vegetation dessert. LWT-Food Sci Technol 2004; 37: 461–6.
107. Rivera-Espinoza Y, Gallardo-Navorro Y. Non-dairy probiotic products. Food Microbiol 2010; 27: 1–11.
108. Boke H, Aslim B, Alp G. The role of resistance to bile salts and acid tolerance of exopolysaccharides (EPSS) produced by yogurt starter bacteria. Arch Biol Sci, Belgrade 2010; 62: 323–8.
109. Lourens-Hattingh A, Viljoen BC. Yogurt as probiotic carrier food. Int Dairy J 2001; 11: 1–17.
110. Bandiera NS, Carneiro I, Da Silva AS, Honjoya ER, Helena E. Viability of probiotic Lactobacillus casei in yoghurt: defining the best processing step to its addition. Arch Lat de Nutr 2013; 63: 58–63.
111. Collins J, Thornton G, Sullivan G. Selection of probiotic strains for human applications. Int Dairy J 1998; 8: 487–90.
112. Dunne C, O'mahony L, Murphy L, Thornton G, Morrissey D, O'halloran S, et al. In vitro selection criteria for probiotic bacteria of human origin: correlation with in vivo findings. Am J Clin Nutr 2001; 73: 386S–92S.
113. Ammor M, Mayo B. Selection criteria for lactic acid bacteria to be used as functional starter cultures in dry sausage production: an update. Meat Sci 2007; 76(1): 138–46.
114. Mourad K, Nour-Eddine K. *In vitro* preselection criteria for probiotic lactobacillus plantarum strains of fermented olives origin. Int J Probiotics Prebiotics 2006; 1: 27–32.
115. Grover S, Rashmi HM, Srivastava AK, Batish VK. Probiotics for human health -new innovations and emerging trends. Gut Pathogens 2012; 4: 1–14.
116. Tomasik PJ, Tomasik P. Probiotics and prebiotics. Cereal Chem J 2003; 80: 113.
117. Kostinek M, Specht I, Edward V, Schillinger U, Hertel C, Holzapfel W, et al. Diversity and technological properties of predominant lactic acid bacteria from fermented cassava used for the preparation of Gari, a traditional African food. Syst Appl Micr 2005; 28: 527–40.
118. Bacha K, Mehari T, Ashenafi M. Microbiology of the fermentation of *shamita*, a traditional Ethiopian fermented beverage. Ethiopian J Sci 1999; 22: 113–26.
119. Osvik R, Sperstad S, Breines E, Hareide E, Godfroid J, Zhou Z, et al. Bacterial diversity of *amasi*, a South African fermented milk product, determined by clone library and denaturing gradient gel electrophoresis analysis. Afr J Microbiol Res 2013; 7: 146–4158.
120. Nyambane B, Thari W, Wangoh J, Njage P. Lactic acid bacteria and yeasts involved in the fermentation of amabere amaruranu, a Kenyan fermented milk. Food Sci Nutr 2014; 2: 692–9.
121. Muyanja CMBK, Narvhus JA, Treimo J, Langsrud T. Isolation, characterisation and identification of lactic acid bacteria from *bushera*: a Ugandan traditional fermented beverage. Int J Food Microbiol 2003; 80: 201–10.
122. Katongole JN. The microbial succession in indigenous fermented maize products. Bloemfontein, South Africa: Masters of Science in Agriculture, University of Free State, 2008.
123. Bhardwaj P, Krishnappa S. Various approaches for prevention of dental caries with emphasis on probiotics: a review. IOSR J Dent Med Sci 2014; 13: 62–7.
124. Delzenne NM, Neyrinck AM, Backhed F, Cani PD. Targeting gut microbiota in obesity: effects of prebiotics and probiotics. Nat Rev Endcrinol 2011; 7: 639–46.

*Mduduzi Paul Mokoena
Discipline of Microbiology
School of Life Sciences
College of Agriculture, Engineering and Science
University of KwaZulu-Natal (Westville Campus)
Private Bag X54001, Durban 4000
South Africa
Email: mokoenap@ukzn.ac.za

10

Effects of spinach nitrate on insulin resistance, endothelial dysfunction markers and inflammation in mice with high-fat and high-fructose consumption

Ting Li[1,2], Xinshan Lu[1], Yanfei Sun[1] and Xingbin Yang[1]*

[1]Shaanxi Engineering Laboratory for Food Green Processing and Safety Control, College of Food Engineering and Nutritional Science, Shaanxi Normal University, Xi'an, China; [2]Centre for Cancer and Inflammation Research, School of Chinese Medicine, Hong Kong Baptist University, Hong Kong, China

Abstract

Background: Insulin resistance, which is associated with an increased risk of cardiovascular morbidity and mortality, has become a leading nutrition problem. Inorganic nitrate enriched in spinach has been demonstrated to reverse the pathological features of insulin resistance and endothelial dysfunction. However, the effects of a direct intake of nitrate-enriched spinach on insulin resistance and endothelial dysfunction have not been studied.
Objective: To investigate the effects of spinach nitrate on insulin resistance, lipid metabolism, endothelial function, and inflammation in mice fed with a high-fat and high-fructose diet.
Design: A diet intervention of spinach with or without nitrate was performed in mice. A high-fat and high-fructose diet was used to cause insulin resistance, endothelial dysfunction, and inflammation in mice. The impacts of spinach nitrate on lipid profile, insulin resistance, markers of endothelial function, and inflammation were determined in mice.
Results: Spinach nitrate improved the vascular endothelial function of the mice with high-fat and high-fructose consumption, as evidenced by the elevated plasma nitrite level, increased serum nitric oxide (NO) level and decreased serum ET-1 level after spinach nitrate intervention. Spinach nitrate also reduced serum triglycerides, total cholesterol, and low-density lipoprotein-cholesterol levels and elevated serum high-density lipoprotein-cholesterol levels in the mice fed with a high-fat and high-fructose diet. Mice receiving spinach with 60 mg/kg of nitrate (1.02 ± 0.34) showed a significantly low homeostasis model assessment-insulin resistance index as compared with the model mice (2.05 ± 0.58), which is indicating that spinach nitrate could effectively improve the insulin resistance. In addition, spinach nitrate remarkably decreased the elevated serum C-reactive protein, tumor necrosis factor α, and interleukin-6 levels induced by a high-fat and high-fructose diet.
Conclusions: The intake of spinach nitrate can augment NO status, improve lipid homeostasis, relieve inflammation, and enhance endothelial function, suggesting that spinach is promising dietary supplements for insulin resistance prevention.

Keywords: *spinach*; *nitrate*; *dyslipidemia*; *endothelial function*; *inflammation*; *NO*

Responsible Editor: Per Ole Iversen, University of Oslo, Norway.

Insulin resistance is one of the powerful risk factors for the development of cardiovascular disease (CVD) and type 2 diabetes (1). The prevalence of insulin resistance is increasing, especially in developing countries and in younger populations, with approximately 20 to 40% of prevalence in different populations (2, 3). Increasing evidences support that the presence of insulin resistance, characterized as impaired insulin-stimulated glucose and/or lipid metabolism, represents early events in individuals at high risk for developing CVD (4). Insulin resistance was shown to be associated with increased production of pro-inflammatory cytokines, which are predictors of cardiovascular events (5). Insulin resistance is also linked to endothelial dysfunction in that hyperinsulinemia causes the release of the potent vasoconstrictor endothelin (6). Previous studies have demonstrated that pro-oxidative and pro-inflammatory processes play a pivotal role in endothelial dysfunction (4, 7).

Vascular damage resulting from lipid deposition and oxidative stress to the vessel wall triggers an inflammatory reaction, which can worsen the insulin resistance and endothelial dysfunction (4).

Diet exerts important long-term effects on body functions and also plays a vital role in body health and disease development. Indeed, compelling epidemiological evidence suggests that increasing consumption of vegetables reduces the risk of CVD, and the potential cardiovascular benefits of vegetables may be attributed to the high content of inorganic nitrate (8, 9). Several clinical and experimental studies have reported that oral consumption of inorganic nitrate can reduce blood pressure, protect against ischemia–reperfusion injury, prevent endothelial dysfunction, and reverse pathological features of metabolic syndrome including visceral fat accumulation and elevated triglyceride levels, thereby preventing the occurrence and development of CVD (10–13). In addition, dietary nitrate is thought to enhance the production of bioactive nitric oxide (NO) in the body, which is a critical regulator of vascular homeostasis (9). Green leafy vegetables, such as spinach, are among the richest sources of nitrate in the diet and account for approximately 80–85% of the average daily dietary nitrate exposure (14, 15). Although there are some investigations about the protective effects of dietary intake of inorganic nitrate on insulin response and endothelial function, few studies report the influences of a direct intake of nitrate-enriched vegetables on insulin resistance in mice. Therefore, the present study for the first time established a diet intervention method using spinach with or without nitrate to evaluate the impacts of different contents of spinach nitrate on insulin resistance, endothelial dysfunction, and inflammation in mice. More specifically, the effects of spinach nitrate on the lipid metabolism, lipid peroxidation, insulin resistance, endothelial dysfunction markers, and inflammation were evaluated *in vivo*.

Materials and methods

Materials and chemicals

The fresh spinach, which was harvested from the greenhouse in winter, was purchased from a local vegetable market of the Xi'an region of Shaanxi Province, China. Pentafluorobenzyl bromide (PFB-Br) and tetraoctylammonium bromide (TOA-Br) were purchased from Sigma (Sigma–Aldrich GmbH, Sternheim, Germany). Sodium nitrate and sodium nitrite were bought from Cambridge Isotope (Andover, MA, USA). Assay kits of serum total-cholesterol (TC), triglycerides (TG), high-density lipoprotein-cholesterol (HDL-C), low-density lipoprotein-cholesterol (LDL-C), and glucose were the products of Huili of Biotechnology (Changchun, China). The commercially diagnostic kit of NO and nitric oxide synthase (NOS) were obtained from the Jiancheng Institute of Biotechnology (Nanjing, China). The ELISA kits of insulin, F_2-isoprostanes, interleukin 6 (IL-6), tumor necrosis factor α (TNF-α), C-reactive protein (CRP), and endothelin 1 (ET-1) were obtained from the Lantu Biotech Co. Ltd (Fujian, China). Deionized water was prepared using a Millipore Milli Q-Plus system (Millipore, Bedford, MA). HPLC grade acetonitrile and methanol were purchased from Honeywell (Morristown, NJ, USA). Other chemicals used in the study were of analytic grade and commercially available.

Sample preparation

To remove the nitrate from spinach, clean fresh spinach was boiled thrice with warm water at 70°C (40 min each time), filtered, and freeze-dried with a lyophilizer. The residue was freeze-dried using a lyophilizer to make the nitrate-removed spinach. To obtain the intact spinach rich in nitrate, clean fresh spinach was directly homogenized and freeze-dried. Finally, the samples were shattered by a disintegrator and saved as a standby (Voucher specimens of the plant materials were deposited at College of Food Engineering and Nutritional Science, Shaanxi Normal University, China).

Derivatization of NO_2^- and NO_3^-

Aqueous standard solutions ($NaNO_2$ and $NaNO_3$) or spinach samples (300 μL) were treated with 500 μL of 8.0 mM TOA-Br in acetone and 50 μL of 20% PFB-Br in acetone at 50°C for 30 min (16). Samples were evaporated under N_2 to remove acetone. The reaction products were extracted from the remaining aqueous phase with toluene (1.0 mL) and then centrifuged at 3,000*g* for 10 min at 4°C. A volume of 200 μL of supernatant was extracted with 1 mL acetonitrile again after removing the toluene. Finally, the organic phase was collected for HPLC analysis (16).

HPLC quantification of NO_2^- and NO_3^-

The HPLC analysis of nitrite and nitrate was performed on a Shimadzu LC-2010A HPLC system. The analytical column used was a RP-C_{18} column (4.6 mm i.d. × 250 mm, 5 μm, Venusil, Wilmington, DE, USA), and the separation was performed at 30°C. A gradient elution was performed by varying the proportion of solvent A (acetonitrile) to solvent B (water). The gradient program was as follows: 0–10 min from 75 to 60% B, 10–30 min from 60 to 40% B, and 30–40 min from 40 to 10% B. Elution was carried out at a flow rate of 1.0 mL/min, and the wavelength for UV detection was 218 nm. The injection volume was 20 μL.

Animal experiment

In total, 40 healthy male Swiss-Kunming mice (weighing 22 ± 2 g) were purchased from the Experimental Animal Center of the Fourth Military Medical University (Xi'an, China). The mice were housed in cages in a standardization animal laboratory, which was maintained at a temperature of 22–24°C and a humidity of 50–55% under a 12:12 light–dark cycle, with free access to water and rodent chow (40% corn flour, 26% wheat flour, 10% bran, 10% fish meal, 10% bean cake, 2% mineral, 1% coarse, and 1% vitamin complex; Qianmin Feed Factory, Xi'an, China). The experimental animal procedures were in accordance with the Regulations of Experimental Animal Administration of the Fourth Military Medical University Committee on Animal Care and Use (approval number XJYYLL-2015689).

After a 1-week acclimation period, mice were given high-fructose (20% fructose-deionized water) and a high-fat diet (93.8% rodent chow, 1% cholesterol, 5% lard, and 0.2% bile salt complex; Qianmin Feed Factory). Simultaneously, mice were randomly divided into four groups to receive different concentrations of nitrate with eight mice in each group: model group (0 mg/kg NO_3^-, 0.5 mL of solution consisting of 100% nitrate-removal spinach), low-dose group (15 mg/kg NO_3^-, 0.5 mL of solution containing 75% nitrate-removed spinach and 25% intact spinach rich in nitrate), medium-dose group (30 mg/kg NO_3^-, 0.5 mL of solution containing 50% nitrate-removed spinach and 50% intact spinach rich in nitrate), and high-dose group (60 mg/kg NO_3^-, 0.5 mL of solution consisting of 100% intact spinach rich in nitrate). Mice which were given a normal diet and 0 mg/kg NO_3^- were used as the normal group. The powder of spinach dissolved in 5% carboxymethylcellulose sodium (CMC-Na, 0.4 mL, m/v) was administered by oral gavage once daily (9:00 a.m.) for 28 consecutive days. At the end of the experiment, all the animals were euthanized and sacrificed to obtain the blood and livers. The blood was collected by cardiac puncture.

Ozone-based chemiluminescence assay of NO_2^-

The plasma nitrite was detected by gas-phase chemiluminescence assay using our previously described method (16, 17). Blood was collected into chilled tubes containing 50 μL of the mixed NEM/EDTA (10/2.0 mM) and immediately mixed and centrifuged at 3,000*g* for 5 min at 4°C. Fresh plasma was kept on ice in the dark and was analyzed within an hour. The tri-iodide solution (2 mL) and glacial acetic acid (6 mL) were delivered into a glass purge vessel with a rubber septum-covered injection inlet and connected to a gas ice-trap cooler with 15 mL of 0.5 M NaOH solution in the outlet. The resulting I_3^- solution reduces NO_2^- to NO gas, which can be detected by a sensitive ozone-based chemiluminescence analyzer (CLD66, Eco Physics, Duernten, Switzerland). The tri-iodide solution was prepared by dissolving 1.0 g KI and 0.4 g I_2 in 20 mL H_2O. A volume of 300 μL of the tested samples or nitrate standard solutions was quickly injected into the purge vessel under NO-free N_2 atmosphere. Fresh plasma was spiked with 10% antifoam before injection. The concentration of nitrite was quantified by the NO signal peak area. All containers were adequately washed with Milli-Q water to remove NO_2^- contamination.

Determination of blood biochemical indexes

The serum levels of TC, TG, HDL-C, LDL-C, GLU, NO, and NOS were assessed with commercially available diagnostic kits, and the results were expressed in mmol/L (for TC, TG, HDL-C, LDL-C, and NO), μmol/L (for GLU), and U/mL (for NOS). The serum concentrations of insulin, F_2-isoprostanes, IL-6, CRP, TNF-α, and ET-1 were measured using the ELISA kits, and the results were expressed in μU/mL (for insulin), pg/mL (for F_2-isoprostanes and IL-6), ng/mL (for CRP), and ng/L (for TNF-α and ET-1). The atherogenic index (AI) was calculated by the following formula (18):

$$AI = (TC - HDL\text{-}C)/HDL\text{-}C$$

The homeostasis model assessment-insulin resistance (HOMA-IR) index was computed from the glucose (mmol/L) and insulin (μU/mL) levels:

$$HOMA\text{-}IR = glucose(mmol/L) \times insulin(\mu U/mL)/22.5$$

Histopathological examination

Histology of liver was studied using hematoxylin and eosin (H&E) and Oil Red O staining (19, 20). The fresh liver samples were rapidly dissected, and the liver tissue sections (5 mm) were fixed by immersing in a 10% neutral formalin solution at room temperature for 24 h. The fixed tissues were embedded in paraffin, and sectioned (5–6 μm thick) and stained with H&E. For Oil Red O staining, the frozen liver samples were processed using a cryostat and then fixed and stained. The histopathological changes in the sections were observed by a light photomicroscope.

Statistical analysis

All experiments were performed at least in triplicate, and the results were expressed as mean ± SD (standard deviation). Data obtained were analyzed using one-way analysis of variance (ANOVA) and Duncan's multiple range tests. The difference is considered statistically significant if $p < 0.05$ (SPSS, version 16.0).

Results

The nitrate and nitrite content in spinach

The analytical results of the nitrate and nitrite content in spinach after different processing were showed in Table 1. In fresh spinach, the nitrate content (1,913.1 ± 182.4 mg/kg) was 10,000 times higher than the nitrite content (189.3 ± 72.1 μg/kg). After boiling in water for three times, the contents of nitrate and nitrite in spinach were sharply dropped to 3.1 ± 0.6 mg/kg and 69.4 ± 17.3 μg/kg, respectively. The significant decrease in nitrate levels

Table 1. The content of NO_3^- and NO_2^- in spinach with different processing

Spinach	Fresh[a]	Boiled dried[b]
Nitrate (mg/kg)	1913.1 ± 182.4	3.1 ± 0.6
Nitrite (μg/kg)	189.3 ± 72.1	69.4 ± 17.3

[a]Clean fresh spinach was directly homogenized and freeze-dried; [b]clean fresh spinach was boiled with warm water at 70°C for three times (40 min each time), and then the residue was freeze-dried.

confirmed that the process of boiling with water combined with further filtration could effectively remove excessive amounts of nitrate from spinach.

Effect of spinach nitrate ingestion on plasma nitrite, serum ET-1, NO levels, and NOS activity

Figure 1 shows the plasma nitrite levels in mice receiving the processed spinach with different doses of nitrate measured by gas-phase chemiluminescence assay. The chemiluminescence signal area exhibited a strict linear correlation with the amount of NO_2^- in a certain range (0–20 μmol), with the linear equation of $Y = 18.495X - 0.1628$ ($R^2 = 0.9994$) (Fig. 1a). As shown in Fig. 1b, the plasma nitrite content in mice was elevated by the intake of spinach nitrate in a dose-dependent manner, and the mice receiving spinach containing 60 mg/kg of nitrate showed a significant higher level (2.11 ± 0.47 μmol/L) than the mice treated with nitrate-removed spinach (0.72 ± 0.26 μmol/L, $p < 0.05$). Furthermore, the influences of dietary spinach nitrate on serum ET-1, NO levels, and NOS activity in mice were shown in Fig. 2d, e, and f, respectively. In comparison with the normal mice, a high-fat and high-fructose diet remarkably elevated the serum ET-1 levels and reduced the NO levels and NOS activity in the model mice. However, both the serum NO level and NOS activities were raised by spinach nitrate ingestion in a dose-dependent manner, where the mice given spinach with 30 and 60 mg/kg of nitrate showed significantly higher NO levels and NOS activities than the model mice, respectively ($p < 0.05$ and < 0.01). Moreover, the serum ET-1 level in mice decreased after giving nitrate-rich spinach for 28 days, where it dropped from 5.18 ± 0.88 ng/L for the model group to 4.34 ± 0.86 ng/L($p > 0.05$), 4.01 ± 0.57 ng/L ($p < 0.05$), and 3.50 ± 0.69 ng/L ($p < 0.01$) for the low-, medium-, and high-dose groups, respectively. Notably, no significant differences were observed between the body weight of nitrate-enriched spinach-treated mice and the nitrate-removed model mice (Fig. 3).

Effects of spinach nitrate on the levels of serum TG, TC, LDL-C, HDL-C, and AI

To determine whether spinach nitrate caused changes of serum lipid profile in mice, the serum levels of TG, TC, LDL-C, and HDL-C were assessed. As depicted in Table 2, the mice in model group exhibited significantly high levels of serum TG, TC, and LDL-C ($p < 0.05$, < 0.01, and < 0.01), and low levels of serum HDL-C ($p < 0.01$), in comparison with the normal mice. Spinach nitrate dose-dependently reduced the elevated serum TG, TC, and LDL-C levels of mice with high-fat and high-fructose consumption, and the differences between high-dose group (60 mg/kg) and model group (0 mg/kg) were statistically significant ($p < 0.05$). It was noteworthy that all the spinaches containing 15, 30, and 60 mg/kg of nitrate led to a remarkable increase in the serum HDL-C levels, with values of 0.41 ± 0.05, 0.43 ± 0.09, and 0.47 ± 0.07

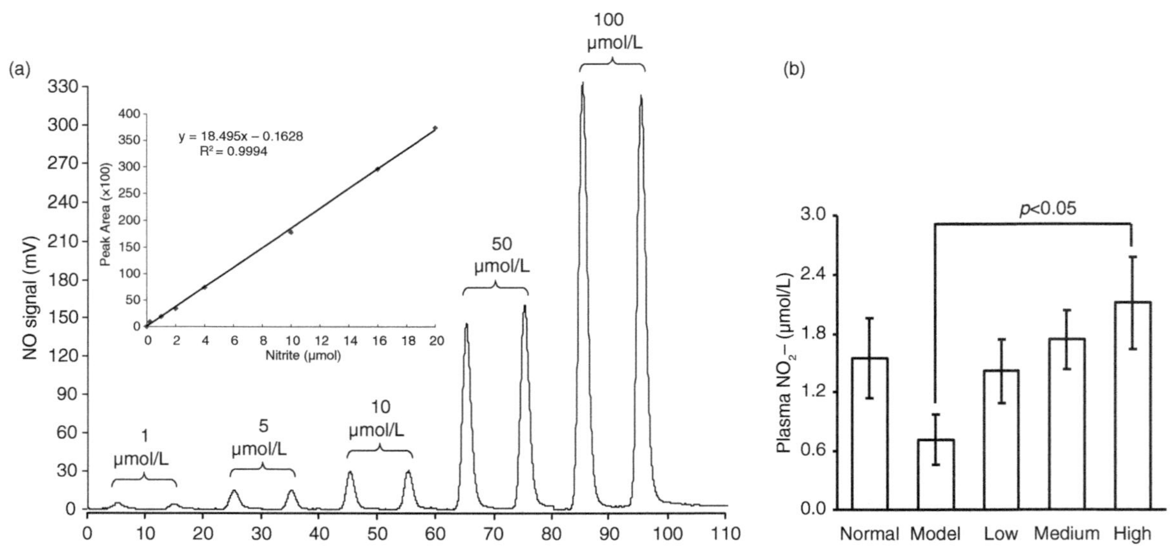

Fig. 1. The effect of dietary spinach nitrate on the plasma NO_2^- levels. (a) The NO signal intensity of different concentrations of NO_2^- and the corresponding standard curve. (b) The plasma NO_2^- concentration in mice treated with spinach at different dosages of nitrate. Results are expressed as means ± SD of eight mice in each group.

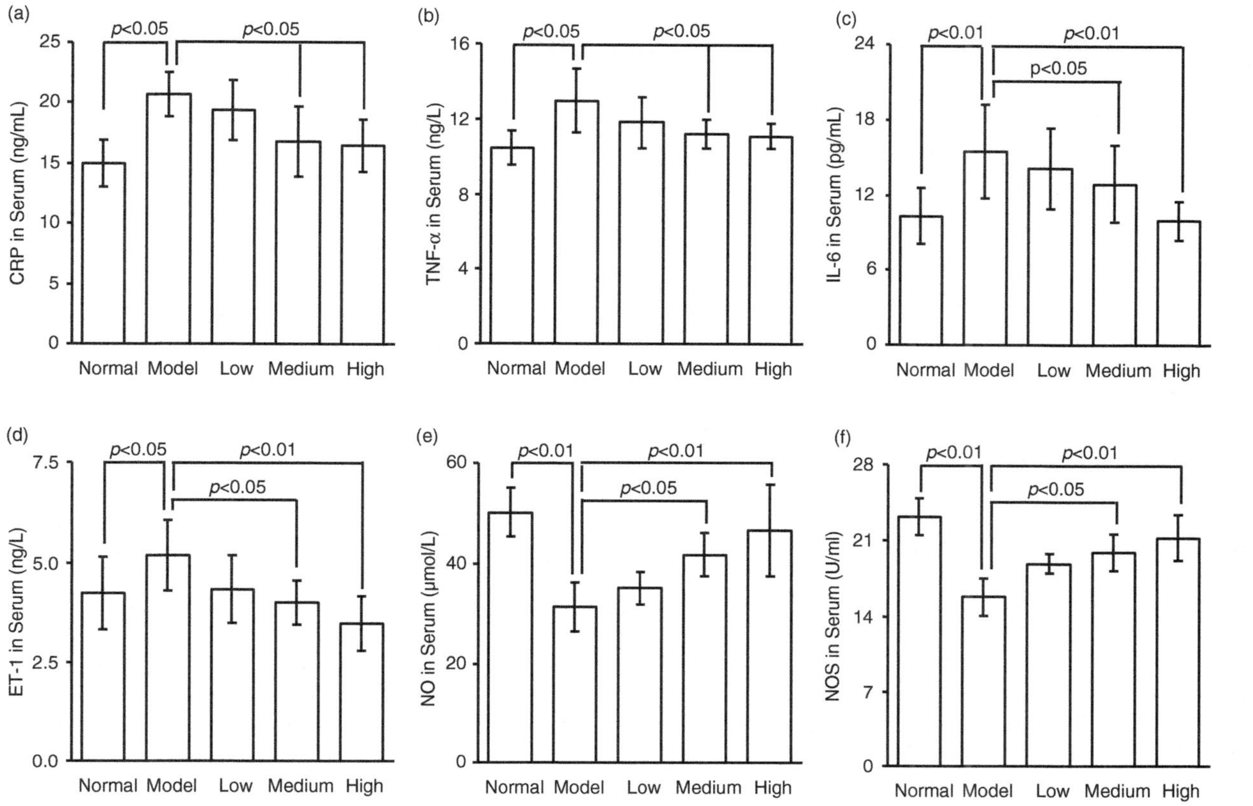

Fig. 2. The effect of dietary spinach nitrate on the serum CRP (a), TNF-α (b), IL-6 (c), ET-1 (d), and NO (e) levels and the NOS activity (f) in mice. Data are means ± SD, $n = 8$.

mmol/L, respectively ($p < 0.05$, < 0.05, and < 0.01), as compared to the model mice (0.30 ± 0.04 mmol/L). Furthermore, AI of high-fat and high-fructose diet-fed mice receiving spinach containing 0, 15, 30, and 60 mg/kg of nitrate was 5.13 ± 1.18, 3.84 ± 0.92, 3.19 ± 1.04, and 2.73 ± 0.76, respectively. The marked drop of AI caused by nitrate-enriched spinach suggested that spinach nitrate had the ability to alleviate hyperlipidemia.

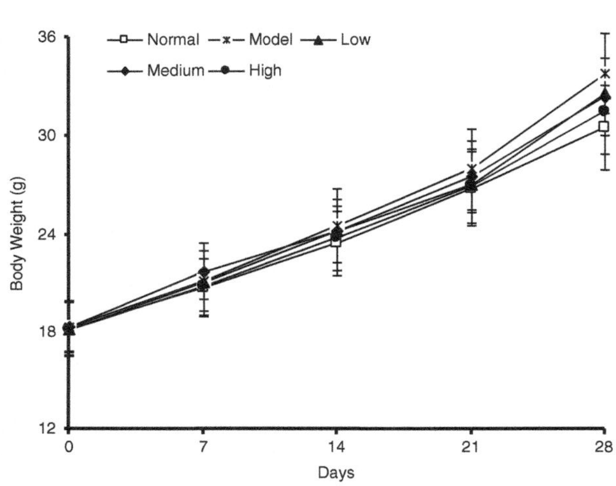

Fig. 3. Effect of spinach nitrate on body weight. Results are expressed as means ± SD of eight mice in each group.

Effects of spinach nitrate on the serum levels of glucose, insulin, and HOMA

The serum glucose and insulin concentrations in mice given spinach with or without nitrate were presented in Table 2. Administration of high-fat and high-fructose diet caused a significant increase in serum glucose levels ($p < 0.01$) and insulin levels ($p < 0.01$), as compared with the normal mice. After spinach nitrate intervention, both the serum glucose and insulin levels of high-fat and high-fructose diet-fed mice decreased. Spinach with 30 and 60 mg/kg of nitrate caused evident fall in the serum glucose levels from 9.12 ± 2.20 mmol/L of the model group to 7.08 ± 1.63 mmol/L ($p < 0.05$) and 6.13 ± 1.86 mmol/L ($p < 0.01$), respectively. Similarly, the insulin level sharply declined to 4.19 ± 0.33 μU/mL ($p < 0.05$) for the mice given spinach containing 30 mg/kg of nitrate, and 3.75 ± 0.17 μU/mL ($p < 0.01$) for the mice given spinach with 60 mg/kg of nitrate, in contrast to the model mice (5.01 ± 0.55 μU/mL). To quantify the insulin sensitivity, HOMA was used. As depicted in Table 2, the HOMA-IR index was tremendously decreased from 2.05 ± 0.58 of the model group (0 mg/kg) to 1.62 ± 0.33, 1.32 ± 0.37, and 1.02 ± 0.34 of the low-dose (15 mg/kg), medium-dose (30 mg/kg), and high-dose (60 mg/kg) groups, respectively ($p < 0.05$, < 0.01, and < 0.01), indicating that spinach nitrate could effectively improve the insulin resistance.

Table 2. The effect of dietary intake of spinach nitrate on serum markers in mice

Group	Normal (0 mg/kg)	Model (0 mg/kg)	Low (15 mg/kg)	Medium (30 mg/kg)	High (60 mg/kg)
Serum TG (mmol/L)	2.17±0.39	2.83±0.46#	2.69±0.42	2.51±0.50	2.23±0.41*
Serum TC (mmol/L)	1.61±0.30	2.13±0.41##	1.96±0.45	1.80±0.38	1.68±0.32**
Serum LDL-C (mmol/L)	0.85±0.10	1.16±0.17##	1.09±0.09	0.98±0.09*	0.90±0.09**
Serum HDL-C (mmol/L)	0.49±0.06	0.30±0.04##	0.41±0.05*	0.43±0.09*	0.47±0.07**
Atherogenic index (AI)	2.48±0.71	5.13±1.18##	3.84±0.92*	3.19±1.04*	2.73±0.76**
F_2-isoprostanes (pg/mL)	14.25±5.91	26.75±7.95##	22.51±8.57	19.64±8.30	16.89±6.76*
Serum GLU (mmol/L)	6.26±1.21	9.12±2.20##	7.97±1.74	7.08±1.63*	6.13±1.86**
Serum INS (μU/mL)	3.27±0.41	5.01±0.55##	4.65±0.46	4.19±0.33*	3.75±0.17**
HOMA-IR	0.91±0.26	2.05±0.58##	1.62±0.33*	1.32±0.37**	1.02±0.34**

Values are expressed as means ± SD of eight mice in each group. #$p < 0.05$ and ##$p < 0.01$, relative to the normal group. *$p < 0.05$ and **$p < 0.01$, relative to the model group.

Effect of spinach nitrate on the serum F_2-isoprostanes levels

To further evaluate the effect of spinach nitrate on the degree of lipid peroxidation, we examined the serum F_2-isoprostanes level, which is considered as the gold standard for quantifying lipid peroxidation/oxidative stress *in vivo* (21). High-fat and high-fructose diet caused a remarkable increase in F_2-isoprostanes levels from 14.25 ± 5.91 pg/mL of normal mice to 26.75 ± 7.95 pg/mL ($p < 0.01$). Our results demonstrated that supplementation with nitrate-rich spinach could effectively lower the serum concentration of F_2-isoprostanes. The serum F_2-isoprostanes level of the model mice was 26.75 ± 7.95 pg/mL, whereas for the mice given spinach containing 15, 30, and 60 mg/kg of nitrate, the levels decreased to 22.51 ± 8.57, 19.64 ± 8.30, and 16.89 ± 6.76 pg/mL ($p < 0.05$), respectively (Table 2), implying a subdued oxidative stress and lipid peroxidation in mice administrated with nitrate-enriched spinach.

Effects of spinach nitrate on the serum CRP, IL-6, and TNF-α levels

Figure 2a–c illustrates the serum CRP, TNF-α, and IL-6 concentrations of mice supplemented with spinach containing different dosages of nitrate, respectively. High-fat and high-fructose diet significantly elevated the serum levels of CRP, IL-6, and TNF-α in mice. However, it was found that spinach nitrate decreased the elevated serum CRP, TNF-α, and IL-6 levels in dose-dependent manners. More specifically, the CRP levels of mice treated with spinach containing 30 and 60 mg/kg of nitrate (16.79 ± 2.94 and 16.50 ± 2.13 pg/mL, $p < 0.05$ and < 0.05, respectively) were significantly lower than that of the model mice (20.68 ± 1.86 pg/mL), but the decrease caused by spinach with 15 mg/kg of nitrate was not distinct ($p > 0.05$). Similar trends were observed in the serum TNF-α and IL-6 levels after spinach nitrate intervention.

Histopathological examination of mouse liver

The histopathological observation of mouse liver was performed to further support the results of the serum biochemical analysis. Representative photomicrographs of liver tissues with Oil Red O and H&E staining are shown in Figs. 4 and 5, respectively. Significant lipid accumulation was observed in the liver tissues of the model mice (Fig. 4a), whereas the hepatic fat deposit induced by the high-fat and high-fructose diet was evidently ameliorated after spinach nitrate intervention (Fig. 4b–d). The spinach with 60 mg/kg of nitrate exhibited a much higher efficacy than spinach containing with 15 and 30 mg/kg of nitrate. The H&E-stained liver specimen showed that the acute administration of the high-fat and high-fructose diet led to severe cellular degeneration, hepatocyte necrosis, and cytoplasmic vacuolation in mice (Fig. 5a). However, the hepatic histopathological changes were apparently improved by the treatment with nitrate-rich spinach, and the mice treated with spinach containing 60 mg/kg of nitrate showed well-preserved cytoplasm, prominent nuclei, and legible nucleoli (Fig. 5b–d). The results of the histopathological examination well supported the consequences of serum biochemical markers and lipid peroxidation.

Discussion

Dietary inorganic nitrate (NO_3^-) and nitrite (NO_2^-) have been considered to be toxic constituents in our diet for half a century because of their proposed association with the development of gastric cancer and other malignancies, and the concentrations of them are strictly limited in food and drinking water (22, 23). However, scientific and medical interest has grown exponentially in the beneficial effects of dietary or inorganic nitrate on cardiovascular health in recent years (24). NO was shown to modulate insulin sensitivity, and a decreased bioavailability of NO contributes to endothelial dysfunction (25). Lundberg et al. reported that dietary inorganic nitrate exerted robust NO-like effects in our human body including lowering blood pressure, inhibiting platelet aggregation, preventing endothelial dysfunction, and protecting vascular function (22). Diet is a major source of nitrate, and the content of naturally occurring nitrate is particularly high in certain

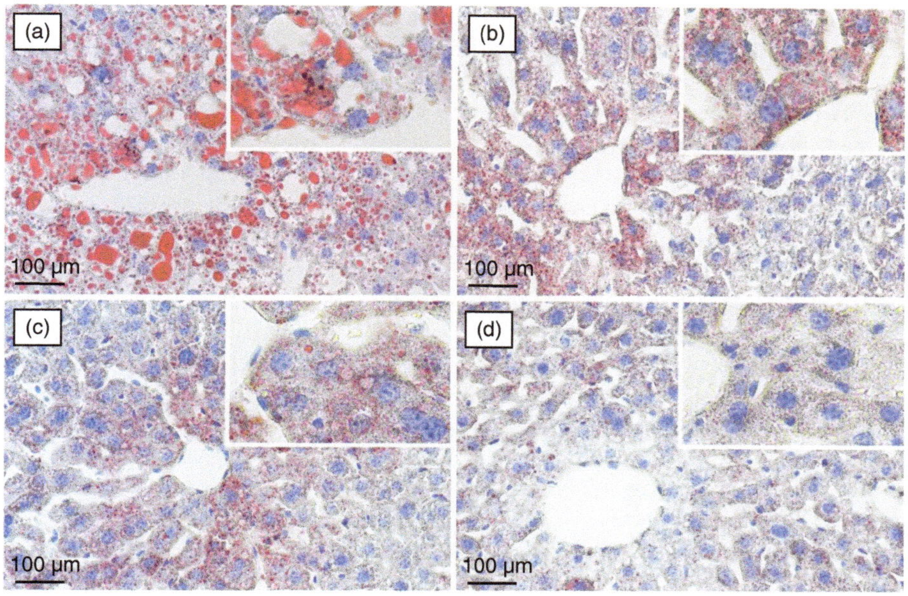

Fig. 4. Lipid staining of the liver sections from high-fat and high-fructose treated mice using Oil Red O staining: (a) model group (0 mg/kg), (b) low-dose group (15 mg/kg), (c) medium-dose group (30 mg/kg), and (d) high-dose group (60 mg/kg).

green leafy vegetables, including spinach, rocket, lettuce, beetroot, and Chinese cabbage (26). Therefore, this study was designed to elucidate the influences of dietary nitrate on insulin resistance, endothelial dysfunction, and inflammation in mice. To achieve this goal, spinach as a source of dietary nitrate was administered to mice for 28 days. As a result, the nitrate-rich spinach positively regulated glucose and lipid metabolism, insulin resistance, inflammation, and endothelial dysfunction markers in mice.

Spinach, a common green leafy vegetable, has been reported to have a high content of nitrate (27). Dietary nitrate is mostly transformed into nitrite by oral symbiotic bacterial nitrate reductases and then converted into NO in the gastrointestinal tract and vascular smooth muscle cells under the action of key enzymes including nitrite reductase, xanthine oxidoreductase, aldehyde oxidase, deoxidized hemoglobin, myoglobin, and cytochrome *c* oxidase, thereby exhibiting regulative effects

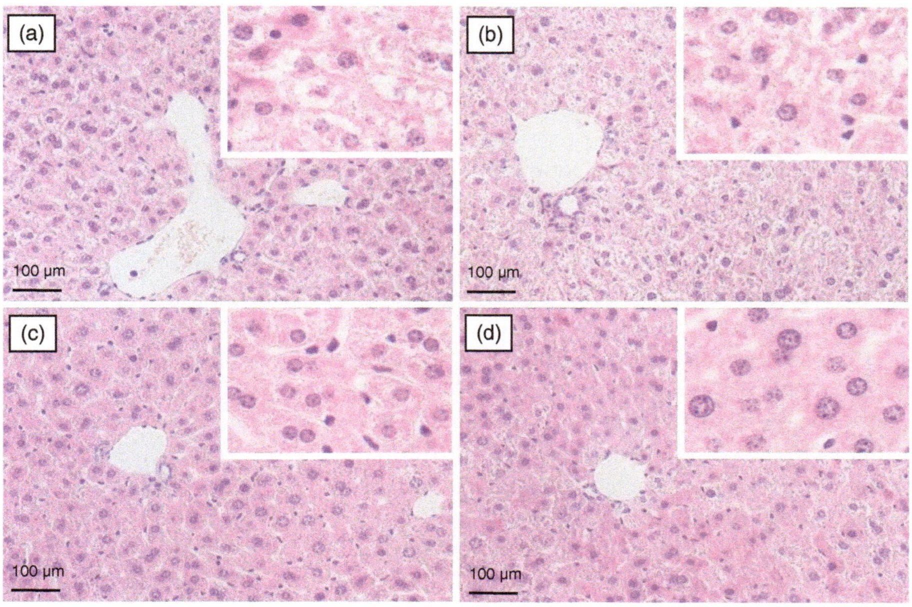

Fig. 5. The effect of spinach nitrate on histopathological changes of liver hepatocytes stained with H&E in high-fat and high-fructose fed mice: (a) model group (0 mg/kg), (b) low-dose group (15 mg/kg), (c) medium-dose group (30 mg/kg), and (d) high-dose group (60 mg/kg).

on endothelial function in the body (28). In this study, to illustrate the metabolism of dietary nitrate *in vivo*, we determined the plasma nitrite content using ozone-based chemiluminescence assay. It was found that the nitrite concentration in plasma was dose-dependently increased by administration of spinach with different doses of nitrate, indicating that the nitrate from spinach was metabolized to nitrite in the body of mice. In addition, no significant differences were found in the body weight between nitrate-rich spinach treated mice and model mice (Fig. 3), suggesting the non-toxic property of spinach nitrate at the dose of 60 mg/kg on mice.

Emerging evidences have showed that a combined use of a high-fat and high-fructose diet may predispose to insulin resistance in animals, such as abdominal fat deposition, glucose tolerance, dyslipidemia, hyperinsulinemia, and hypertension (29–31). In recent years, high-fructose consumption has been confirmed to effectively cause insulin resistance, hypertriglyceridemia, hepatic steatosis, non-alcoholic fatty liver, hypertension, and metabolic disorders, as well as vascular lesions (18, 32). High fat feeding was also considered as a good manner for hyperlipidemia animal model establishment (33). Furthermore, the high-fat and high-fructose diet increases the excessive reactive oxygen species (ROS) generated by the renin–Ang II system and mitochondrial dysfunction (34). ROS generation mediates a pro-inflammatory cascade, which can cause an increase of adipogenesis, release of inflammatory cytokines, and decrease in adiponectin, leading to insulin resistance and vascular endothelial dysfunction (34, 35). In this study, spinach samples with different concentrations of nitrate were given intragastrically to the mice fed with high-fructose (20%, w/v) and high-fat (1% cholesterol and 5% lard, w/w) diet for 28 consecutive days. Our results showed that the high-fat and high-fructose diet induced significant reduction of serum HDL-C level and elevation of serum TG, TC, LDL-C, glucose, and insulin levels in mice (Table 2). However, ingestion of spinach nitrate significantly lowered the elevation of TG, TC, LDL-C, glucose, and insulin levels, and remarkably enhanced the decrease of HDL-C level in the mice fed with the high-fat and high-fructose diet. Furthermore, the calculated AI and HOMA-IR values of nitrate-enriched spinach-treated mice were significantly lower than that of the model mice, suggesting that spinach nitrate effectively improved the impairment of lipid and glucose metabolism, as well as the insulin resistance of mice receiving the high-fat and high-fructose diet. The improvement effect of spinach nitrate on lipid homeostasis was further confirmed by the results of the histopathological observation, where treatment of spinach rich in nitrate effectively ameliorated the hepatic fat deposit, severe cellular degeneration, hepatocyte necrosis, and cytoplasmic vacuolation triggered by the high-fat and high-fructose diet (Fig. 4). F_2-isoprostanes, which are formed by free radical-catalyzed peroxidation of phospholipid-bound arachidonic acid *in vivo* and *in vitro*, are considered as the most reliable markers of oxidative stress and lipid peroxidation (21, 36). In our hands, it was found that nitrate-enriched spinach obviously inhibited the elevation of serum F_2-isoprostanes induced by the high-fat and high-fructose diet, indicating the improving effect of spinach nitrate on oxidative stress and lipid peroxidation in mice (Table 2).

CRP, a stable downstream marker of the inflammatory process, has been reported to be an independent predictor of the risk of atherosclerosis, cardiovascular events, and myocardial infarction (26). In addition, IL-6 and TNF-α can play a pivotal role in inflammation-associated disturbances in glucose and insulin metabolism, lipid homeostasis, endothelial dysfunction, and accelerated atherosclerosis (37–39). Herein, our results revealed that the administration of nitrate-enriched spinach resulted in the decreases in serum CRP, IL-6, and TNF-α levels, which were evidently elevated by a high-fructose and high-fat diet in mice (Fig. 2). It is well known that the increasing production of inflammatory cytokines can contribute to endothelial dysfunction (4). IL-6 and TNF-α, which can be elevated in obesity and insulin resistance, have been confirmed to inhibit endothelial-dependent vasodilatation (40), and the degenerative endothelial vasodilatation in response to IL-6 and TNF-α can result in the reduction of NO availability (41). NO is an important protective molecule in the vasculature, and a defect in the production or activity of NO leads to endothelial dysfunction (42), whereas ET-1 is a peptide secreted mostly from vascular endothelial cells with profound vasoconstriction, pro-inflammatory action, stimulation of free radical formation, and platelet activation (43). As a result, ET-1 and NO are natural counterparts in vascular function, and an imbalance between these two mediators is the characteristic of endothelial dysfunction (42). Herein, it was found that the high-fat and high-fructose diet induced a significant increase in serum ET-1 level and a decrease in serum NO level in mice, suggesting a certain degree of endothelial injury. However, supplementation with spinach nitrate remarkably lowered serum ET-1 level and simultaneously raised serum NO level in mice with vascular endothelial injury, suggesting the potential vascular endothelial protective efficacy of spinach nitrate. Moreover, serum NOS activity was dose-dependently enhanced by spinach nitrate in mice. These results suggested that the nitrate-enriched spinach could stimulate the vascular endothelial cell to produce NO via the upregulation of NOS activity. Taken together, this finding indicates that the improvement of vascular NO status by nitrate-enriched spinach may play an important role in remittance of insulin resistance. However, the specific mechanisms underlying these effects need to be explored in the future.

Conclusions

The present study for the first time restores the prototype of spinach food and establishes a diet intervention with four nitrate content-matched treatments (spinach with or without low, medium, and high dose of nitrate) in high-fat and high-fructose treated mice, highlighting the significant differences in the contents of the nitrate ingredient to be evaluated. This study for the first time showed the ameliorative effects of spinach nitrate on lipid metabolism, insulin resistance, endothelial function, and inflammation in high-fat and high-fructose diet-fed mice. Our findings also suggest that spinach is a promising nitrate resource of dietary supplements for insulin resistance prevention, and provide basic information for exploring the potential benefits of dietary spinach against chronic diseases induced by high fat or high fructose.

Acknowledgements

This study was supported by the grants from the National Natural Science Foundation of China (C31671823).

Conflict of interest and funding

The authors have not received any funding or benefits from industry or elsewhere to conduct this study.

References

1. Brown AE, Walker M. Genetics of insulin resistance and the metabolic syndrome. Curr Cardiol Rep 2016; 18: 1–8.
2. Prasad DS, Kabir Z, Dash AK, Das BC. Prevalence and risk factors for metabolic syndrome in Asian Indians: a community study from urban eastern India. J Cardiovasc Dis Res 2012; 3: 204–11.
3. Ford ES, Li C, Zhao G, Pearson WS, Mokdad AH. Prevalence of the metabolic syndrome among US adolescents using the definition from the International Diabetes Federation. Diabetes Care 2008; 31: 587–9.
4. Cersosimo E, DeFronzo RA. Insulin resistance and endothelial dysfunction: the road map to cardiovascular diseases. Diabetes Metab Res Rev 2006; 22: 423–36.
5. Dandona P, Aljada A, Chaudhuri A, Mohanty P, Garg R. Metabolic syndrome: a comprehensive perspective based on interactions between obesity, diabetes, and inflammation. Circulation 2005; 111: 1448–54.
6. Steinberg HO, Chaker H, Leaming R, Johnson A, Brechtel G, Baron AD. Obesity/insulin resistance is associated with endothelial dysfunction. Implications for the syndrome of insulin resistance. J Clin Invest 1996; 97(11): 2601–10.
7. Sola S, Mir MQ, Cheema FA, Khan-Merchant N, Menon RG, Parthasarathy S, et al. Irbesartan and lipoic acid improve endothelial function and reduce markers of inflammation in the metabolic syndrome: results of the irbesartan and lipoic acid in endothelial dysfunction (ISLAND) study. Circulation 2005; 111: 343–8.
8. Lundberg JO, Feelisch M, Björne H, Jansson EA, Weitzberg E. Cardioprotective effects of vegetables: is nitrate the answer? Nitric Oxide 2006; 15: 359–62.
9. Machha A, Schechter AN. Inorganic nitrate: a major player in the cardiovascular health benefits of vegetables? Nutr Rev 2012; 70: 367–72.
10. Kapil V, Milsom AB, Okorie M, Maleki-Toyserkani S, Akram F, Rehman F, et al. Inorganic nitrate supplementation lowers blood pressure in humans: role for nitrite-derived NO. Hypertension 2010; 56: 274–81.
11. Bryan NS, Calvert JW, Elrod JW, Gundewar S, Ji SY, Lefer DJ. Dietary nitrite supplementation protects against myocardial ischemia-reperfusion injury. Proc Natl Acad Sci USA 2007; 104: 19144–9.
12. Carlström M, Larsen FJ, Nyström T, Hezel M, Borniquel S, Weitzberg E, et al. Dietary inorganic nitrate reverses features of metabolic syndrome in endothelial nitric oxide synthase-deficient mice. Proc Natl Acad Sci USA 2010; 107: 17716–20.
13. Gilchrist M, Shore AC, Benjamin N. Inorganic nitrate and nitrite and control of blood pressure. Cardiovasc Res 2011; 89: 492–8.
14. Hord NG, Tang Y, Bryan NS. Food sources of nitrates and nitrites: the physiologic context for potential health benefits. Am J Clin Nutr 2009; 90: 1–10.
15. Santamaria P. Nitrate in vegetables: toxicity, content, intake and EC regulation. J Sci Food Agric 2006; 86: 10–17.
16. Yang X, Bondonno CP, Indrawan A, Hodgson JM, Croft KD. An improved mass spectrometry-based measurement of NO metabolites in biological fluids. Free Radic Biol Med 2013; 56: 1–8.
17. Bondonno CP, Yang X, Croft KD, Considine MJ, Ward NC, Rich L. Flavonoid-rich apples and nitrate-rich spinach augment nitric oxide status and improve endothelial function in healthy men and women: a randomized controlled trial. Free Radic Biol Med 2012; 52: 95–102.
18. Makni M, Fetoui H, Garouiel M, Gargouri NK, Jaber H, Makni J, et al. Hypolipidemic and hepatoprotective seeds mixture diet rich in ω-3 and ω-6 fatty acids. Food Chem Toxicol 2010; 48: 2239–46.
19. Tappy L, Lê KA, Tran C, Paquot N. Fructose and metabolic diseases: new findings, new questions. Nutrition 2010; 26: 1044–9.
20. Jaya C, Anuradha CV. *Cissus quadrangularis* stem alleviates insulin resistance, oxidative injury and fatty disease in rats fed high fat plus fructose diet. Food Chem Toxicol 2010; 48: 2021–9.
21. Comporti M, Signorini C, Arezzini B, Vecchio D, Monaco B, Gardi C. F_2-isoprostanes are not just markers of oxidative stress. Free Radic Biol Med 2008; 44: 247–56.
22. Lundberg JO, Carlström M, Larsen FJ, Weitzberg E. Roles of dietary inorganic nitrate in cardiovascular health and disease. Cardiovasc Res 2011; 89: 525–32.
23. Mirvish SS. Role of N-nitroso compounds (NOC) and N-nitrosation in etiology of gastric, esophageal, nasopharyngeal and bladder cancer and contribution to cancer of known exposures to NOC. Cancer Lett 1995; 93: 17–48.
24. Kevil CG, Lefer DJ. Review focus on inorganic nitrite and nitrate in cardiovascular health and disease. Cardiovasc Res 2011; 89: 489–91.
25. Sydow K, Mondon CE, Cooke JP. Insulin resistance: potential role of the endogenous nitric oxide synthase inhibitor ADMA. Vasc Med 2005; 10(Suppl 1): S35–43.
26. Lidder S, Webb AJ. Vascular effects of dietary nitrate (as found in green leafy vegetables and beetroot) via the nitrate–nitrite–nitric oxide pathway. Br J Clin Pharmacol 2012; 75: 677–96.

27. Correia M, Barroso Â, Barroso MF, Soares D, Oliveirab M, Delerue-Matos C. Contribution of different vegetable types to exogenous nitrate and nitrite exposure. Food Chem 2010; 120: 960–6.
28. Lundberg JO, Weitzberg E, Gladwin MT. The nitrate-nitrite-nitric oxide pathway in physiology and therapeutics. Nat Rev Drug Discov 2008; 7: 156–67.
29. Zhang ZH, Wang ZQ, Yang Z, Niu YX, Zhang WW, Li XY, et al. A novel mice model of metabolic syndrome: the high-fat–high-fructose diet-fed ICR mice. Exp Anim 2015; 64(4): 435–42.
30. Poudyal H, Panchal S, Brown L. Comparison of purple carrot juice and β-carotene in a high-carbohydrate, high-fat diet-fed rat model of the metabolic syndrome. Br J Nutr 2010; 104: 1322–32.
31. Wada T, Kenmochi H, Miyashita Y, Sasaki M, Ojima M, Sasahara M, et al. Spironolactone improves glucose and lipid metabolism by ameliorating hepatic steatosis and inflammation and suppressing enhanced gluconeogenesis induced by high-fat and high-fructose diet. Endocrinology 2010; 151: 2040–9.
32. Miatello R, Vázquez M, Renna N, Cruzado M, Zumino AP, Risler N. Chronic administration of resveratrol prevents biochemical cardiovascular changes in fructose-fed rats. Am J Hypertens 2005; 18: 864–70.
33. Axelsen LN, Pedersen HD, Petersen JS, Holstein-Rathlou NH, Kjølbye AL. Metabolic and cardiac changes in high cholesterol–fructose-fed rats. J Pharmacol Toxicol Methods 2010; 61: 292–6.
34. Chidambaram J, Carani VA. *Cissus quadrangularis* stem alleviates insulin resistance, oxidative injury and fatty liver disease in rats fed high fat plus fructose diet. Food Chem Toxicol 2010; 48: 2021–9.
35. Lehnen AM, Rodrigues B, Irigoyen MC, De Angelis K, Schaan BD. Cardiovascular changes in animal models of metabolic syndrome. J Diabetes Res 2013; 2013: 761314.
36. Stoner L, Lucero AA, Palmer BR, Jones LM, Young JM, Faulkner J. Inflammatory biomarkers for predicting cardiovascular disease. Clin Biochem 2013; 46: 1353–71.
37. Patterson CC, Smith AE, Yarnell JW, Rumley A, Ben-Shlomo Y, Lowe GD. The associations of interleukin-6 (IL-6) and downstream inflammatory markers with risk of cardiovascular disease: the Caerphilly Study. Atherosclerosis 2010; 209: 551–7.
38. Nishida H, Horio T, Suzuki Y, Iwashima Y, Tokudome T, Yoshihara F, et al. Interleukin-6 as an independent predictor of future cardiovascular events in high-risk Japanese patients: comparison with C-reactive protein. Cytokine 2012; 53: 342–6.
39. Al-Aly Z, Pan H, Zeringue A, Xian H, McDonald JR, El-Achkar TM, et al. Tumor necrosis factor-α blockade, cardiovascular outcomes, and survival in rheumatoid arthritis. Transl Res 2011; 157: 10–18.
40. Diamant M, Lamb HJ, van de Ree MA, Endert EL, Groeneveld Y, Bots ML, et al. The association between abdominal visceral fat and carotid stiffness is mediated by circulating inflammatory markers in uncomplicated type 2 diabetes. J Clin Endocrinol Metab 2005; 90: 1495–501.
41. Ritchie SA, Connell JM. The link between abdominal obesity, metabolic syndrome and cardiovascular disease. Nutr Metab Cardiovasc Dis 2007; 17: 319–26.
42. Bourque SL, Davidge ST, Adams MA. The interaction between endothelin-1 and nitric oxide in the vasculature: new perspectives. Am J Physiol Regul Integr Comp Physiol 2011; 300: R1288–95.
43. Böhm F, Pernow J. The importance of endothelin-1 for vascular dysfunction in cardiovascular disease. Cardiovasc Res 2007; 76: 8–18.

***Xingbin Yang**
College of Food Engineering and Nutritional Science
Shaanxi Normal University
Xi'an 710062, China
Email: xbyang@snnu.edu.cn

11

Cpt1a gene expression in peripheral blood mononuclear cells as an early biomarker of diet-related metabolic alterations

Rubén Díaz-Rúa†, Andreu Palou* and Paula Oliver

Laboratory of Molecular Biology, Nutrition and Biotechnology, Universitat de les Illes Balears and CIBER de Fisiopatología de la Obesidad y Nutrición (CIBERobn), Palma de Mallorca, Spain

Abstract

Background: Research on biomarkers that provide early information about the development of future metabolic alterations is an emerging discipline. Gene expression analysis in peripheral blood mononuclear cells (PBMC) is a promising tool to identify subjects at risk of developing diet-related diseases.
Objective: We analysed PBMC expression of key energy homeostasis-related genes in a time-course analysis in order to find out early markers of metabolic alterations due to sustained intake of high-fat (HF) and high-protein (HP) diets.
Design: We administered HF and HP diets (4 months) to adult Wistar rats in isocaloric conditions to a control diet, mainly to avoid overweight associated with the intake of hyperlipidic diets and, thus, to be able to characterise markers of metabolically obese normal-weight (MONW) syndrome. PBMC samples were collected at different time points of dietary treatment and expression of relevant energy homeostatic genes analysed by real-time reverse transcription-polymerase chain reaction. Serum parameters related with metabolic syndrome, as well as fat deposition in liver, were also analysed.
Results: The most outstanding results were those obtained for the expression of the lipolytic gene carnitine palmitoyltransferase 1a (*Cpt1a*). *Cpt1a* expression in PBMC increased after only 1 month of exposure to both unbalanced diets, and this increased expression was maintained thereafter. Interestingly, in the case of the HF diet, *Cpt1a* expression was altered even in the absence of increased body weight but correlated with alterations such as higher insulin resistance, alteration of serum lipid profile and, particularly, increased fat deposition in liver, a feature characteristic of metabolic syndrome, which was even observed in animals fed with HP diet.
Conclusions: We propose *Cpt1a* gene expression analysis in PBMC as an early biomarker of metabolic alterations associated with MONW phenotype due to the intake of isocaloric HF diets, as well as a marker of increased risk of metabolic diseases associated with the intake of HF or HP diets.

Keywords: *dietary markers*; *prevention markers*; *PBMC*; *high-fat diet*; *high-protein diet*; *unbalanced diets*; *metabolic syndrome*; *liver steatosis*

An unbalanced proportion of macronutrients in the diet (mainly fats and proteins) is associated with alterations in body composition, metabolic parameters and different pathologies (1–6). In different animal and human models, alterations in the macronutrient composition of a diet are described as greatly relevant in energy homeostasis and metabolic disorders (7, 8). Increased fat consumption is related to obesity and metabolic complications, even when the subjects do not develop overweight (9). There is a special, and very prevalent, group of individuals, the metabolically obese normal-weight (MONW), who are not obese regarding weight and height (body mass index – BMI), but present higher visceral adiposity with ectopic fat deposition in tissues, such as liver, and alteration in parameters related to metabolic syndrome, such as insulin resistance (9–11). On the other hand, increased protein consumption in detriment of carbohydrates, which has become a popular

†Present address: Rubén Díaz-Rúa, Red Sea Research Center (RSRC), King Abdullah University of Science and Technology (KAUST), Thuwal, 23955-6900, Saudi Arabia.

strategy for body weight control, has also been related to a potential increase in health risk, especially in the long term (5, 6, 12–14).

One of the main efforts in nutritional research is to develop an early intervention for the identification and prevention of diet-related diseases such as diabetes mellitus type 2 and cardiovascular disease (15). For this, the study of new biomarkers of intake of unbalanced diets is very important because they can be used as indicators of metabolic or physiological deviations that may increase the risk of future chronic diseases related to unhealthy dietary habits (16). A fraction of blood cells, the peripheral blood mononuclear cells (PBMC), mainly composed by lymphocytes and monocytes/macrophages, is increasingly being used in nutritional studies as a source of biomarkers (17). These cells are easily obtainable by a simple blood extraction (18) and, in addition to their role in the innate immune system response, they can be used to assess biological responses as their gene expression profile may reflect the pathological and physiological state of the organism in humans and rats (19–21). PBMC travel around the body interacting with serum metabolites, thus they can reflect the gene expression patterns of different organs without needing invasive techniques (22).

We have previously shown that PBMC can reflect nutritional responses of key energy homeostatic tissues as well as metabolic deviations related to obesity development (19, 20, 23, 24). The use of techniques based on transcriptomic analysis can help provide more information on eventual biomarkers of certain physiophatological changes associated with impaired nutrition (25, 26). Recently, using microarray analysis, we have also shown that PBMC can reflect increased health risk due to long-term intake of diets with unbalanced macronutrient composition (14). These results encouraged us to search for early biomarkers in PBMC to detect metabolic deviations and health consequences of diets with an unbalanced macronutrient composition. Our research focused on the identification of early biomarkers to detect increased metabolic risk related to the normal-weight obesity syndrome due to the intake of isocaloric high-fat (HF) or high-protein (HP) diets. To this purpose, we designed a pair-fed isocaloric experiment in rats fed during 4 months with unbalanced HF and HP diets. We collected blood for isolation of PBMC, monthly and at the end of the experiment, in order to evaluate early changes in mRNA expression of key energy metabolism genes which could predict future health risks, before changes in others classical markers could be detected. Fatty liver is a leading cause of later chronic liver disease and is related to increased risk of death (27); however, there is a lack of non-invasive biomarkers for liver steatosis. Thus, we were particularly interested in identifying easily obtainable early biomarkers which could predict increased liver fatty deposition.

Methods and materials

Ethical approval

All experimental procedures followed in this study were reviewed and approved by the Ethical Committee of the University of the Balearic Islands, and guidelines for the use and care of laboratory animals of the university were followed.

Animals

The experiments were conducted with 2-month-old male Wistar rats (Charles River Laboratories España, SA, Barcelona, Spain), single-housed at 22°C with a period of light/dark of 12 h and pair-fed with different experimental diets for 4 months. We chose 2-month-old rats to begin the experiment because our objective was to analyse the effect of the intake of unbalanced diets during adulthood. Two experimental procedures were performed. In the first experiment (Experiment 1), animals were divided into three groups: a control group ($n = 7$), an HF group (HF60, $n = 7$) and an HP group (HP, $n = 6$). Control animals were fed a normolipidic diet (D12450B, Research Diets) containing 70% of energy (Kcal) from carbohydrates, 10% from fats and 20% from proteins. HF60 animals were fed an HF diet (D12492, Research Diets) containing 20% of energy from carbohydrates, 60% from fats (40% saturated and 60% unsaturated fat) and 20% from proteins. HP animals were fed an HP diet (Research Diets) containing 45% of energy from carbohydrates, 10% from fats and 45% from proteins (mainly casein). Diets were purchased from Brogaarden (Gentofte, Denmark). The same set of animals was used in a previous study aimed to characterise the physiological implications of the intake of unbalanced diets on body weight, adiposity, serum parameters and gene expression in key energy homeostatic tissues (28) and to determine by microarray analysis their effect on PBMC gene expression (14). These previous studies only addressed changes found at the end of the study (6-month-old animals), whereas the focus of the present work is on changes seen during the dietary intervention. In addition, we performed a second experiment (Experiment 2) with a new group of animals fed an HF diet but with a lower percentage of fat (45% instead of 60% Kcal). In this second experimental approach, 2-month-old animals were divided into two groups: a control group ($n = 6$) and a HF group (HF45, $n = 5$). Control animals were fed with the same diet used in Experiment 1, and HF45 animals were fed an HF diet (D12451, Research Diets) containing 35% of energy from carbohydrates, 45% from fats and 20% from proteins.

During the experimental trials, food was administered isocalorically. The HF60 and the HP groups in Experiment 1 and the HF45 group in Experiment 2 received an equal amount of Kcal as consumed by their controls the day before. The energy density of the diets used for calculation was as follows: control: 3.85; HF60: 5.24; HF45: 4.73 and HP: 3.85 Kcal per gram. When present, residual food in each cage was weighed, discarded and replaced with fresh diet every 24 h. Food was administered always at the same hour (13:00 h) and was available to the animals over a 24-h period. Food intake of all groups was recorded daily to calculate the daily caloric intake and cumulative caloric intake throughout the experiment; body weight was recorded three times a week.

At the end of the experimental period, animals were sacrificed by decapitation. Anaesthesia was not used in order to avoid interferences, and trunk blood was collected from the neck, stored at room temperature for 1 h and centrifuged at 3,000 rpm for 10 min at 4°C to collect serum. Liver and different white adipose tissue depots, both visceral (epididymal, mesenteric and retroperitoneal) and subcutaneous (inguinal), were rapidly removed and weighed.

Blood extraction and PBMC isolation

After initiation of the experimental trials, blood samples were collected every month during the 4 months of the dietary treatment; thus, a total of four time points were available from each dietary group, corresponding to 3, 4, 5 and 6-month-old animals. Blood samples were obtained from the saphena vein in the post-prandial absorptive state within the two first hours of the light cycle (8.00–10.00 h) to isolate serum and PBMC. We spent around 5–10 min per sample collection and obtained 1–1.5 mL of blood per animal. For PBMC isolation, blood was collected using heparin in NaCl (0.9%) as an anticoagulant, and then cells were obtained by Ficoll gradient separation, according to the instructions indicated by the manufacturer (GE Healthcare Bio Sciences, Barcelona, Spain), with some modifications, as previously described (14). One week prior to sacrifice and at 4 months of age, animals were submitted to a nocturnal 14-h fast to collect serum in fasted conditions to calculate the homeostatic model assessment for insulin resistance (HOMA-IR) index.

Body composition

Body composition (fat and lean mass) was measured every 15 days using an EchoMRI-700™ (Echo Medical Systems, LLC, TX, USA). Animals were not anaesthetised.

Quantification of circulating glucose, insulin, triacylglycerols and non-esterified free fatty acids

Blood glucose was measured using an Accu-Chek Glucometer (Roche Diagnostics, Barcelona, Spain). Serum insulin and tumor necrosis factor (TNF)-alpha were measured using enzyme-linked immunosorbent assay (ELISA) kits from DRG Instruments, Marburg, Germany (insulin) and R&D Systems Europe, Abingdon, UK (TNF-alpha). Commercial enzymatic colorimetric kits were used for the determination of triacylglycerols (TG) (Sigma Diagnostics, St Louis, MO, USA) and non-esterified free fatty acids (NEFA) (Wako Chemicals GmbH, Neuss, Germany).

HOMA-IR analysis

Insulin resistance was assessed by the HOMA-IR in rats submitted to overnight (14 h) fasting using the following formula of Matthews et al. (29). HOMA-IR = fasting glucose (mmol/L) × fasting insulin (mU/L)/22.5.

Liver lipid and triacylglycerol determination

Quantification of total lipid levels was determined by the method of Folch et al. (30). Liver TG content was measured in liver lipid extracts as previously described (31) using the Serum Triglyceride Determination Kit (Sigma Aldrich, Madrid, Spain).

Real-time RT-PCR analysis

Gene expression of key genes involved in energy homeostatic control (mainly lipid metabolism but also carbohydrate metabolism) was determined in the PBMC and liver by real-time reverse transcription-polymerase chain reaction (RT-PCR). Total RNA from PBMC and liver samples was extracted using Tripure Reagent (Roche Diagnostics, Barcelona, Spain). PBMC RNA was purified with Qiagen RNesay Mini Kit spin columns (Izasa SA, Barcelona, Spain), and liver RNA using E.Z.N.A. Total RNA Kit I (Omega Bio-Tek, Norcross, GA, USA) and treated with DNase I (Omega Bio-Tek). RNA yield was quantified on a Nanodrop ND 1000 spectrophotometer (NanoDrop Technologies, Wilmington, DE, USA), and its integrity was measured on an Agilent 2100 Bioanalyzer with RNA 6000 Nano chips (Agilent Technologies, South Queensferry, UK). Fifty nanogram for PBMC and 250 ng for liver of total RNA (in a final volume of 5 μL) were denatured at 65°C for 10 min and then reverse transcribed to cDNA using murine leukaemia virus reverse transcriptase (Applied Biosystems, Madrid, Spain) at 20°C for 15 min, 42°C for 30 min, with a final step of 5 min at 95°C in an Applied Biosystems 2720 Thermal Cycler (Applied Biosystems, Madrid, Spain). PCRs were performed from diluted (1/5 for PBMC and 1/20 for liver) cDNA template, forward and reverse primers (in a final concentration of 0.2 μm each) and Power SYBER Green PCR Master Mix (Applied Biosystems, CA, USA) in a total volume of 11 μL, with the following profile: 10 min at 95°C, followed by a total of 40 temperature cycles (15 sec at 95°C and 1 min at 60°C). Primers for the different genes analysed are described in Supplementary Table 1. All primers were obtained from Sigma Genosys (Sigma Aldrich Química SA, Madrid, Spain). To verify the purity of the products, a melting curve was produced after each run according to the manufacturer's instructions. The threshold cycle (Ct) was calculated by the instrument's software (StepOne Software v2.0), and the relative expression of each mRNA was calculated as a percentage versus control rats, using the $2^{-\Delta\Delta Ct}$ method (32). Data were normalised against the reference genes *beta-actin* and *integrin beta 1*. *Beta-actin* was used in liver because it is a well-known reference gene, and *integrin beta 1* was used in PBMC because microarray analysis performed with these samples at the final point of Experiment 1 (data not shown) showed equal and high expression for this gene in the different experimental groups.

Statistical analysis

All data are expressed as the mean ± SEM. Differences between HF or HP groups with controls were analysed using Student's *t*-test. In addition, a one-way analysis of variance (ANOVA) and least significant difference *post hoc* tests were performed in Experiment 1 to compare the three different experimental groups. The test used for each comparison is indicated in the footnote of the specific figures. Linear relationships between key variables were tested using Pearson correlation coefficients. All analyses were performed with SPSS for Windows (SPSS, Chicago, IL, USA). Threshold of significance was defined at $p < 0.05$ and is indicated when different.

Results

Body weight and adiposity

As expected, at the end of the experimental trial, 6-month-old Wistar rats that had been isocalorically fed with the unbalanced HF diets (HF60 and HF45) for 4 months showed the same body weight as their respective controls (Fig. 1a). However, in spite of no difference in body weight, HF60 animals presented increased fat mass content (mainly due to the increase in visceral fat – data not shown), which was evident soon after the start of the dietary treatment and which became significant since day 134 of age (Fig. 1b). Nevertheless, no increase in fat mass was observed in the HF45 group (Fig. 1b). In the case of the HP group, rats presented a tendency to lower body weight throughout the 4 months of dietary treatment, which became significant since day 149 (Fig. 1a). This lower body weight was not related to any apparent decrease in fat mass (Fig. 1b) but mainly related to lower water content (228 ± 6 g of total water in the HP vs. 253 ± 8 g in the control group at the final time-point, $p < 0.05$, Student's *t*-test). The cumulative energy intake was similar for the HF60 and HF45 animals and their controls, while HP animals showed a lower intake (data not shown).

Indicators of glucose metabolism: circulating glucose, insulin and HOMA-IR index

In *ad libitum* conditions, the intake of both HF diets resulted in higher circulating glucose levels (Fig. 2a). This hyperglycaemia was observed from the beginning, after only 1 month of HF feeding (animals of 3 months of age), and throughout the dietary treatment. In contrast, serum insulin levels were lower for the first 2 months after intake of the HF60 diet, but were not affected in the HF45 group

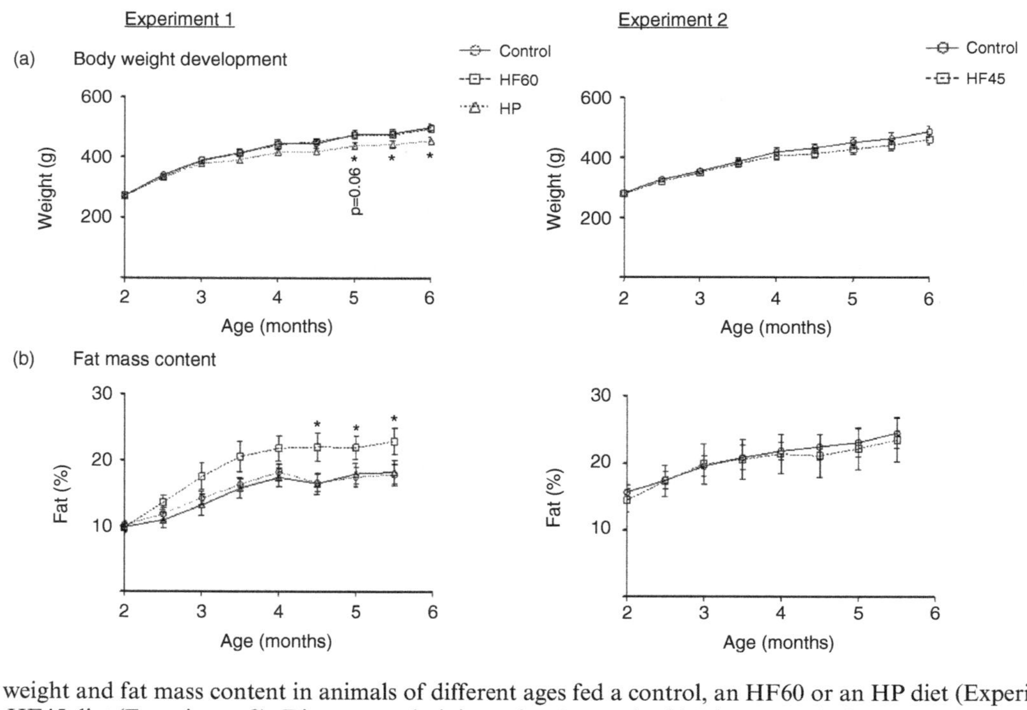

Fig. 1. Body weight and fat mass content in animals of different ages fed a control, an HF60 or an HP diet (Experiment 1), or a control or an HF45 diet (Experiment 2). Diets were administered to 2-month-old Wistar rats during 4 months. HF and HP diets were offered in isocaloric amounts to control animals and water was offered *ad libitum*. Body weight was followed thrice a week. Results represent mean ± SEM ($n = 5$–7). *indicates values significantly different versus control animals (Student's *t*-test, $p < 0.05$ or indicated when different).

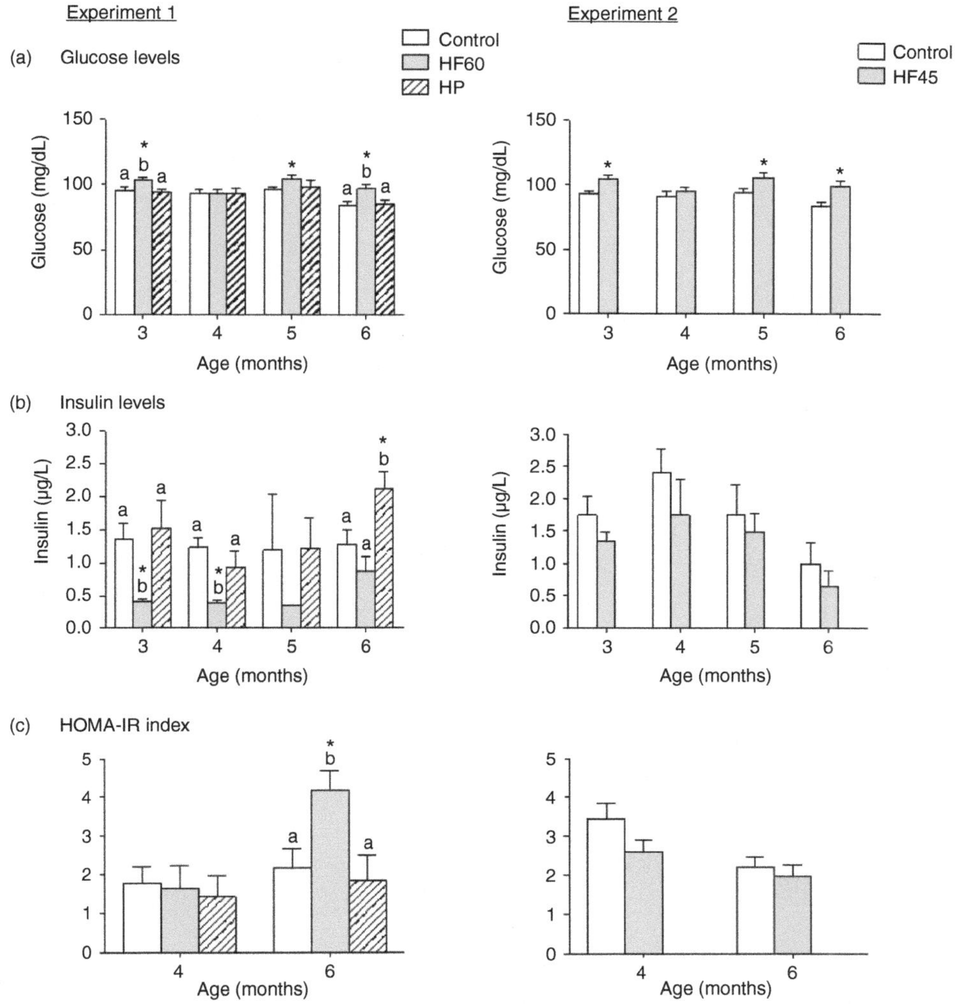

Fig. 2. Circulating glucose, insulin levels and HOMA-IR index measured in the same animals and conditions described in Fig. 1. All parameters were measured in the fed state. Results represent mean ± SEM ($n = 5–7$). Values not sharing a common letter (a, b) are significantly different (one-way ANOVA, $p < 0.05$); no letter indicates no significant differences; *indicates values significantly different versus control animals (Student's t-test, $p < 0.05$).

(Fig. 2b). Regarding the HP group, no changes were observed in circulating glucose or insulin levels, except at the end of the experiment, after 4 months of diet, when insulin levels were increased in the HP-fed animals (Fig. 2a and b). HOMA-IR index, measured at 2 and 4 months of dietary treatment (4- and 6-month-old rats, respectively), was increased only in animals of the HF60 group, and only at the end of the experiment, after 4 months of diet (Fig. 2c). No increase in HOMA-IR index was observed in the HF45 or in the HP groups.

Indicators of lipid metabolism: circulating TG and NEFA, and TG and lipid content in liver

As shown in Fig. 3, both HF diets (HF60 and HF45) decreased serum TG levels in the fed state in the different months analysed. On the other hand, we observed a tendency to higher circulating NEFA levels in the two HF groups, but it did not attain statistical significance. Neither serum TG nor NEFA levels were affected by the HP diet.

Interestingly, the three unbalanced diets (HF60, HF45 and HP) increased TG content in liver, and the HF60 diet also increased total hepatic lipid content (Fig. 4). This is of relevance as fat deposition in liver is linked to systemic insulin resistance and the development of metabolic syndrome (33).

Regulation of Cpt1a mRNA levels in PBMC and liver of rats fed with different unbalanced diets rich in fat or protein

We analysed mRNA expression of different key genes involved in energy homeostasis in PBMC obtained monthly since the beginning of the dietary intervention, but the most outstanding results were those of the key lipolytic gene carnitine palmitoyltransferase 1a (*Cpt1a*),

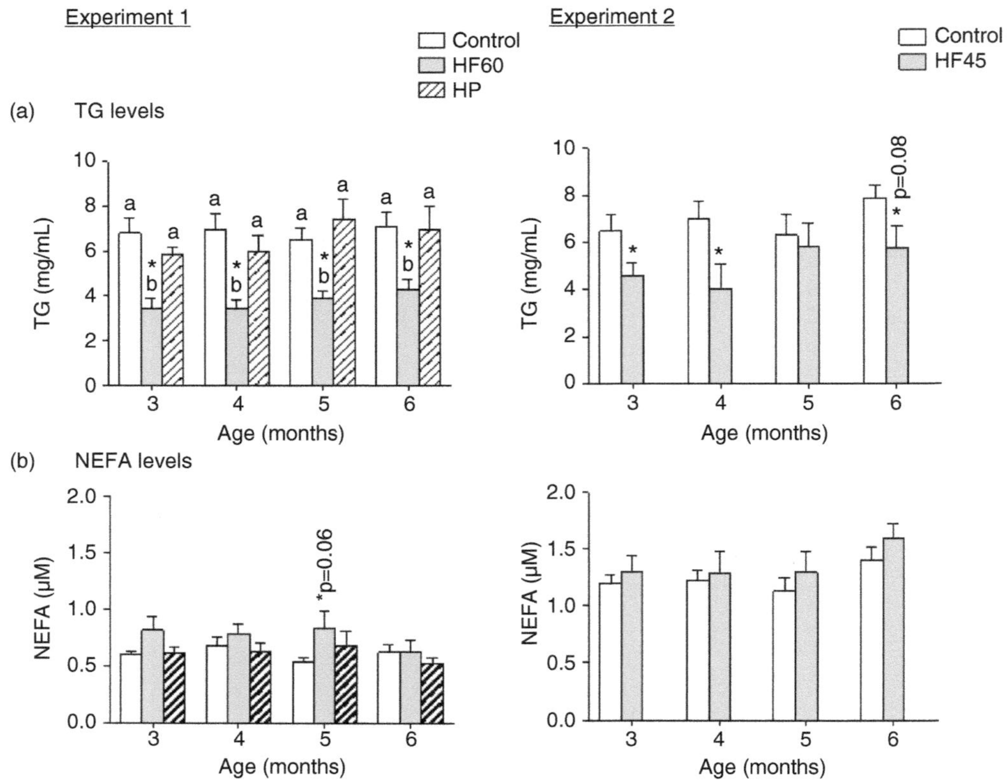

Fig. 3. Circulating triacylglycerols (TG) and non-esterified fatty acids (NEFA) measured in the same animals and conditions described in Fig. 1. All parameters were measured in the fed state. Results represent mean ± SEM ($n = 5$–7). Values not sharing a common letter (a, b) are significantly different (one-way ANOVA, $p < 0.05$); no letter indicates no significant differences; *indicates values significantly different versus control animals (Student's t-test, $p < 0.05$ or indicated when different).

which codes for an enzyme that allows entrance of fatty acids into the mitochondria for their beta-oxidation. In Experiment 1, the two unbalanced diets, rich in fat (HF60) and rich in protein (HP), produced an up-regulation of *Cpt1a* mRNA levels in PBMC obtained at the different months analysed (Fig. 5a). In Experiment 2, the HF45 diet also increased PBMC *Cpt1a* mRNA expression, although statistical significance was not reached in all the months (Fig. 5a), evidencing the relevance of the lower fat proportion. This nutritional regulatory pattern observed in PBMC of rats fed with HF diets coincided to that observed in liver at the end of the experimental period: *Cpt1a* mRNA levels increased in liver of the HF60 and HF45 groups. However, contrary to what observed in PBMC, no increased *Cpt1a* expression was observed in liver of the HP group (Fig. 5b).

Regulation of key energy homeostatic genes in PBMC of rats fed with different unbalanced diets rich in fat or protein

In addition to *Cpt1a*, we also analysed the effect of the unbalanced diets on PBMC expression of other relevant genes involved in lipid metabolism and, in general, no relevant effect was observed (see Fig. 6). Contrary to what happened for *Cpt1a*, dietary treatment did not affect the mRNA expression of another gene involved in fatty acid oxidation, *Mlycd*. This gene codes for malonyl-CoA decarboxylase, which catalyses the breakdown of malonyl-CoA into acetyl-CoA and carbon dioxide, inhibiting fatty acid oxidation. We also analysed the mRNA expression of two genes involved in fatty acid synthesis: *Acc1*, coding for acetyl-CoA carboxylase which catalyses the carboxylation of acetyl-CoA to produce malonyl-CoA, and *Fasn*, coding for fatty acid synthase that forms fatty acids using malonyl-CoA. Moreover, we studied mRNA expression of *Pparg* which codes for a key adipogenic factor PPAR-gamma. HP diet increased *Acc1* and *Pparg* expression in PBMC obtained at different months, the latter only after the first month of diet. However, HF diets did not affect *Acc1* or *Pparg* mRNA levels. Regarding *Fasn*, its PBMC expression was not affected by any of the unbalanced diets. No effect was observed for the expression of *Slc27a2*, coding for a fatty acid transport gene which we have reported to be affected, in PBMC, by the intake of cafeteria diets (20).

Finally, we analysed the potential effects of the diets in PBMC expression of two key genes involved in the maintenance of glucose homeostasis: *Eno1* and *Glut4*, coding for the glycolytic enzyme enolase 1 and for the

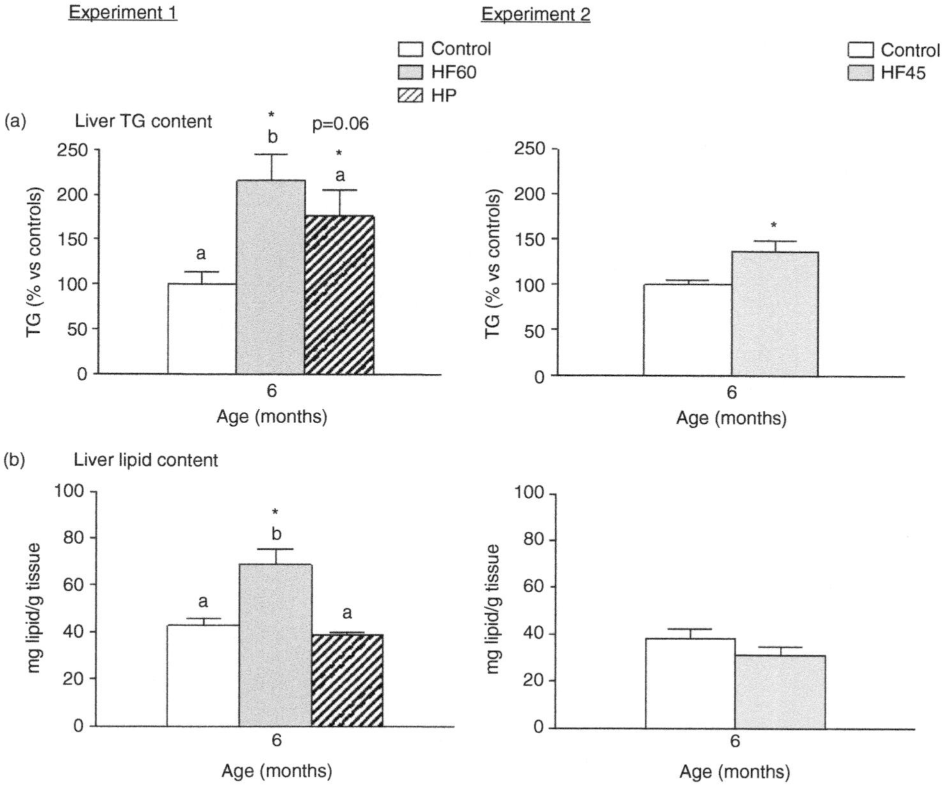

Fig. 4. Liver triacylglycerol (TG) and total lipid content in 6-month-old animals fed during 4 months a control, an HF60 or an HP diet (Experiment 1), or a control or an HF45 diet (Experiment 2). All diets were offered in isocaloric amounts to control animals and water was offered *ad libitum*. Values not sharing a common letter (a, b) are significantly different (one-way ANOVA, $p < 0.05$); no letter indicates no significant differences; *indicates values significantly different versus control animals (Student's *t*-test, $p < 0.05$ or indicated when different).

insulin-responsive glucose transporter, respectively (see Fig. 7). *Enol* mRNA expression resulted affected only by the HF60 diet, which decreased PBMC mRNA levels of the glycolytic gene at different months of dietary treatment; no effect was observed for the HF45 or the HP diets. *Glut4* expression in PBMC was affected by the HF60 and HP diets; both of them decreased its mRNA levels, but the effect was only observed in the first and last month of treatment, while no effect was observed for the HF45 diet. Thus, this gene was not so relevant to be considered a biomarker as the previously mentioned *Cpt1a,* whose expression was affected by all the dietary treatments and at the different time-points analysed.

Correlation of Cpt1a mRNA in PBMC and liver with serum and liver parameters

To have a better comprehension of the relation of *Cpt1a* gene expression changes with the metabolic status of the animals, we performed Pearson correlation analysis between *Cpt1a* mRNA levels in PBMC and liver with body weight, adiposity and the measured indicators of glucose and lipid metabolism. The most relevant correlations are shown in Table 1. To be able to compare the correlations obtained for *Cpt1a* mRNA expression in PBMC with that of liver, we considered parameters obtained at the final time-point (6-month-old animals that followed 4 months of dietary treatment). Statistical correlations were found mainly taking into account HF60 and control animals from Experiment 1. *Cpt1a* mRNA expression in PBMC correlated positively with HOMA-IR index, and with TG and total lipid content of liver. Interestingly, these correlations were maintained even after considering fat mass (which was higher in the HF60 group) as a confounding factor. It is worth to note that the positive correlation between HOMA-IR index and *Cpt1a* mRNA in PBMC was also observed when using data obtained during the experiment (at 4 and 6 months of age), and also a negative correlation with TG was seen when considering all the data – from animals of 3, 4, 5 and 6 months of age – ($r = -0.348$, $p = 0.013$). Surprisingly, correlations were less evident for liver *Cpt1a* mRNA expression; we observed a positive correlation with hepatic TG content and a negative correlation with circulating TG, but no relation was found with HOMA-IR or total lipid content. The effect of the HF diet on *Cpt1a* expression was dependent on the percentage of fat,

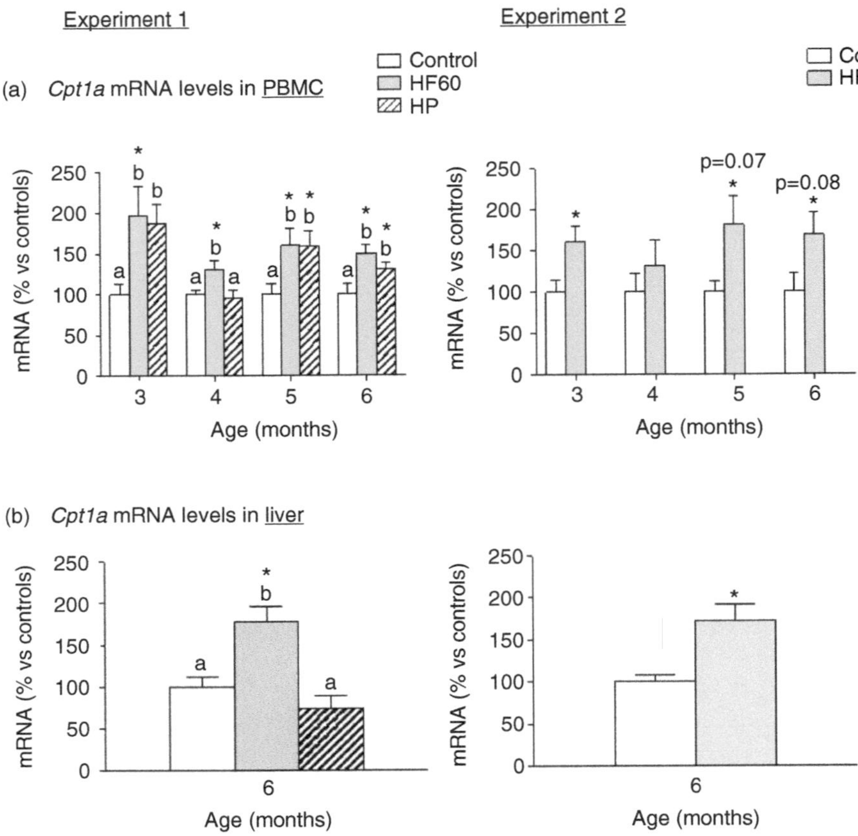

Fig. 5. *Cpt1a* mRNA gene expression in PBMC (a) in animals of different ages and (b) in liver of 6-month-old animals. *Cpt1a* mRNA was measured by real-time RT-PCR in animals fed a control, an HF60 or an HP diet (Experiment 1), or a control or an HF45 diet (Experiment 2). Diets were administered to 2-month-old Wistar rats during 4 months. HF and HP diets were offered in isocaloric amounts to control animals and water was offered *ad libitum*. Results represent mean ± SEM ($n = 5$–7) of ratios of specific mRNA levels relative to *integrin beta 1* in PBMC and *beta-actin* in liver, and expressed as a percentage of the value of control group at the age of 3 (for PBMC) or 6 months (for liver) that was set to 100%. Values not sharing a common letter (a, b) are significantly different (one-way ANOVA, $p < 0.05$); no letter indicates no significant differences; *indicates values significantly different versus control animals (Student's t-test, $p < 0.05$ or indicated when different).

as no significant correlation was found for the above mentioned parameters using data of HF45 and control animals (Experiment 2). No statistically relevant correlation was detected when considering data of the HP and control animals in Experiment 1.

Discussion

The use of PBMC as a tool to identify nutritional biomarkers is increasing, since this fraction of blood cells has been validated as a good model for dietary intervention studies (17). Our group has previously reported, based on microarray analysis, that PBMC gene expression is affected by the intake of diets with an unbalanced macronutrient composition (14). Here, we aimed to identify, in PBMC, early gene expression biomarkers of diet-related metabolic alterations (mainly those linked to metabolic syndrome and liver steatosis) due to the intake of unbalanced diets (rich in fat or protein). We focused our attention on identifying early biomarkers of normal-weight obesity caused by either an increase in dietary fat intake, but without exceeding caloric needs, or by increased protein intake, simulating the relative overconsumption observed in humans following HP weight-loss diets.

We performed a first experiment (Experiment 1) in which we administered two unbalanced diets: HF (with 60% Kcal as fat vs. 10% in controls) and HP (45% Kcal as proteins vs. 20% in controls), during 4 months to adult Wistar rats. Both diets were administrated in isocaloric conditions to the control diet mainly to avoid hyperphagia and development of overweight/obesity in the HF group. Thus, animals of the HF60 group progressively developed increased adiposity (mainly visceral), due to the higher input of dietetic fat, but did not exhibit overweight. A high level of visceral fat is the principal feature of MONW subjects and is directly associated with alterations in glucose metabolism and other parameters related to metabolic syndrome (34). Accordingly, HF60

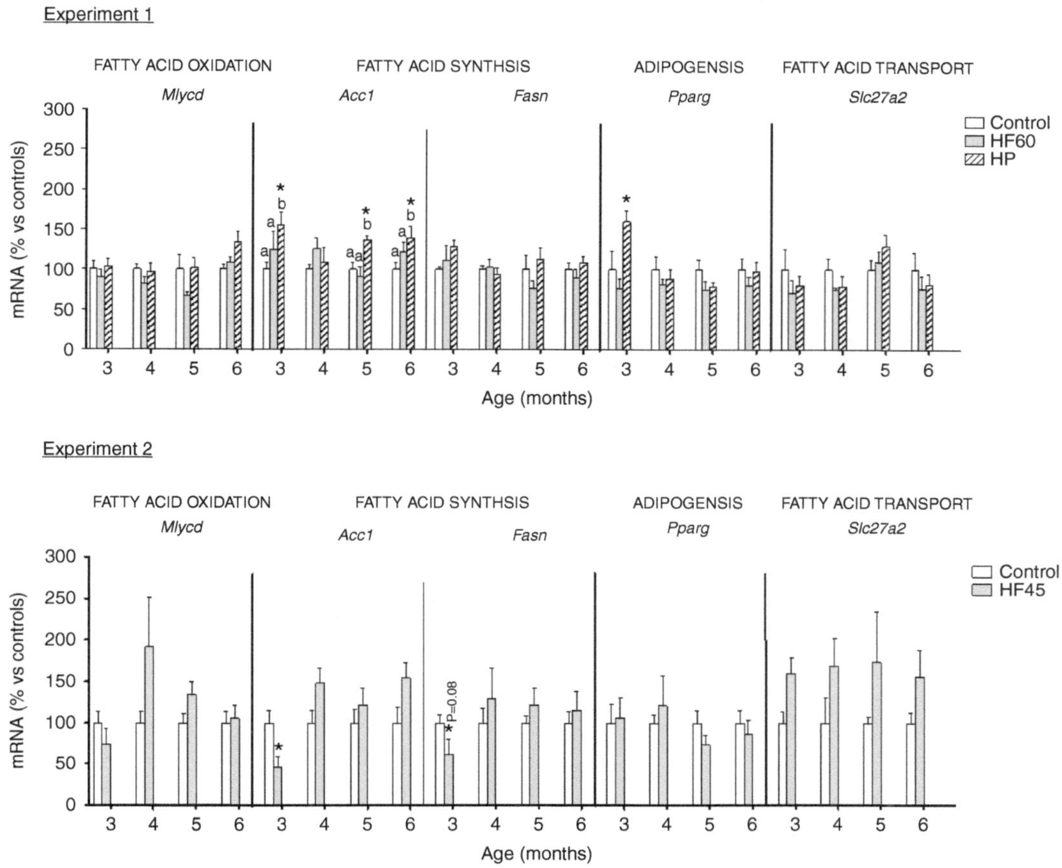

Fig. 6. Gene expression (mRNA) of genes involved in fatty acid oxidation (*Mlycd*), fatty acid synthesis (*Acc1* and *Fasn*), adipogenesis (*Pparg*) and fatty acid transport (*Slc27a2*) in PBMC of the same animals and conditions described in Fig. 1, measured by real-time RT-PCR. Results represent mean $\pm$ SEM ($n = 5$–7) of ratios of specific mRNA levels relative to *integrin beta 1,* expressed as a percentage of the value of control group at the age of 3 months that was set to 100%. Values not sharing a common letter (a, b) are significantly different (one-way ANOVA, $p < 0.05$); no letter indicates no significant differences; *indicates values significantly different versus control animals (Student's t-test, $p < 0.05$ or indicated when different).

animals presented higher serum glucose levels from the first month of intake of the HF diet. However, in spite of the hyperglycaemia, circulating insulin levels were lower the first 2 months of HF diet intake, probably because of the lower carbohydrate content of the diet, as it has been previously shown that low-carbohydrate/HF diets generate hypoinsulinemia (35). Nevertheless, as a result of the sustained intake of the HF diet, animals progressively developed insulin resistance, evidenced by a higher HOMA-IR index at the final point, after 4 months of HF diet feeding. All these alterations evidence an impairment in glucose metabolism and insulin signalling due to increased fat intake, a well-known effect of HF-diet-induced obesity (36), and which is also characteristic of MONW subjects (37). Alterations were also evident for circulating TG; HF60 diet intake produced a decrease in circulating TG from the first month of diet intake until the end of the experiment. These decreased serum TG levels, which are characteristic of HF-diet interventions, have been related to a reduced very low-density lipoprotein production rate and increased TG removal from blood to be used as a source of energy because of the lower carbohydrate content of the diet (28, 38, 39). Other relevant indicators of lipid metabolism, such as circulating NEFA, did not present any significant changes in the HF group at any of the different times analysed.

The HF60 diet was particularly rich in fat; therefore, to increase the robustness of the results, we designed another experiment (Experiment 2) with a new group of rats isocalorically fed with an HF diet containing a lower amount of lipids (45% Kcal of total calories). Development of an MONW phenotype due to sustained intake of this more moderate HF diet would be more similar to the situation which could be occurring in humans. Logically, the alterations found in HF45 animals were less marked than those of the MONW HF60 group. As expected, animals presented the same body weight than controls but, in this case, 4 months of isocaloric intake of the HF45 diet

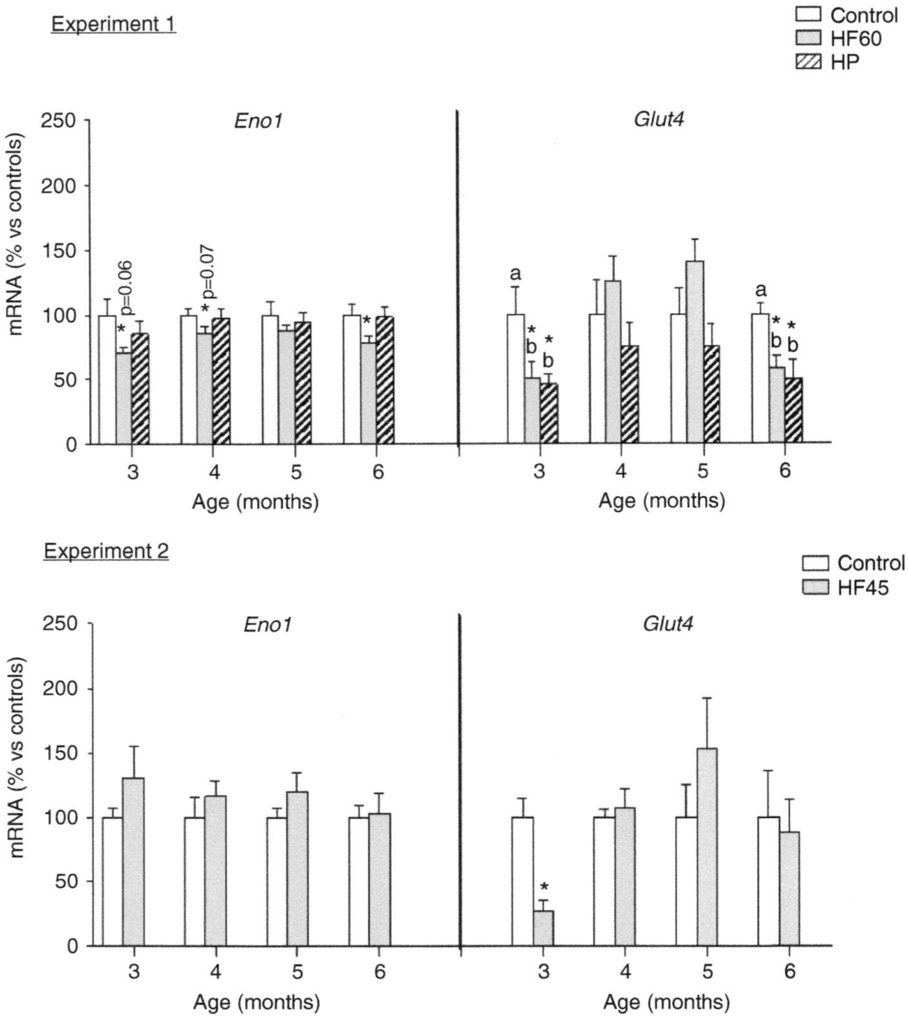

Fig. 7. Gene expression (mRNA) of the glycolytic gene *Eno1* and of the glucose transporter *Glut4* in PBMC of the same animals and conditions described in Fig. 1, measured by real-time RT-PCR. Results represent mean ± SEM ($n = 5$–7) of ratios of specific mRNA levels relative to *integrin beta 1,* expressed as a percentage of the value of control group at the age of 3 months that was set to 100%. Values not sharing a common letter (a, b) are significantly different (one-way ANOVA, $p < 0.05$); no letter indicates no significant differences; *indicates values significantly different versus control animals (Student's *t*-test, $p < 0.05$ or indicated when different).

was not enough to increase fat mass of the animals. However, animals presented some alterations such as increased serum glucose levels, which were observed after only 1 month of dietary intake. In spite of this, HOMA-IR index (measured after 2 and 4 months of diet intake) was not affected. As seen in the HF60 animals, serum TG levels also decreased at different time points.

Regarding the protein-rich diet, its intake resulted in a progressive decrease in body weight which was not due to a decreased fat mass, which remained unchanged during the experimental trial, but to a lower water content. This HP diet produced a lower alteration in the analysed indicators of glucose and lipid metabolism than the fat-rich diets. We did not observe alterations in serum glucose levels, NEFA or TG and, although higher insulin levels were required to maintain glycaemia in HP-fed animals after 4 months of dietary treatment, HOMA-IR remained unchanged.

One of the most, somehow unexpected, relevant features observed in our three animal models was an alteration in liver lipid composition. Liver is a key tissue, which is involved in energy balance maintenance by appropriate handling of ingested macronutrients (40), and increased TG deposition in this tissue has been associated with a higher risk of metabolic syndrome, different hepatic pathologies and death (27, 41). Notably, we found an increased TG content in liver of the different dietary groups studied: HF60, HF45 and HP. We have previously described in detail, based on microarray data analysis, the potential mechanisms involved in TG accumulation in liver due to the intake of isocaloric HF (42) or HP diets

Table 1. Correlations of *Cpt1a* mRNA expression in PBMC and liver with HOMA-IR and lipid parameters, either considering fat as a confounding factor or not

	PBMC		Liver	
	Cpt1a	*Cpt1a*	*Cpt1a*	*Cpt1a*
Confounding factor	None	Fat	None	Fat
Experiment 1 (data of the HF60 and control groups)				
HOMA-IR	$r=0.671$*	$r=0.692$*	$R=0.502$	$R=0.477$
	$p=0.024$	$p=0.027$	$P=0.116$	$P=0.164$
Circulating TG	$r=-0.431$	$r=-0.325$*	$R=-0.660$*	$R=-0.601$*
	$p=0.124$	$p=0.023$	$P=0.010$	$P=0.030$
Liver TG content	$r=0.670$*	$r=0.602$*	$R=0.559$*	$R=0.488$
	$p=0.012$	$p=0.038$	$P=0.031$	$P=0.107$
Liver lipid content	$r=0.748$**	$r=0.580^{+}$	$R=0.487$	$R=0.335$
	$p=0.005$	$p=0.061$	$P=0.126$	$P=0.315$
Experiment 2 (data of the HF45 and control groups)				
HOMA-IR	$r=-0.408$	$r=-0.062$	$R=0.153$	$R=-0.213$
	$p=0.315$	$p=0.896$	$P=0.673$	$P=0.583$
Circulating TG	$r=0.318$	$r=-0.545$	$R=-0.570$	$R=-0.566$
	$p=0.487$	$p=0.263$	$P=0.085$	$P=0.112$
Liver TG content	$r=0.386$	$r=0.735$	$R=0.425$	$R=0.381$
	$p=0.393$	$p=0.096$	$P=0.220$	$P=0.312$
Liver lipid content	$r=-0.250$	$r=0.682$	$R=0.339$	$R=-0.337$
	$p=0.550$	$p=0.092$	$P=0.308$	$P=0.341$

r = Pearson correlation coefficients; $^{+}p=0.06$; $^{*}p<0.05$, $^{**}p<0.01$; HOMA-IR, homeostatic model assessment for insulin resistance; PBMC, peripheral blood mononuclear cells, TG, triacylglycerol.

(article submitted). Because fatty liver is a serious health concern, it would be of great interest to identify easily obtainable non-invasive biomarkers of increased fat accumulation in this relevant organ, which could help to predict future metabolic diseases.

To deal with the identification of PBMC biomarkers, and based on our previous experience showing that PBMC reflect with particular accuracy lipid metabolism gene expression in response to nutritional interventions (19, 20, 22, 23), we selected key genes involved in fatty acid oxidation (*Cpt1a* and *Mlycd*), fatty acid synthesis (*Acc1* and *Fasn*), adipogenesis (*Pparg*) and fatty acid transport (*Slc27a2*), to be tested as potential early markers of health risk related to dietary interventions. In addition, the HF and HP diets, as those used in our experiment, usually imply a decrease in carbohydrate content; therefore, we also analysed the expression of a key glycolytic gene (*Eno1*) and of a relevant glucose transporter (*Glut4*) to be considered as potential early biomarkers of dietary imbalance in PBMC. We analysed these genes in PBMC samples obtained monthly from the different animal models during the 4 months of the dietary intervention.

The most outstanding results were those obtained for *Cpt1a*, involved in long-chain fatty acids transport across the inner mitochondrial membrane. We had previously reported that *Cpt1a* mRNA expression in PBMC is a good indicator of gene expression patterns typical of key energy homeostatic tissues such as liver and adipose tissues in response to changes in dietary patterns (fasting/refeeding) or *ad libitum* intake of HF diets (19, 22, 24). Interestingly, our data show that *Cpt1a* mRNA levels increased in animals isocalorically fed with the two different HF diets (HF60 and HF45) and also in animals fed with the HP diet. The increase was observed after only 1 month of the dietary treatment, when animals had not yet developed changes in body weight, fat mass or HOMA-IR index. This increase in *Cpt1a* expression was also observed in the following 3 months of the experimental trial. In the case of the HF groups, increased *Cpt1a* expression, which was statistically stronger in the HF60 than in the HF45 group, reflected higher levels of this gene in liver, and thus evidenced the expected higher fatty acid oxidative capacity. However, the sustained increase in *Cpt1a* expression observed in PBMC of the HP group did not correlate with an increased expression in liver of the animals.

To have a better comprehension of the utility of *Cpt1a* expression analysis in PBMC as a dietary biomarker of health risk, we performed correlations with the different analysed parameters at the end of the experiment. Relevant correlations were obtained considering the HF60 animals (those that presented strongest metabolic alterations) and controls. Interestingly, we found positive correlations between *Cp1a* mRNA in PBMC and HOMA-IR, liver TG and total liver lipid content, as well as a negative correlation with circulating TG. These correlations were maintained even after correcting by fat mass (which was higher in HF60 animals than in controls) as a confounding factor. This is relevant, since altered (increased) *Cpt1a* expression in PBMC of MONW animals is not only a reflection/consequence of higher adiposity in the animals but also provides additional information, such as increased risk of developing insulin resistance or accumulating fat in liver. Moreover, analysis of *Cpt1a* analysed in PBMC provided better correlations than in liver; hepatic *Cpt1a* mRNA expression, taking into account HF60 and control animals, correlated positively with liver TG content, but not with total liver lipid content or HOMA-IR. No relevant correlations were obtained in PBMC or liver in the case of HF45 or HP animals, probably due to the fact that the alterations observed in these animals were not as strong as those in HF60 ones. However, all the groups presented higher TG accumulation in liver (i.e. increased metabolic risk) at the end of the experiment as well as increased PBMC *Cpt1a* expression not only at the final point, but since the first month of unbalanced dietary treatment. Thus, based on the observed correlations, we could consider this gene as an early risk marker of diet-related liver damage and insulin resistance, of interest to identify dietary imbalances that can affect health, particularly lipid accumulation in liver, when animals are still healthy.

Gene expression analysis of the rest of pre-selected potential biomarkers did not report relevant results. It is well known that PBMC can reflect metabolic adaptations to the intake of HF/high energy diets by inhibition of lipogenic and enhancement of lipolytic genes (19, 22, 24). Interestingly, in our study, apart from *Cpt1a*, the other lipid metabolism-related genes were not importantly affected, probably because our diets were offered in isocaloric conditions to controls, not *ad libitum.* This is an additional evidence of the robustness of *Cpt1a* as a biomarker, as its gene expression reflected expected liver behaviour in response to a lighter dietary stimulus: isocaloric HF diets non-related to overweight. In addition, we observed changes in gene expression of the two studied genes involved in glucose homeostasis, the glycolytic gene *Eno1* and the insulin-responsive glucose transporter *Glut4*. According to the lower carbohydrate content of the diet, *Eno1* mRNA levels decreased at different ages, but the decrease did not always reach statistical significance and was only observed in the HF60 group. On the other hand, *Glut4* expression greatly decreased in the HF and HP groups, but only the first and the last month of dietary treatment, while *Cpt1a* altered expression was observed at all the different months studied.

In summary, in HF-diet pair-fed animals that developed an MONW phenotype, *Cpt1a* gene expression increased in PBMC, reflecting the nutritional response that takes place in liver aimed to increase the usage of fatty acids as energy and preserve glucose, as an adaptation to the higher fat and decreased carbohydrate content of the diet. These results evidence the usefulness of PBMC as a surrogate tissue to study nutritional effects on other internal organs. Moreover, the same adaptation (increased *Cpt1a* expression) was observed in PBMC of HP-fed animals, even if *Cpt1a* did not increase in liver of these animals. These higher *Cpt1a* mRNA levels were observed after only 1 month of dietary intervention with both unbalanced diets and were maintained thereafter. Thus, *Cpt1a* gene expression analysis in PBMC could be used as a blood marker of dietary macronutrient intake to report nutritional imbalances. The use of molecular dietary biomarkers provides a more objective and accurate measure of intake in comparison to traditional questionnaires used in dietetic studies and will improve the assessment of the relationship between diet and chronic metabolic alterations or diseases. *Cpt1a* expression in PBMC positively correlated with HOMA-IR and with liver fat and TG content using data of HF60 MONW animals (those presenting the strongest metabolic alterations). Based on this, the results of this work suggest that *Cpt1a* can be used, not only as a nutritional biomarker, but as an early marker of future alterations such as liver fat deposition, which is a common feature of animals fed with both the HF and the HP unbalanced diets. At present, development of overweight and alterations of classical blood parameters are used to identify metabolic syndrome. However, a high percentage of the population currently present a high risk to develop metabolic syndrome in the future, even with a normal BMI (11, 43). Moreover, according to our data, unbalanced diets can result in increased metabolic syndrome risk (measured as fat liver accumulation), not only in the absense of overweight/obesity but also in the absense of increased adiposity or signs of insulin resistance, as seen in the animals fed with the moderate HF diet (HF45) or the HP diet. For this reason, it is important to identify robust early markers which could help detect dietary imbalances and therefore act in consequence.

Conclusions

Our results reinforce the use of PBMC as a tool in nutritional studies and clearly show that *Cpt1a* analysis in PBMC could be used as an early biomarker of future complications related to the intake of unbalanced diets, such as insulin resistance and increased liver fat deposition. At this point, it would be of interest to confirm the usefulness of this biomarker in humans.

Acknowledgements

CIBER de Fisiopatología de la Obesidad y Nutrición is an initiative of the Instituto de Salud Carlos III (ISCIII). This work was supported by the Spanish Government (Ministerio de Economía y Competitividad, INTERBIOBES, AGL2015-67019-P) and by the University of the Balearic Islands (IBIFLEX, FA38/2016). The Laboratory of Molecular Biology, Nutrition and Biotechnology is a member of the European Research Network of Excellence NuGO (The European Nutrigenomics Organisation). RDR was recipient of a fellowship from the Spanish Government.

Conflict of interest and funding

The authors declare no conflict of interest.

References

1. Galgani J, Ravussin E. Energy metabolism, fuel selection and body weight regulation. Int J Obes (Lond) 2008; 32: S109–19.
2. Hill JO, Melanson EL, Wyatt HT. Dietary fat intake and regulation of energy balance: implications for obesity. J Nutr 2000; 130: 284S–8S.
3. Juraschek SP, Appel LJ, Anderson CA, Miller ER, 3rd. Effect of a high-protein diet on kidney function in healthy adults: results from the OmniHeart trial. Am J Kidney Dis 2013; 61: 547–54.
4. Labayen I, Ruiz JR, Ortega FB, Huybrechts I, Rodriguez G, Jimenez-Pavon D, et al. High fat diets are associated with higher abdominal adiposity regardless of physical activity in adolescents; the HELENA study. Clin Nutr 2014; 33: 859–66.
5. Hernández-Alonso P, Salas-Salvadó J, Ruiz-Canela M, Corella D, Estruch R, Fitó M, et al. High dietary protein intake is associated with an increased body weight and total death risk. Clin Nutr 2016; 35: 496–506.
6. Wu G. Dietary protein intake and human health. Food Funct 2016; 7: 1251–65.
7. Krauss RM, Eckel RH, Howard B, Appel LJ, Daniels SR, Deckelbaum RJ, et al. AHA dietary guidelines: revision 2000: a statement for healthcare professionals from the Nutrition Committee of the American Heart Association. Circulation 2000; 102: 2284–99.
8. Linn T, Santosa B, Gronemeyer D, Aygen S, Scholz N, Busch M, et al. Effect of long-term dietary protein intake on glucose metabolism in humans. Diabetologia 2000; 43: 1257–65.
9. Lopez-Miranda J, Perez-Martinez P. It is time to define metabolically obese but normal-weight (MONW) individuals. Clin Endocrinol (Oxf) 2013; 79: 314–15.
10. Wang B, Zhuang R, Luo X, Yin L, Pang C, Feng T, et al. Prevalence of metabolically healthy obese and metabolically obese but normal weight in adults worldwide: a meta-analysis. Horm Metab Res 2015; 47: 839–45.
11. Kelishadi R, Cook SR, Motlagh ME, Gouya MM, Ardalan G, Motaghian M, et al. Metabolically obese normal weight and phenotypically obese metabolically normal youths: the CASPIAN study. J Am Diet Assoc 2008; 108: 82–90.
12. Schwingshackl L, Hoffmann G. Long-term effects of low-fat diets either low or high in protein on cardiovascular and metabolic risk factors: a systematic review and meta-analysis. Nutr J 2013; 12: 48.
13. Abete I, Astrup A, Martinez JA, Thorsdottir I, Zulet MA. Obesity and the metabolic syndrome: role of different dietary macronutrient distribution patterns and specific nutritional components on weight loss and maintenance. Nutr Rev 2010; 68: 214–31.
14. Diaz-Rua R, Keijer J, Caimari A, van Schothorst EM, Palou A, Oliver P. Peripheral blood mononuclear cells as a source to detect markers of homeostatic alterations caused by the intake of diets with an unbalanced macronutrient composition. J Nutr Biochem. 2015; 26: 398–407.
15. Graham I, Atar D, Borch-Johnsen K, Boysen G, Burell G, Cifkova R, et al. European guidelines on cardiovascular disease prevention in clinical practice: executive summary. Atherosclerosis 2007; 194: 1–45.
16. Brennan L. Metabolomics in nutrition research: current status and perspectives. Biochem Soc Trans 2013; 41: 670–3.
17. de Mello VD, Kolehmanien M, Schwab U, Pulkkinen L, Uusitupa M. Gene expression of peripheral blood mononuclear cells as a tool in dietary intervention studies: what do we know so far? Mol Nutr Food Res 2012; 56: 1160–72.
18. Bouwens M, Afman LA, Muller M. Fasting induces changes in peripheral blood mononuclear cell gene expression profiles related to increases in fatty acid beta-oxidation: functional role of peroxisome proliferator activated receptor alpha in human peripheral blood mononuclear cells. Am J Clin Nutr 2007; 86: 1515–23.
19. Caimari A, Oliver P, Keijer J, Palou A. Peripheral blood mononuclear cells as a model to study the response of energy homeostasis-related genes to acute changes in feeding conditions. OMICS. 2010; 14: 129–41.
20. Caimari A, Oliver P, Rodenburg W, Keijer J, Palou A. Slc27a2 expression in peripheral blood mononuclear cells as a molecular marker for overweight development. Int J Obes (Lond). 2010; 34: 831–9.
21. Rudkowska I, Raymond C, Ponton A, Jacques H, Lavigne C, Holub BJ, et al. Validation of the use of peripheral blood mononuclear cells as surrogate model for skeletal muscle tissue in nutrigenomic studies. OMICS 2011; 15: 1–7.
22. Oliver P, Reynes B, Caimari A, Palou A. Peripheral blood mononuclear cells: a potential source of homeostatic imbalance markers associated with obesity development. Pflugers Arch. 2013; 465: 459–68.
23. Reynes B, Diaz-Rua R, Cifre M, Oliver P, Palou A. Peripheral blood mononuclear cells as a potential source of biomarkers to test the efficacy of weight-loss strategies. Obesity (Silver Spring). 2015; 23: 28–31.
24. Reynes B, Garcia-Ruiz E, Palou A, Oliver P. The intake of high-fat diets induces an obesogenic-like gene expression profile in peripheral blood mononuclear cells, which is reverted by dieting. Br J Nutr. 2016; 115: 1887–95.
25. Wittwer J, Rubio-Aliaga I, Hoeft B, Bendik I, Weber P, Daniel H. Nutrigenomics in human intervention studies: current status, lessons learned and future perspectives. Mol Nutr Food Res 2011; 55: 341–58.
26. Muller M, Kersten S. Nutrigenomics: goals and strategies. Nat Rev Genet 2003; 4: 315–22.
27. Dam-Larsen S, Franzmann M, Andersen IB, Christoffersen P, Jensen LB, Sorensen TI, et al. Long term prognosis of fatty liver: risk of chronic liver disease and death. Gut 2004; 53: 750–5.
28. Diaz-Rua R, Garcia-Ruiz E, Caimari A, Palou A, Oliver P. Sustained exposure to diets with an unbalanced macronutrient proportion alters key genes involved in energy homeostasis and obesity-related metabolic parameters in rats. Food Funct. 2014; 5: 3117–31.
29. Matthews DR, Hosker JP, Rudenski AS, Naylor BA, Treacher DF, Turner RC. Homeostasis model assessment: insulin resis-

tance and beta-cell function from fasting plasma glucose and insulin concentrations in man. Diabetologia 1985; 28: 412–19.
30. Folch J, Lees M, Sloane Stanley GH. A simple method for the isolation and purification of total lipides from animal tissues. J Biol Chem 1957; 226: 497–509.
31. Caimari A, del Bas JM, Crescenti A, Arola L. Low doses of grape seed procyanidins reduce adiposity and improve the plasma lipid profile in hamsters. Int J Obes (Lond). 2013; 37: 576–83.
32. Livak KJ, Schmittgen TD. Analysis of relative gene expression data using real-time quantitative PCR and the 2(-Delta Delta C(T)) method. Methods 2001; 25: 402–8.
33. Marchesini G, Brizi M, Bianchi G, Tomassetti S, Bugianesi E, Lenzi M, et al. Nonalcoholic fatty liver disease: a feature of the metabolic syndrome. Diabetes 2001; 50: 1844–50.
34. Thomas EL, Parkinson JR, Frost GS, Goldstone AP, Dore CJ, McCarthy JP, et al. The missing risk: MRI and MRS phenotyping of abdominal adiposity and ectopic fat. Obesity (Silver Spring) 2012; 20: 76–87.
35. Bielohuby M, Menhofer D, Kirchner H, Stoehr BJ, Muller TD, Stock P, et al. Induction of ketosis in rats fed low-carbohydrate, high-fat diets depends on the relative abundance of dietary fat and protein. Am J Physiol Endocrinol Metab 2011; 300: E65–76.
36. Liu Z, Patil IY, Jiang T, Sancheti H, Walsh JP, Stiles BL, et al. High-fat diet induces hepatic insulin resistance and impairment of synaptic plasticity. PLoS One 2015; 10: e0128274.
37. Dvorak RV, DeNino WF, Ades PA, Poehlman ET. Phenotypic characteristics associated with insulin resistance in metabolically obese but normal-weight young women. Diabetes 1999; 48: 2210–14.
38. Adam-Perrot A, Clifton P, Brouns F. Low-carbohydrate diets: nutritional and physiological aspects. Obes Rev 2006; 7: 49–58.
39. Fukao T, Lopaschuk GD, Mitchell GA. Pathways and control of ketone body metabolism: on the fringe of lipid biochemistry. Prostaglandins Leukot Essent Fatty Acids 2004; 70: 243–51.
40. Otero YF, Stafford JM, McGuinness OP. Pathway-selective insulin resistance and metabolic disease: the importance of nutrient flux. J Biol Chem 2014; 289: 20462–9.
41. Koo SH. Nonalcoholic fatty liver disease: molecular mechanisms for the hepatic steatosis. Clin Mol Hepatol 2013; 19: 210–15.
42. Diaz-Rua R, van Schothorst EM, Keijer J, Palou A, Oliver P. Isocaloric high-fat feeding directs hepatic metabolism to handling of nutrient imbalance promoting liver fat deposition. Int J Obes (Lond). 2016; 40: 1250–9.
43. Choi KM, Cho HJ, Choi HY, Yang SJ, Yoo HJ, Seo JA, et al. Higher mortality in metabolically obese normal-weight people than in metabolically healthy obese subjects in elderly Koreans. Clin Endocrinol (Oxf) 2013; 79: 364–70.

*Andreu Palou
Laboratory of Molecular Biology
Nutrition and Biotechnology
Universitat de les Illes Balears
Cra. Valldemossa Km 7.5
ES-07122 Palma de Mallorca
Spain
Email: andreu.palou@uib.es

12

Production and evaluation of mineral and nutrient contents, chemical composition, and sensory properties of ice creams fortified with laboratory-prepared peach fibre

Filiz Yangılar*

Department of Nutrition and Dietetics, Faculty of Health Sciences, Erzincan University, Erzincan, Turkey

Abstract

Background: In the coming years, a nutraceutical food may provide both physical and mental benefits that are commonly attributed to the active components of the food.

Objective: In this study, we determined the nutrient and mineral contents, sensory properties, and physical and chemical characteristics of ice creams manufactured using peach fibre at different concentrations (1 and 2%).

Method: A total of five experimental groups were formed: two types (from peach peel and pulp) of flour, two fibre concentrations (1 and 2%), and a control group without fibres.

Results: Flour obtained from peach pulp and peel was found to have a significant ($p < 0.05$) effect on the chemical composition and elemental composition of ice cream samples, especially the rates of Ca, K, Mg, and P, which increased in the samples depending on the content of peach fibre. Sensory ratings and acceptability of ice creams decreased significantly with increasing peach peel fibre, whereas ice creams made with C (control) and B1 (ice creams made from 1% peach pulp fibre) was the highest scored by the panellists.

Conclusions: Peach fibre concentrates might be used as a good source of nutraceutical ingredients.

Keywords: *ice cream*; *peach fibre*; *chemical composition*

Peach (*Prunus persica* L.) fruits have high economic and nutritional value. Carbohydrates, organic acids, minerals, and dietary fibre (DF) are among the major components of peach fruit, which contribute to the nutritional quality of both fruits and juices (1, 2). Peach fruits have aperient properties, are appropriate to prevent costiveness, and are used for the treatment of duodenum ulcers. Phenolic acids, flavonoids, and anthocyanin compounds serve as major sources of potential antioxidants in peach fruit, which might be responsible for these therapeutic functions (2). Peaches are a tropical fruit, which means that the ripening process is triggered and driven by a plant hormone called ethylene. This is responsible for its short shelf-life and represents a serious constraint for its efficient handling and transportation (3, 4).

DF can provide a multitude of functional properties when they are incorporated into food systems (5). But, there are little data dealing with the study of the functionality of DF in ice creams (6). To the best of our knowledge, no data have been published regarding the effect of drying technique on physicochemical characteristics of fibre obtained from peach or about possible differences on physical properties and functionality of peach fibre because of the type of tissue used (peel or pulp) (7). Fibre addition contributes to the modification and improvement of the texture, sensory characteristics, and shelf-life of food because of its water-binding capacity, gel-forming ability, and fat mimetic, antisticking, anticlumping, texturising, and thickening effects (6).

Peach fibre is a valuable nutrition component and its non-use for human diet constitutes a real nutritional loss because peach fibres contain extractable bioactive compounds which can be used as value-added materials. The objective of the present study is to evaluate the functional properties of fibres obtained from peach peel and pulp for possible enrichment of the quality and nutritional contents of ice creams.

Materials and methods

Materials

Cow's milk and cream were purchased from the Research and Application Farm of Atatürk University, Erzurum, Turkey. The peach fruits were purchased from a supermarket in Erzurum, Turkey, and classified visually for colour and physical damage. Sugar, salep, and emulsifier (mono- and diglycerides) were obtained from the local market. Skimmed milk powder was purchased from a commercial company (Pınar Dairy Products Co., Istanbul, Turkey).

Preparation of peach peel and pulp fibre

The total weight of the peaches used was 4 kg, and the average diameter of each peach was 7 cm. Pulp and peel were stripped off after each peach fruit was dipped in water and washed. Pulp and peel were submitted to a juice extraction using a domestic appliance with the purpose of eliminating a great part of the water content and its solubility. The remaining solids were contacted with ethanol (96%, v/v) and stirred (600 rpm) for 15 min. Finally, ethanol was discarded and a portion of each remnant (pulp remnant or peel remnant) was dried under 30°C forced air convection for 7 h. As a result of the process, two types of flour were produced: type A flour, obtained from peach peel, and B flour, obtained from peach pulp. The two types of flour were milled in a Mill Laboratory at 2,890 rpm and then at 5,000 rpm until they could pass through a 0.2-mm sieve to recover the peach fibre concentrates and stored at −18°C for subsequent analyses and incorporation studies (7).

Flour yield

Yield was calculated by dividing the amount of flour produced by the amount of peach used, and the results were converted to g/kg (g of flour per kg of peach).

Chemical and physical composition of DFs

Moisture content was measured according to the Association of Official Analytical Chemists (AOAC) method (8). Ash was analysed by combusting the sample in a muffle furnace at 550°C for 4 h. The residue was dissolved in HNO_3 and the mineral constituents (Ca, K, Na, Mg, P, and Fe) were determined using an inductively coupled plasma optical emission spectrophotometer (Optima 2100 DV, ICP/OES, Perkin-Elmer, Shelton, CT). The Kjeldahl method was used to evaluate the protein content (9). The flour's pH was determined using a pH meter (Mettler-Toledo AG 8603, Schwerzenbach, Switzerland) (10). The colour of the flour was monitored using a Minolta colorimeter (Chroma Meter CR-200, Osaka, Japan). DF, that also accounts for structural variability and associated health benefits, has recently been defined by CODEX Alimentarius to be 'carbohydrate polymers', which have been obtained from food raw material by physical, enzymatic, or chemical means and which have been shown to have a physiological effect of benefit to health as demonstrated by generally accepted scientific evidence to competent authorities (11, 12). Insoluble dietary fibres (IDFs) and soluble dietary fibres (SDFs) were assessed using the method of Prosky et al. (13). In this method, samples were enzymatically digested under the same conditions as used in the AOAC official method, and the total dietary fibre (TDF) was calculated as the sum of IDFs and SDFs. Total phenolic content was determined for peach peel and pulp flour according to Bunzel et al. (14). The total phenolic contents were evaluated using the Folin–Ciocalteu method (15).

Water- and oil-holding capacity

A volume of 25 mL of distilled water or commercial olive oil was mixed with 1 g of dry sample. The mixture tubes were centrifuged at 3,000*g* for 20 min and then the supernatant was poured out. After that, the tubes were drained for 10 min by putting them at an angle of 45°. The residue was weighed and water-holding capacity (WHC, g of water per 100 g of sample) and oil-holding capacity (OHC, g of oil per 100 g of sample) were calculated according to Gould et al. (16) and Caprez et al. (17), respectively.

Manufacture of ice creams

The ice cream samples were prepared at the Seref patisserie, Erzurum, Turkey. First, the fat content of cow's milk was adjusted to 6% by adding cream, and the prepared milk was separated into five equal amounts of 2 kg each. Skimmed milk powder (125 g), sugar (405 g), a stabiliser (salep; 16.2 g), and emulsifiers (mono- and diglycerides; 6.75 g) were added to these milk samples. Flour samples obtained both from peach peel and pulp were also added to the milk samples (65°C) at two different mass fractions (1 and 2%). The mixtures were subjected to pasteurisation at 85°C for 25 min and stored at 4°C for 24 h, after which they were placed in an ice cream machine to freeze and then hardened at −22°C for 24 h. They remained at −18°C during all physical, chemical, mineral, and sensory analyses.

Ice cream analysis

Dry matter, fat and ash contents, acidity (°SH), and pH of ice cream samples were determined using the method of Demirci and Gündüz (18). Mineral contents (Ca, K, Na, P, S, Mg, Fe, Mn, Zn, and Ni) of ice cream samples were described by Guler (19). Overrun was detected by the method proposed by Jimenez et al. (20) and calculated using the following equation:

$$\text{Overrum} = [V\,(\text{ice cream}) - V(\text{mix})/V\,(\text{mix})] \times 100$$
$(V\text{: volume})$

Time period (sec) from the initial dripping to complete melting was determined using the method of Güven and Karaca (21). Samples of 25 g were heated to melt at room temperature (20°C) by putting them in a beaker capped with a 0.2-cm wire mesh screen. Initial dripping and complete melting times of the samples were calculated in seconds. Viscosity of the ice cream samples was measured at 4°C using a digital Brookfield viscometer (22).

The colour parameters of ice cream samples were obtained by measuring L^* (brightness, 0: black, 100: white), a^* (+: red, −: green), and b^* (+: yellow, −: blue) values using the method of described in (23).

Sensory assessment

Eight professional panellists participated in the study and evaluated the ice cream samples using a score test for flavour, body and texture, colour and appearance, resistance to melting, and general acceptability. Hardened ice cream samples were tested at a serving temperature of −10°C and given scores for their sensory characteristics using a scale ranging from 1 (poor) to 9 (excellent). All panellists were preferred to be non-smokers (24).

Statistical analysis

In total, five experimental groups were formed: two types (from peach peel and pulp) of flour, two fibre concentrations (1 and 2%), and a control group without fibres. Statistical analysis was carried out using SPSS 15.0 (SPSS, Inc., Chicago, IL) (25) software. Data were subjected to a multiple analysis of variance, and the average values were compared using Duncan's multiple range test.

Results and discussion

The mean yield of peach peel and peach pulp flour was calculated to be 57.1 and 100.5 g/kg, respectively. Pulp was found to give a larger amount of flour than peel.

Chemical and physical characteristics of DFs

Chemical compositions of fibre samples produced from peach peel and pulp are given in Table 1. Peach pulp flour was found to have higher moisture content (11.36%) than peach peel flour (9.21%). Abdul Aziz et al. (26) stated that mango pulp flours have consistently higher moisture content than mango peel flours, and moisture content increased in the pulp as the ripening process progressed and are in agreement with our report.

As observed in Table 1, the ash content of peach peel and pulp flour was found to be 4.3 and 4.11%, respectively. Rodríquez-Ambriz et al. (27) found that banana flour had an ash content of 4.4%, whereas Juarez-Garcia et al. (28) found this rate to be 4.7%. These findings were in agreement with the findings of the present study.

The WHC value obtained for the peach peel flour was lower than that obtained for the peach pulp flour, and that found (21.87 g water per g dry sample) in the present study was lower than that reported by Grigelmo-Miguel and Martín-Belloso (29) in peach DF (between 9.2 and 12.1 g of water per g of dry sample). de Escalada Pla et al. (7) found that the WHC value of peach pulp fibre was 24 g water per g dry sample, whereas the WHC value of peach peel fibre was 25 g water per g dry sample. OHC is among the important functional properties of peach flour and was found in the peach peel (2.88 g oil per g dry sample) and pulp flour samples (1.76 g oil per g dry sample) in our study. When compared with the results of previous studies, the peach pulp flour values were lower than the value of 2.2 g of oil per g of dry sample found in the study of Rodríquez-Ambriz et al. (27). It was stated by de Escalada Pla et al. (7) that the OHC value in peach pulp fibre was 1.81 g oil per g dry sample and in peach peel fibre was 2.03 g oil per g dry sample. Calvache et al. (30) reported high values of OHC in DF from peach bagasse *P. persica* L., which is in agreement with the results obtained in this study.

The mean L^*, a^*, and b^* values were found to be 58, 11.42, and 37.49 in peach peel flour, and 79.7, 6.99, and 28.71 in peach pulp flour, respectively. It was found by monitoring the samples in the present study that the flour obtained from peach peel had a darker colour than that produced from pulp. Because of the possible existence of some browning contributor enzymes, such as polyphenol oxidase, and the occurrence of the Maillard reaction (31), a significant colour change was observed during the peel drying process in the present study, from which dark brown powder was produced from the peel. The L^*, a^*, and b^* values were found to be 76, 5.5, and 29.39 in peach pulp flour, and 56, 12.2, and 34 in peach peel flour, respectively (7), and these results are in agreement with the results of the present study.

Table 1. The chemical and physical properties of peach peel and pulp flour

	Peach peel (type A)	Peach pulp (type B)
Chemical analysis		
Moisture (g/100 g)	9.21 ± 0.50	11.36 ± 0.20
Ash (g/100 g)	4.3 ± 0.28	4.11 ± 0.37
pH	4.21 ± 0.43	3.58 ± 0.64
Protein (g/100 g)	7.51 ± 0.71	6.90 ± 0.20
Total phenolic content[c]	1002 ± 1.91	1566 ± 0.91
Total dietary fibre (g/100 g)	57.48 ± 0.25	51.05 ± 0.24
Insoluble dietary fibre (g/100 g)	53.15 ± 0.41	46.21 ± 0.63
Soluble dietary fibre (g/100 g)	12.00 ± 1.10	8.53 ± 0.72
Minerals (mg/kg)		
Ca	88.36 ± 0.18	53.60 ± 0.37
K	1269 ± 0.83	1744 ± 0.03
Mg	97.72 ± 0.15	55.30 ± 0.43
Zn	0.54 ± 0.27	0.27 ± 0.52
Fe	7.14 ± 0.29	2.43 ± 0.50
Physical analysis		
L^*	58 ± 1.00	79.7 ± 0.06
a^*	11.42 ± 0.17	6.99 ± 0.10
b^*	37.49 ± 0.71	28.71 ± 0.46
WHC[a]	13.10 ± 0.92	21.87 ± 0.70
OHC[b]	2.88 ± 0.64	1.76 ± 0.32

L^*, lightness; a^*, redness (+); b^*, blueness (−).
[a]Water-holding capacity (g water per g sample).
[b]Oil-holding capacity (g oil per g sample).
[c]mg/100 g of fibre concentrates.

Antioxidants play an important role in the prevention of oxidative stress-related diseases (32). Quantitatively, the main dietary antioxidants are polyphenols, followed by vitamins, and carotenoids (33). Goñi et al. (34) stated that polyphenols associated with polysaccharides and proteins in cell walls are significant constituents of DF. Table 1 shows the polyphenol contents of the peach peel and pulp flour types. The pulp flour (1,566 mg/100 g) was found to have the highest content of polyphenols. The total phenolics of the pulp and peel of three different peach fruit varieties (Golden, Shireen, and Shahpasand) was determined by Manzoor et al. (2). Among the different peach varieties tested, the peel and pulp of cv. Golden exhibited the highest phenolic contents (1,354.5 and 881.3 mg gallic acid equivalents (GAE) per 100 of DW, respectively). The findings given above are in accordance with those found in the present study.

As observed in Table 1, peach peel fibres are rich in protein (7.51 g/100 g). Grigelmo-Miguel and Martín-Belloso (29) reported that the protein content (5.44–6.29%) of peach fibre concentrate was also low and that it was the only component, among those studied, that decreased throughout the peach harvest time. Ahmed et al. (35) reported that the sodium content was significantly lower than other minerals (55–86 mg/kg); however, the fibres were rich in potassium.

TDF content in the peach peel flour was found to be 57.48% (Table 1), the majority of which was represented by IDF (53.15%) and the rest by SDF (12.00%). Compared with this finding, in a fibre-rich fraction of chia (*Salvia hispanica*), Alfredo et al. (36) reported TDF, IDF, and SDF contents to be 56.46, 53.45, and 3.01 g per 100 g respectively, whereas in orange peel were found, determined by Chau and Huang (37), to be 57, 47.6, and 9.4 g per 100 g, respectively. These rates were 64.1, 55.2, and 8.9 g per 100 g, respectively, found by Ruales and Zumba (38) in guava and were 66.8, 58.6, and 8.2 g per 100 g, respectively, found by Yangılar (39) in green banana flour. The findings given above are in agreement with those found in the present study.

Physical and chemical characteristics of ice cream samples

The results of some physical and chemical analyses and mineral contents of ice cream samples are given in Tables 2 and 3. The dry matter content of the control sample was lower than that of other samples at significant levels ($p < 0.05$). The dry matter rate of ice creams increased with the addition of peach fibre. As observed in Table 2, the addition of DF significantly affected the fat and acidity values ($p < 0.05$). The pH values of ice cream samples ranged from 5.89 to 6.51 in samples with fibre.

Viscosity, accepted to be among the significant characteristics of an ice cream mixture, may result in good body and texture properties in the production process of ice cream. From this point of view, it is important to measure viscosity to determine how peach flour may affect the characteristics of an ice cream mixture. As shown in Fig. 1, a lowest viscosity value was obtained in the control sample (3,100 cP) and the highest in sample A (with 2% of peach peel flour added; 4,600 cP). These findings are in agreement with the results of Hwang et al. (40) for ice cream samples with grape wine lees, Dervisoglu and Yazici (5) for ice cream samples with citrus fibre, Cakmakci et al. (41) for ice creams with oleaster (*Elaeagnus angustifolia* L.) flour, and Yangılar (42) for ice cream samples containing date fibre.

The lightness (L^*) values of ice cream samples were close to each other, but they were significantly higher for the A1 and A2 samples than for others (Table 2). All of the samples taken into consideration were found to have negative greenness rates, whereas B1 and B2 samples seemed to be similar to and sometimes higher than the others. The colour rates of the samples were affected favourably by an increase in the concentration of peach fibre ($p < 0.05$). Samples had negative a^* (greenness) values, and the A2 (4.13) sample was significantly higher than the other samples. The b^* values were increased by the

Table 2. Some chemical and physical properties of ice cream samples with peach fibre

Analysis	C	A1	A2	B1	B2
Dry matter (%)	40.01 ± 0.01^a	40.45 ± 0.04^a	41.21 ± 0.16^b	40.33 ± 0.30^a	41.05 ± 0.05^b
Ash (%)	0.98 ± 0.00^a	1.01 ± 0.02^{ab}	1.14 ± 0.03^d	1.07 ± 0.02^{bc}	1.11 ± 0.02^{cd}
Fat (%)	6.55 ± 0.07^b	6.11 ± 0.01^a	5.98 ± 0.02^a	6.00 ± 0.03^a	6.06 ± 0.08^a
Acidity (%)	0.30 ± 0.00^{ab}	0.31 ± 0.02^c	0.34 ± 0.03^d	0.28 ± 0.01^a	0.30 ± 0.00^{ab}
pH	6.51 ± 0.02^c	6.10 ± 0.14^b	6.15 ± 0.04^b	6.04 ± 0.04^{ab}	5.89 ± 0.04^a
L^*	87.17 ± 0.24^e	78.18 ± 0.28^b	74.85 ± 0.37^a	83.87 ± 0.98^d	80.30 ± 0.43^c
a^*	3.26 ± 0.09^a	4.02 ± 0.03^{bc}	4.13 ± 0.01^c	3.81 ± 0.10^b	4.00 ± 0.00^{bc}
b^*	9.69 ± 0.05^a	10.84 ± 0.09^c	11.07 ± 0.21^d	10.12 ± 0.17^{ab}	10.55 ± 0.57^{bc}

*Mean values followed by different letters in the same row are significantly different ($p < 0.05$).

C, control without fibre; A1, ice cream made with 1% (w/w) peach peel fibre; A2, ice cream made with 2% (w/w) peach peel fibre; B1, ice cream made with 1% (w/w) peach pulp fibre; B2, ice cream made with 2% (w/w) peach pulp fibre.

Table 3. Elemental composition (mg/kg) of the ash in ice creams with peach fibre

Concentrations of minerals	C	A1	A2	B1	B2
Ca	1981.11 ± 7.96^{a}	2157 ± 26.82^{c}	2256 ± 8.57^{d}	2101 ± 2.18^{b}	2104 ± 5.65^{b}
K	2050 ± 14.14^{a}	2174.05 ± 25.18^{b}	2435.33 ± 49.96^{e}	2263 ± 36.76^{c}	2372.82 ± 32.97^{d}
Na	488.30 ± 3.81^{d}	463.24 ± 4.58^{c}	438.78 ± 0.82^{b}	413.96 ± 5.60^{a}	459.49 ± 2.24^{c}
P	1038.45 ± 9.12^{a}	2224.21 ± 7.19^{b}	2342.78 ± 37.85^{c}	2518.21 ± 36.18^{d}	2618.67 ± 29.25^{e}
S	541.32 ± 1.87^{c}	628.60 ± 2.12^{e}	590.18 ± 1.61^{d}	494.32 ± 4.70^{a}	513.56 ± 4.73^{b}
Mg	124.65 ± 0.49^{a}	161.45 ± 1.47^{b}	188.01 ± 2.80^{d}	179.35 ± 0.91^{c}	192.85 ± 2.04^{d}
Fe	10.47 ± 0.16^{a}	12.18 ± 0.26^{b}	12.58 ± 0.18^{c}	11.01 ± 0.04^{a}	14.43 ± 1.72^{d}
Mn	0.46 ± 0.01^{a}	0.54 ± 0.03^{b}	0.69 ± 0.01^{c}	0.55 ± 0.05^{ab}	0.66 ± 0.04^{bc}
Zn	73.54 ± 0.65^{a}	99.85 ± 0.21^{b}	112.21 ± 3.12^{d}	100.52 ± 0.29^{b}	106.77 ± 3.50^{c}
Ni	1.59 ± 0.01^{a}	1.60 ± 0.02^{a}	1.69 ± 0.02^{c}	1.61 ± 0.04^{b}	1.70 ± 0.01^{c}

*Mean values followed by different letters in the same row are significantly different ($p < 0.05$).
C, control without fibre; A1, ice cream made with 1% (w/w) peach peel fibre; A2, ice cream made with 2% (w/w) peach peel fibre; B1, ice cream made with 1% (w/w) peach pulp fibre; B2, ice cream made with 2% (w/w) peach pulp fibre.

addition of peach peel fibre. Samples C (9.69) gave the lowest b^* rate, whereas the highest rate was received from the A2 (11.07) samples. Dervisoglu and Yazici (5) reported that the addition of citrus fibre increased the colour properties; these results are in agreement with the results of the present study.

Overrun and melting are associated with the volume of air involved in the manufacturing process. This property can shape the structure of the final product because the air present in the ice cream can provide it with a light texture and affect some physical properties, such as melting and hardness (43). All of the ice cream samples in the present study showed much lower overrun values (31.8–42.35%) compared with the values reported in the literature (80–120%). Although the addition of peach fibre lowered the overrun rate of the ice cream samples ($p > 0.05$), the control samples showed higher overrun rates than the peach flour samples (Fig. 2). Because the viscosity of the ice cream increased with fibre samples, it was possible that less air was incorporated into the ice cream mixture with fibre during batch freezing, which resulted in a lower overrun compared with the control (without fibre). The results of the study carried out by El-Samahy et al. (44) showed that overrun decreased in ice cream as cactus pulp was added, which could be dependent on the increase in the viscosity of the mixture. Hwang et al. (40) reported that the overrun values of ice cream samples decreased significantly with the addition of grape wine lees. It was found by Sun-Waterhouse et al. (45) that the overrun rate of ice cream containing green

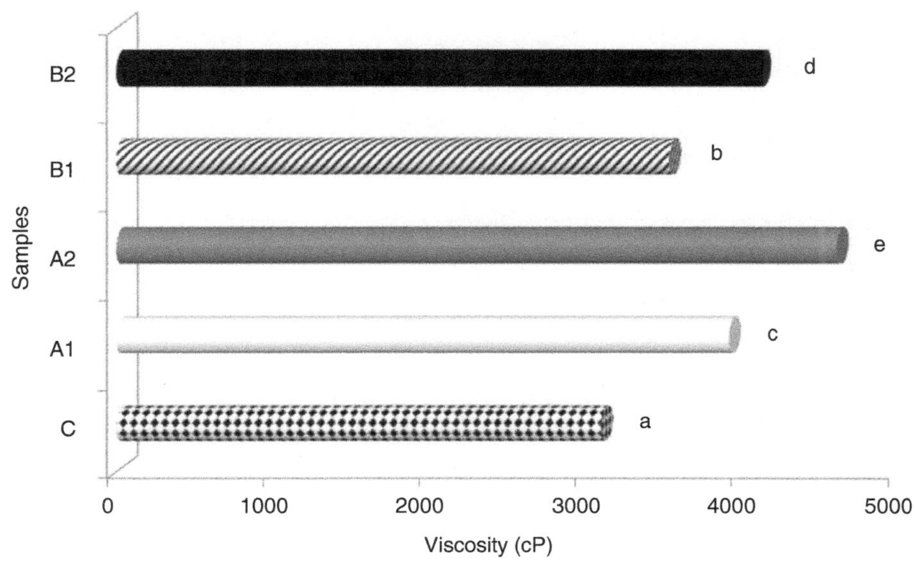

Fig. 1. Viscosity values (20 rpm) of ice cream mixes produced using peach fibre. Different letters above the bars indicate significant differences by Duncan multiple comparison test ($p < 0.05$).

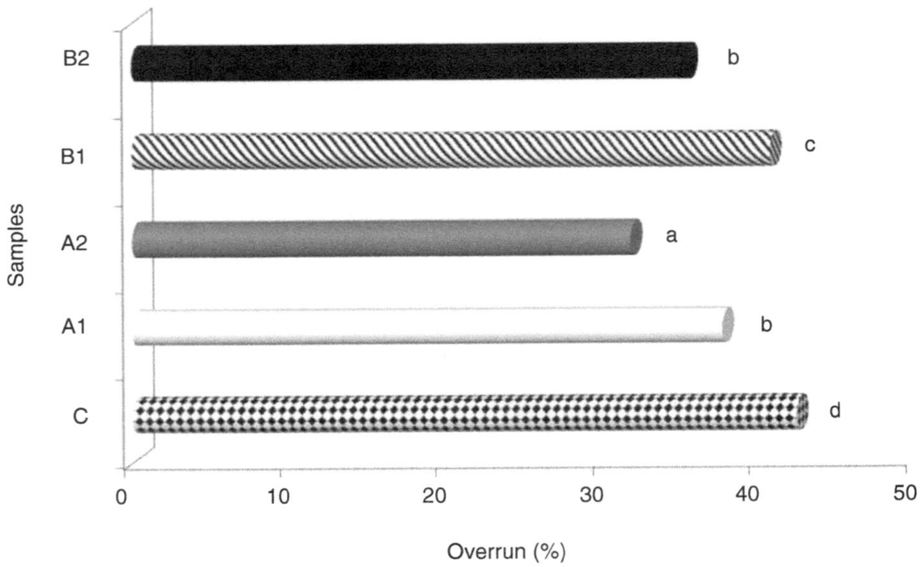

Fig. 2. Overrun values of ice cream mixes produced using peach fibre. Different letters above the bars indicate significant differences by Duncan multiple comparison test ($p < 0.05$).

kiwifruit was 90.5%, which is higher than that in the present study. Results similar to those found in the present study were found by Cakmakci et al. (41) who studied producing ice cream with oleaster (*E. angustifolia* L.) flour.

As observed in Fig. 3, the length of the time period required for the melting process to be completed was found to be significantly longer in B2 samples with the addition of fibre content. Such a situation may result from the addition of some components with the ability to absorb water in B. The ice cream with B2 revealed the longest complete melting time (0.43 g/min), whereas the shortest complete melting time (0.37 g/min) was shown by the A1 sample. It was stated by Akin et al. (22) that the reason for a decrease in the melting rate of ice cream with added inulin might be because of the ability of inulin to prevent water molecules from moving freely. B (1 and 2%) concentrations affected the initial dripping time positively (Table 2).

The results of the present study indicate that the length of the time period until the initial dripping became prolonged as the fibre content of the ice cream samples

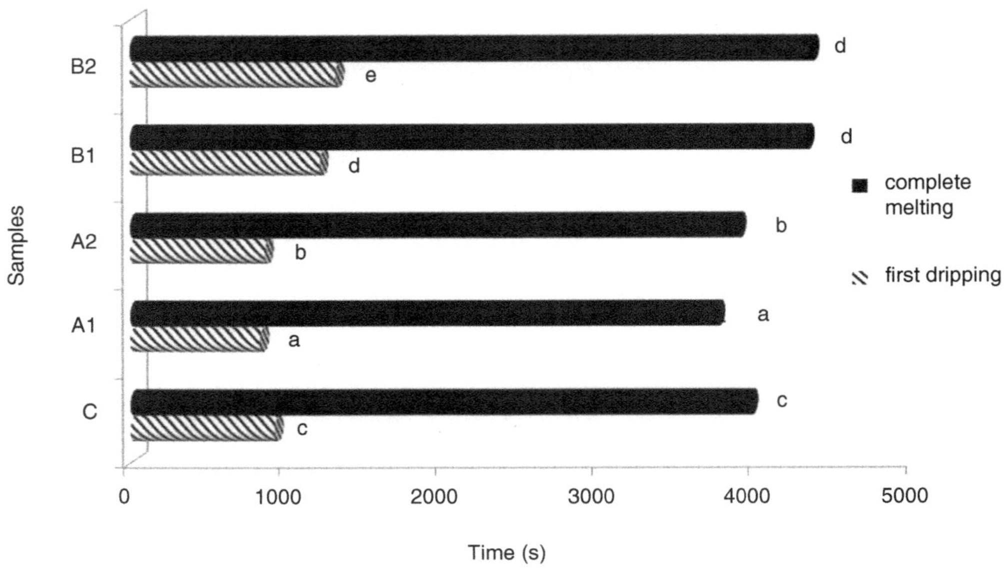

Fig. 3. First dripping and complete melting times of ice cream samples with added peach fibre. Different letters above the bars indicate significant differences by Duncan multiple comparison test ($p < 0.05$).

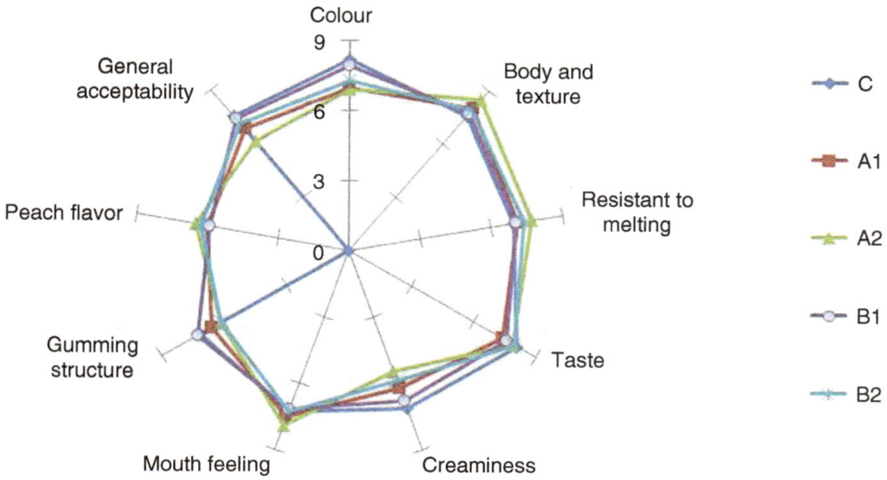

Fig. 4. Some sensorial properties of ice cream samples.

increased ($p < 0.05$). Dervisoglu and Yazici (5) reported that ice cream samples with citrus fibre had longer dripping times and a similar result was also reported by Yangılar (39) in ice cream with green banana peel flour.

Table 3 shows the changes in the mineral contents of the ice cream samples. The contents of K, Mg, and P in ice cream samples significantly increased, and statistically significant differences were found in terms of the major element contents, such as Ca, K, P, and Mg, between the samples, except for the S concentration in all ice cream samples. The increase in these mineral contents may be because of the high K, Mg, and P concentrations in peach fruit. As observed in Table 3, the K content of peach peel was between 2174.05 and 2435.33 mg/kg, and the A2 sample in the present study revealed the highest K rate. Manzoor et al. (2) reported that mineral analysis results were in agreement with those of Basar (46) who reported that K was the most abundant nutrient in fruits of different peach varieties, followed by Mg, Ca, Fe, Zn, and Mn. The A1 sample gave the highest S rate (628.60 mg/kg), whereas the B1 sample had the lowest (494.32 mg/kg). In our study, the Na values of ice cream were found to be decreased in peach fibre-added samples. If we evaluate the results only in the study, we see that the decrease is seen in the fibre additive rather than in the control; however, the highest increase is seen in the Na rate coming from the peel flour. A similar result was reported by Dağdemir (47) for vegetable marrow (*Cucurbita pepo* L.) added to ice cream. Decreasing Na in the human diet may provide protection from hypertension in people who are sensitive to high levels of Na. A2 revealed the highest Zn content (112.21 mg/kg). It was stated by Wu et al. (48) that Zn could play some vital roles by serving as a non-enzymatic antioxidant and protecting cells from oxidative damage. Even if peach fibre contains small doses of Fe, Zn, Ni, and Mn, which carry the capability of contributing to the antioxidant activity of fruit (49), in the present study, when added, fibre seems to rise significantly the Fe, Zn, and Mn contents of the ice cream samples ($p < 0.05$). Similar results were reported for Cape gooseberry (*Physalis peruviana* L.) added to ice cream by Erkaya et al. (50) and for the ice cream samples with date fibre by Yangılar (42).

Sensory evaluation of ice creams

The results of the sensory evaluation of the ice cream samples on a scale from 1 (poor) to 9 (excellent) are shown in a radar plot in Fig. 4. Fortifying ice cream with DF had a significant effect on all sensory properties overall. All of the fibre-enriched samples received higher scores for total evaluation in terms of sensory characteristics ($p < 0.05$). Colour scores were significantly different, between 6.95 and 8.20. The lowest score was determined for sample A2. Peach fibre gave a slight yellowish colour to ice cream samples. The A1 and A2 samples containing peach peel fibre showed relatively high scores in terms of organoleptic characteristics such as body and texture, resistance to melting, and mouth feeling compared with the control group. The B2 sample had a similar mouth feeling, showed resistance to melting, and gave the same generally acceptable ratings as the control sample. The highest values for general acceptability belonged to the C, B1, B2, A1, and A2 samples. Processing of peach into fibre presents an excellent opportunity for use as a functional ingredient to ensure its extended consumption and reduce wastage.

Conclusions

The enrichment of ice cream with peach fibre is an effective way to enhance nutritional and physiological aspects by influencing the rheological and thermal properties of the final product. Peach fibre alone or with ice cream stabilisers was successfully used in ice cream production. The addition of peach peel fibre affected moisture, fat, acidity, ash, and viscosity positively; on the contrary, meltdown, colour, and overrun were affected negatively. Given peach fibre's nutritive value and pleasant flavour, it may be used as a suitable source of natural additive in ice cream production to enhance nutritional values. In our study, among the two parts (peel and pulp) analysed, the present results also revealed that peach pulp exhibited higher moisture, phenolic content, and WHC value compared with that of the peel, indicating that removal of peel from such fruits may induce significant nutrient losses. Therefore, the intake of functional foods along with their fibres can be more beneficial to increased nutritional properties of foods such as ice cream. Therefore, our study may provide a base of knowledge for future research.

Conflict of interest and funding
There is no conflict of interest to declare.

References

1. Versari A, Castellari M, Parpinello GP, Riponi C, Galassi S. Characterization of peach juices obtained from cultivars Redhaven, Suncrest and Maria Marta grown in Italy. Food Chem 2002; 76: 181–5.
2. Manzoor M, Anwar F, Mahmood Z, Rashid U, Ashraf M. Variation in minerals, phenolics and antioxidant activity of peel and pulp of different varieties of peach (*Prunus persica* L.) fruit from Pakistan. Molecules 2012; 17(6): 6491–506.
3. Hussain PR, Meena RS, Dar MA, Wani AM. Studies on enhancing the keeping quality of peach (*Prunus persica* Bausch) Cv. Elbert a by gamma-irradiation. Radiat Phys Chem 2008; 77(4): 473–81.
4. Kim KH, Kim MS, Kim HG, Yook HS. Inactivation of contaminated fungi and antioxidant effects of peach (*Prunus persica* L. Batsch cv Dangeumdo) by 0.5–2 kGy gamma irradiation. Radiat Phys Chem 2010; 79(4): 495–501.
5. Dervişoğlu M, Yazıcı F. Note. The effect of citrus fibre on the physical, chemical and sensory properties of ice cream. Food Sci Technol Int 2006; 12(2): 159–64.
6. Soukoulis C, Lebesi D, Tzia C. Enrichment of ice cream with dietary fibre: effects on rheological properties, ice crystallisation and glass transition phenomena. Food Chem 2009; 115(2): 665–71.
7. de Escalada Pla MF, González P, Sette P, Portillo F, Rojas AM, Gerschenson LN. Effect of processing on physico-chemical characteristics of dietary fibre concentrates obtained from peach (*Prunus persica* L.) peel and pulp. Food Res Int 2012; 49(1): 184–92.
8. AOAC (1997). Official methods of analysis. Washington, DC: Association of Official Analytical Chemists.
9. AOAC (1990). Official methods of analysis (15th ed.). Washington, DC: Association of Official Analytical Chemists.
10. Suntharalingam S, Ravindran G. Physical and biochemical properties of green banana flour. Plant Foods Hum Nutr 1993; 43(1): 19–27.
11. McCleary BV, DeVries JW, Rader JI, Cohen Gerald, Prosky leon C, Mugford D, et al. Collaborative study report: determination of insoluble, soluble, and total dietary fibre (Codex definition) by an enzymatic-gravimetric method and liquid chromatography, Cereal Food World, 2011; 56(6): 238.
12. Jones JM. Dietary fiber future directions: integrating new definitions and findings to inform nutrition research and communication. Adv Nutr 2013; 4(1): 8–15.
13. Prosky L, Asp NG, Schweizer TF, DeVries JW, Furda I. Determination of insoluble, soluble, and total dietary fibre in foods and food products: inter laboratory study. J Assoc Off Anal Chem 1988; 71(5): 1017–23.
14. Bunzel M, Ralph J, Marita J, Steinhart H. Identification of 4-O-5′-coupled diferulic acid from insoluble cereal fibre. J Agric Food Chem 2000; 48(8): 3166–9.
15. Singleton VL, Rossi JA. Colorimetry of total phenolics with phosphomolybdic-phosphotungstic acid reagents. Am J Enol Viticul 1965; 16(3): 144–58.
16. Gould JM, Jasberg BK, Dexter LB, Hsu JT, Lewis SM, Fahey GC. High-fibre, noncaloric flour substitute for baked foods. Properties of alkaline peroxide-treated lignocellulose. Cereal Chem 1989; 66(3): 201–5.
17. Caprez A, Arrigoni E, Amado R, Zeukom H. Influence of different types of thermal treatment on the chemical composition and physical properties of wheat bran. J Cereal Sci 1986; 4(3): 233–9.
18. Demirci M, Gündüz H. Süt teknolojisi el kitabı. Hasad Yayıncılık, Istanbul, Turkey; 1997, p. 66.
19. Güler Z. Levels of 24 minerals in local goat milk, its strained yoghurt and salted yoghurt (tuzlu yoğurt). Small Ruminant Res 2007; 71(1–3): 130–7.
20. Jimenez-Florez R, Klipfel NJ, Tobias J. Ice cream and frozen desserts. In: Hui YH, ed. Dairy science and technology handbook: 2. Product manufacturing. New York: VCH Publishers; 1993, p. 57.
21. Güven M, Karaca OB. The effects of varying sugar content and fruit concentration on the physical properties of vanilla and fruit ice-cream-type frozen yogurts. Int J Dairy Technol 2002; 55(1): 27–31.
22. Akın MB, Akın MS, Kırmacı Z. Effects of inulin and sugar levels on the viability of yogurt and probiotic bacteria and the physical and sensory characteristics in probiotic ice-cream. Food Chem 2007; 104(1): 93–9.
23. Anonymous. Farbmetrische Bestimmung von Farbabstanden bci Korperfarben nach der CIELAB Formol. Beuth-Vertrieb GMbH, Berlin, Germany; 1979, p. 30.
24. Roland AM, Phillips LG, Boor KJ. Effects of fat content on the sensory properties, melting, colour, and hardness of ice cream. J Dairy Sci 1999; 82(1): 32–8.
25. SAS. SAS/STAT guide for personal computers, version 6.12 ed. Cary, NC: SAS Institute; 1998.
26. Abdul Aziz NA, Wong LM, Bhat R, Cheng LH. Evaluation of processed green and ripe mango peel and pulp flours (*Mangifera indica* var. *Chokanan*) in terms of chemical composition, antioxidant compounds and functional properties. J Sci Food Agric 2012; 92(3): 557–63.
27. Rodríguez-Ambriz SL, Islas-Hernández JJ, Agama-Acevedo E, Tovar J, Bello-Pérez LA. Characterization of a fibre-rich powder prepared by liquefaction of unripe banana flour. Food Chem 2008; 107(4): 1515–21.
28. Juarez-Garcia E, Agama-Acevedo E, Sáyago-Ayerdi SG, Rodrìguez-Ambriz SL, Bello-Pèrez LA. Composition, digestibility and application in bread making of banana flour. Plant Foods Hum Nutr 2006; 61(3): 131–7.
29. Grigelmo-Miguel N, Martín-Belloso O. Comparison of dietary fibre from by-products of processing fruits and greens and from cereals. LWT-Food Sci Technol 1999; 32: 503–8.
30. Calvache JEN, Fissore EN, Latorre ME, Soria M, Pla MFDE, Gerschenson LN. Obtention of dietary fibre enriched fractions from peach bagasse using ethanol pre-treatment and microwave drying. LWT-Food Sci Technol 2015; 62(2): 1169–76.

31. Thipayarat A. Quality and physiochemical properties of banana paste under vacuum dehydration. Int J Food Eng 2007; 3(4): 1556–3758.
32. Uttara B, Singh AV, Zamboni P, Mahajan RT. Oxidative stress and neurodegenerative diseases: a review of upstream and downstream antioxidant therapeutic options. Curr Neuropharmacol 2009; 7: 65.
33. Pérez-Jiménez J, Arranz S, Tabernero M, Díaz-Rubio ME, Serrano J, Goñi I, et al. Updated methodology to determine antioxidant capacity in plant foods, oils and beverages: extraction, measurement and expression of results. Food Res Int 2008; 41(3): 274–85.
34. Goñi I, Díaz-Rubio ME, Pérez-Jiménez J, Saura-Calixto F. Towards an updated methodology for measurement of dietary fibre, including associated polyphenols, in food and beverages. Food Res Int 2009; 42(7): 840–6.
35. Ahmed J, Almusallam A, Al-Hooti SN. Isolation and characterization of insoluble date (*Phoenix dactylifera* L.) fibres. LWT-Food Sci Technol 2013; 50(2): 414–19.
36. Alfredo VO, Gabriel RR, Luis CG, David BA. Physicochemical properties of a fibrous fraction from chia (*Salvia hispanica* L.). LWT-Food Sci Technol 2009; 42(1): 168–73.
37. Chau C, Huang Y. Comparison of the chemical composition and physicochemical properties of different fibres prepared from the peel of *Citrus sinensis* L. Cv. Liucheng. J Agric Food Chem 2003; 51(9): 2615–18.
38. Ruales J, Zumba J. Cuantificación y caracterización de fibra dietética en frutas y hortalizas ecuatorianas. Temas en Tecnología de Alimentos 1998; 2: 55–9 (in Spanish).
39. Yangılar F. Effects of green banana flour on the physical, chemical and sensory properties of ice cream. Food Technol Biotechnol 2015; 53(3): 315–23.
40. Hwang JY, Shyu YS, Hsu CK. Grape wine lees improves the rheological and adds antioxidant properties to ice cream. LWT-Food Sci Technol 2009; 42(1): 312–18.
41. Çakmakçı S, Topdaş EF, Kalın P, Han H, Şekerci P, Köse LP, et al. Antioxidant capacity and functionality of oleaster (*Elaeagnus angustifolia* L.) flour and crust in a new kind of fruity ice cream. Int J Food Sci Technol 2015; 50(2): 472–81.
42. Yangılar F. Mineral contents and physical, chemical, sensory properties of ice cream enriched with date fibre. Italian J Food Sci 2015; 27(3): 397–406.
43. Sofjan RP, Hartel RW. Effects of overrun on structural and physical characteristics of ice cream. Int Dairy J 2004; 14(3): 255–62.
44. El-Samahy SK, Youssef KM, Moussa-Ayoub TE. Producing ice cream with concentrated cactus pear pulp: a preliminary study. J Prof Assoc Cactus 2009; 11: 1–12.
45. Sun-Waterhouse D, Edmonds L, Wadhwa SS, Wibisono R. Producing ice cream using a substantial amount of juice from kiwifruit with green, gold or red flesh. Food Res Int 2013; 50: 647–56.
46. Başar H. Elemental composition of various peach cultivars. Sci Hort 2006; 107(3): 259–63.
47. Dağdemir E. Effect of vegetable marrow (*Cucurbita pepo* L.) on ice cream quality and nutritive value. Asian J Chem 2011; 23(10): 4684–8.
48. Wu SJ, Ng LT, Huang YM, Lin DL, Wang SS, Huang SN, et al. Antioxidant activities of *Physalis peruviana*. Biol Pharm Bull 2005; 28(6): 963–6.
49. Puente LA, Pinto-Muñoz CA, Castro ES, Cortés M. *Physalis peruviana* Linnaeus, the multiple properties of a highly functional fruit: a review. Food Res Int 2011; 44(7): 1733–40.
50. Erkaya T, Dağdemir E, Sengül M. Influence of cape gooseberry (*Physalis peruviana* L.) addition on the chemical and sensory characteristics and mineral concentrations of ice cream. Food Res Int 2012; 45(1): 331–5.

***Filiz Yangılar**
Department of Nutrition and Dietetics
Erzincan University
TR-24000 Erzincan
Turkey
Email: fyangilar@erzincan.edu.tr and f_yangilar@hotmail.com

Food as a tool for learning in everyday activities at preschool – an exploratory study from Sweden

Hanna Sepp* and Karin Höijer

Food and Meal Science, School of Education and Environment, Kristianstad University, Kristianstad, Sweden

Abstract

Background: There is a need for research both in relation to food education at preschools and in relation to how the individual teacher can handle and relate to the many different scientific facts and paradigms that are prevalent in relation to food, health, and a sustainable lifestyle.

Objective: The aim of this study was to explore the experiences and meanings that preschool teachers associate with involving food as a tool for learning in planned educational activities.

Design: An exploratory study was conducted in 14 preschools with 131 teachers. Twenty semi-structured individual or group interviews with 45 preschool staff were conducted, and 10 interviews were selected for analysis.

Results: According to participants, both children and teachers developed a sensory language; children became more positive towards tasting and teachers discovered new possibilities for interdisciplinary work. However, the results also show that an allowing system, with both an interested and confident teacher who recognises the competent child and a supportive organisation, is needed in order to make food a meaningful tool for learning in preschool.

Discussion: According to previous studies, food has the potential to play an important part in everyday activities at preschool, both in planned educational activities as well as at meal situations. Our results imply that a holistic understanding of food in preschool is required for long-term work with food as a natural part of the everyday activities.

Conclusion: The results imply that it is fun and meaningful for both children and teachers, and quite possible, to work with food as a tool for learning in everyday activities at preschool. In order to include food as a way to work with the preschool curriculum for a sustainable lifestyle, an allowing system is needed.

Keywords: *preschool*; *teacher*; *meal education*; *food education*; *Sapere*; *cooking*

According to the European Food Information Council (EUFIC), children's education concerning a healthy lifestyle is one of the most important keys to good health and to helping children reach their potential as the prevalence of health-related problems associated with food among children has increased during the last decades (1). Although food habits are not stable and do change during a person's lifetime, a base for healthy food habits can be established in early childhood (2). There are many preschool- and school-based interventions (aimed at decreasing obesity and increasing consumption of fruits and vegetables), systematically reviewed in several articles (3–10). Even though the studies have had different approaches, there is a clear common result; the effects of the interventions are limited. Common to the few cases where some change has actually been studied, is a collaboration of several different approaches, such as increased availability of fruits and vegetables, involvement of the home, as well as increased education on healthy food (3, 10, 11). This approach was, for example, employed in a comprehensive European study, the ToyBox study, which also pinpointed preschool teachers as key persons in obesity prevention work among children (12–14). In a recently published review by Mikkelsen et al. (8), 26 healthy-eating interventions in preschools were analysed. The review found that healthy-eating interventions in day-care facilities increased nutrition-related knowledge among the children as well as fruit and vegetable consumption. The conclusion was that preschools have the potential to influence children's food choice at an early age, which several other researchers also suggest (15–17) as well as the American Diet Association (18).

A great deal of learning about food and eating occurs early in life, especially regarding preferences for taste and attitudes towards food (19). As of 1998, Sweden has a specific curriculum for preschool with goals that specify the orientation of the work (20). The curriculum is comprehensive, and the expected developments are very detailed, but it does not specifically include food or meals, either from a health or a sustainable lifestyle perspective. In Sweden, most children aged 1–5 years are enrolled in preschool (21), where they have at least one meal per day and may consume as much as 70% of their daily energy and nutrient intake (22). The preschool and parents, thus, share the responsibility for children's food habits. Consequently, food, eating practices, and meals culture are experienced by young children both at home, in the private sphere, and at preschool, in the public sphere. Despite this, Swedish preschool teachers have very little theoretical and practical knowledge about preschool's role and responsibility for children's food habits (23).

Although, there are a lot of intervention studies which conclude that it is important to educate preschool children about food and health, little attention has been aimed at understanding preschools from the perspective of the teachers. There are several studies in the Nordic countries however, in which meals from a learning perspective are studied, for example in relation to gender (24), language skills (25–27), social interaction (28, 29), and care (30), but to our knowledge there is no research exploring conditions around food as part of planned educational activities in preschool either from a health perspective or from the perspective of teachers. This implies that there is a need for research both in relation to food education at preschools and in relation to how the individual teacher can handle and relate to the many different scientific facts and paradigms that are prevalent in relation to food, health, and a sustainable lifestyle. The aim of this study was to explore the experiences and meanings that preschool teachers associate with involving food as a tool for learning in planned educational activities.

Methodology

The study design chosen to study teacher's experiences associated with involving food in planned educational activities was exploratory and had three stages. The first involved introducing participants to the study and to pedagogic methods. The second involved teachers working on their own by involving food in planned educational activities in their preschools during 1 year. The last involved data collection with qualitative interviews.

The first author was involved in a larger Leader project (31) called 'The children's best table' involving both preschools and schools with children aged 1–12. During fall 2012, county dietary managers and principals at these preschools were informed about the study of this article and invited to participate, and those who were interested enrolled. All teachers at these preschools were orally invited to participate in this study, and 125 decided to accept. In addition to these, one additional preschool was orally invited to participate and accepted, making the total number of participating preschools 14, with 131 teachers. All preschools were located in the south of Sweden.

In order to make it easier for the teachers to know what they can do with food, two books based on two specific pedagogic methods – Sensory education, the so-called Sapere (32), and Cook and learn step-by-step (33) – were introduced during the oral information. These were chosen based on availability and their self-instructive design. It was thus assumed that the participants did not need specific training to involve food in the planned educational activities. Sapere, which has proven to be a successful method (34–39), was developed for training and developing children's sensory abilities and language, where children are encouraged to experience food with all their senses and then put words to their experiences when they taste, smell, listen to, and touch different foods and meals. The step-by-step method was developed for baking and cooking with preschool children and means that children bake or cook something with the help of a sequence of cards with images and text (33, 40). What distinguishes the step-by-step method from other pedagogic image recipes is that only one portion is cooked; the children only make one scone or one smoothie. These methods gave the participants the opportunity to work with food as an educational instrument, with the help of concrete methods. Teachers at participating preschools worked with food in planned educational activities during 2013.

For this study, 20 semi-structured individual or group interviews with 45 preschool staff were conducted in 2014 during preschool hours, held in 10 different pre-schools, and all participants were women with a preschool-teaching degree. The interviews were conducted by the first author, who was trained in interview techniques and group interview methodology, as described by Patton (41). Interviews revolved around three themes about working with children in preschool: food in general at preschool, the curriculum in relation to food, and working with food in planned educational activities. Each teacher was interviewed on one occasion, either individually (for practical reasons) or in a group of 2–5 participants. The interviews lasted from 40 to 60 min and were video recorded.

The preliminary analysis began during the interview, and a pattern of teachers experiencing education with and about food as fun (possibilities) although hard to execute (barriers) emerged. Because saturation thus was experienced in the preliminary analysis of the interviews, a decision was made to transcribe verbatim one of two interviews per preschool, in total 10 group interviews with 23 teachers, using the qualitative software programme Transana, version 2.42. The transcripts were read through several times by both authors separately and sorted into codes using the analysis software Atlas.ti, version 7.5.

It is the experiences and the meanings that preschool teachers associate with involving food in their educational activities that are of interest in this article. Therefore, a social constructionist perspective was chosen because it provides an analytical framework through which it is possible to see how preschool teachers make sense of teaching about food. Wortham and Jackson (42) have described education as a 'set of processes that occur in events and institutions that involve both informal socialization and formal learning' (p. 107). This means that from a social constructionist perspective, education is a process in which various objects are (re)constructed, such as the role of the teacher. By adopting this theoretical perspective, it was possible to make visible how teachers make sense of teaching about food in relation to themselves, children, and preschool.

The codes were discussed and sorted into a matrix in which both the object that was being constructed (what) and the social relationship in which it was being constructed (how) were captured (42). According to Wortham and Jackson (42), an analysis presupposes, or assumes, that some things are solid. In the analysis of the preschool teacher interviews, it was apparent that the informants primarily made their experiences meaningful in relation to perceived barriers or possibilities. This meant that in the analysis, we assumed that the objects (barriers and possibilities) and mechanisms (teachers, children, and organisation) were stable aspects of the social world (see Fig. 1).

Ethical considerations

The Ethical Regional Board at Lund University vetted the project protocol, and the requirements identified by the Swedish Research Council (2011) were followed. In addition to this, both selected pedagogical methods were based upon a foundational view that participation is

		What is constructed (object)	
		Education with and about food as fun (possibilities)	Education with and about food hard to execute (barriers)
How is it constructed (mechanism)	Teacher	*The interested and confident teacher*	*The uncertain teacher*
	Child	*The competent child*	*The "little" child*
	Organisation		*The unsupportive organisation*
Final themes		*The allowing system*	*The reluctant system*

Fig. 1. Matrix for social constructionist analysis of 10 interviews with 23 preschool teachers.

voluntary and that all children have a right to their own taste and a right not to taste or participate.

Results

Although the research questions for this study were focused on which experiences preschool teachers associate with involving food in *planned educational activities*, it soon became apparent that it was impossible for the preschool teachers to talk about food without bringing in the whole meal situation, that is, *all everyday activities* at preschool. Thus, the two main themes of the analysis, the allowing system and the reluctant system, should be understood in a broad perspective. In this section, we will explain these themes based upon the main categories.

The allowing system

The interested and confident teacher

A majority of the participants did point out the possibilities and advantages of integrating food into educational activities as well as during meal times, mostly because it has been fun and because it has provided a new way of learning, even for the youngest. The methods have been experienced as inspiring, concrete, and easy to work with, and they have stimulated more cooking and baking with the children. The project made the teachers aware that they lack knowledge, but as they reflect on this they say that they've also learned a great deal. To use cooking as part of educational activities in preschool was new to most of them and has opened up new possibilities for interdisciplinary work.

> Teacher: That you can use food for pedagogical purposes and have a lot of fun with different projects is to me a great benefit. And the joy of baking with children, well it doesn't have to be just baking, it can be something else that they appreciate, it's very, well to participate and help, they feel that they learn a lot. Many of them didn't know the measuring spoons at first, and there I've noticed a big change that they actually know now. They used to just say cup or something, and now it's 'now we'll take this much'. They didn't use to know what it was or how much, and that it involves maths. For example you can tell them that this is maths – teaspoon, tablespoon and decilitre and things like that. We don't have to just do it with water as we used to; now we can do it with flour or sugar instead.

It appears as if the teachers hadn't considered preschool's potential to play an active role in working with food and good food habits before taking part in the project. However, it becomes apparent that preschool does have an important part to play in providing children with basic skills, and food habits are one part of this.

The competent child

The Sapere method's basic assumptions that all individuals have a right to their own taste and a right not to taste have been described as very positive starting points and have made the teachers reflect on their own part as role models and what rules they implement during regular meals. Many of the teachers also state that they learned a lot about their own taste and to put words to their experiences.

Another result is that the children are competent when it comes to food – more so than the teachers expected. The teachers have faith in the children's abilities but were still surprised at just how much the children were able to do themselves while they worked with the project.

> Teacher: Just to have a recipe, that the child can interpret the recipe on its own is fantastic! They have learned that they can have a recipe to follow, that children can do things on their own. Because before we were the ones who decided that now we'll make buns and we need such and such. But here they can actually do it on their own and, as you say, the process changes completely.

Another effect of the project is that the children talk more about food. The Sapere method is described as a completely different way of working, giving the children the ability to put words to their experiences and develop a sensory language. Many teachers also mention the children's ability to say no and to justify why as a positive effect of the project. The children bring their new skills with them to the meal situations and are more positive towards tasting new things. Now the children consider what food tastes like and discuss with each other and have also become more conscious about and interested in food.

With the step-by-step method, the children have been given the opportunity to see and learn the whole process. The older children have helped the younger children, and they have all learned from each other. The children thought it was fun to cook and/or bake with the step-by-step recipes, and the teachers have perceived them as easy to read and follow. The results show that the teachers believe that food can be a means to gain understanding about other areas that can be hard to grasp, such as science.

The reluctant system

The uncertain teacher

A majority of the participants did point out the possibilities and advantages of integrating food into educational activities; however, there were a few obstacles, for example, ignorance, either conscious or unconscious, and lack of interest that were constructed as absence of support. Conscious ignorance was, for example, when the teachers felt unsure about how they can work with food and children and experienced a lack of requisite skills and knowledge, which made them unable to turn a theory of methods into practice. Ignorance can also concern how the work should be organised or how many children you can work with in a group. Insecurity was also felt when they were unable to answer questions:

> Teacher A: I had one [child] the other day who was thinking about ketchup and how ketchup was made or where the ketchup came from. We had ketchup that day and I read on the back and he [the child] noted that it was tomato and that they were crushed, and that he understood. So I read on the back what was in it and there was vinegar and some other things so you have to mix it. And then there was someone else who asked where the tomatoes came from and we agreed that it was from seeds. But before the first seed was found, where did they come from?
> Teacher B: And then it became philosophy.
> Teacher A: That's when I changed subject.

Unconscious ignorance was primarily connected to the Sapere method when they were to describe their experiences with the help of their senses; it was hard to verbalise these because they had never done so before. This lack of personal experience or practice led to a construction of the method as being slow and boring to work with.

> Teacher: I think that adults find this hard too because when I have talked to other adults and explained what the children are saying, most of them think it is a bit funny. But it is actually quite hard to say if it is sweet or sour or bitter, we don't talk much about that. Many times you just say that something tastes good or not, not how. You don't describe taste very often, at least I don't.

A few informants expressed a lack of interest because they found it hard to see any benefits, stating that it needs enthusiasts with a significant interest to integrate food in the educational activities. None of the interviewed teachers mention that they have defined a purpose *before* the activities, and few reflect upon what the children have learned based on the goals of the curriculum; instead these were added in retrospect when compiling the documentation. The different parts of the curriculum were mentioned in general terms but also in the form of typical school subjects.

> Teacher: Yes, there's a lot of maths in everything, it becomes integrated in all of it sort of. Chemistry and physics also become part of what you do.

The missing connection with the curriculum is especially apparent among the teachers who lack knowledge or interest concerning the integration of food into educational activities.

The 'little' child

The children's young age and limited experience were constructed as barriers by some informants. It is sometimes hard for them to remember, which makes it difficult to apply their knowledge to new situations. It can also be hard for the children to describe tastes and to have an individual taste preference; if one child says that a vegetable is bitter, other children tag along and say the same. The smallest children also generally lack language skills, while the older children lack the vocabulary to describe what they're experiencing in relation to food.

> Teacher: We were tasting carrots. And it is hard for them, because they are not comfortable with seeing how it is; they are not comfortable with thinking about how they feel, with pausing to think about what they're doing. Because now we tasted the carrot when it was on a plate, when it was grated and when it was cut into smaller pieces, and they were given a carrot to nibble on, to see if they experienced any difference. It was new to them to approach it this way, to think and feel.

The unsupportive organisation

The most crucial barrier is the absence of a supporting organisation, both concerning pedagogical leadership and especially in the non-existing cooperation between the preschool units and the kitchens. Teaching staff and kitchen staff at all participating preschools had different managers, which means, for example, that regulations for purchases are unclear. The kitchens normally order their goods 2 weeks in advance, while the teachers make detailed plans of their activities weekly, making ordering ingredients via the kitchen difficult. Teachers also felt resistance from the kitchens to placing orders, because these purchases were charged to the kitchen's budget and not the unit's. In order to be able to work with the project, teachers at some preschools had to go shopping themselves or even bring the ingredients from their own homes.

Shortage of time was mentioned as an obstacle, both when working with documentation and preparations, and also that the children's young age called for extra time. The small number of staff was also mentioned in conjunction with the lack of time, which has meant that it is the teacher's own interest that decides whether or not they are going continue to work with food.

Discussion

The results show that an allowing system, with both an interested and confident teacher who recognises the competent child and a supportive organisation, is needed in order to make food a meaningful tool for learning in preschool. Although there are several studies, in which meal situations from a learning perspective are studied (24–30), there is a lack of research exploring how food can be included as a key part in everyday activities at preschool in Sweden in a health and sustainable lifestyle perspective. Several studies (8, 15–17) and influential institutions as the EUFIC (1) and the American Diet Association (18) argues that children's education concerning a healthy lifestyle is an important key to good health. This study shows that food can be included as a key part in everyday activities at preschool, both in planned educational activities as well as at meal situations which means that both understanding and awareness of food in preschool is required.

Studies show that children dare to try more new foods and dishes when they have worked with sensory training (43, 44) and the Sapere method (34–38). This is in accordance with our results as well as a recently published dissertation from the Netherlands (39), where both teachers and children (4–12 years) experienced the laboratory learning with sensory exercises as very positive. The study revealed that children's knowledge about healthy eating habits increased with the help of sensory training – especially in combination with other methods of cooking and field trips. However, our result shows that there is a need for an allowing system in order to make children's education concerning food habits and a sustainable lifestyle feasible and meaningful on a long-term basis. For example, teachers experienced the lack of a supportive organisation, both concerning pedagogical leadership and in cooperation with the kitchen staff. From this, it can be concluded that a supportive manager with clear leadership and a learning organisation is necessary to efficiently plan activities, and our results are in line with Altin et al. (45) who have studied and evaluated the criteria surrounding the implementation process of health promotion preschool environment in a Swedish municipality.

The curriculum does not specifically include food or meals as a tool for learning, either from a health or a sustainable lifestyle perspective. Research implies that even though the Swedish preschool has had a specific curriculum (20) for almost 20 years there is still a need to transform the curriculum into an active document (46, 47). This became apparent in this study when teachers planned and carried out activities involving food without using the curriculum as a supportive framework but rather as a 'hindsight document'. The teachers in this study reported that they usually have confidence in the children's ability, which is in line with the curriculum as well as Swedish research (e.g. 47). Despite this, the teachers were challenged by the step-by-step method which assumes that children can manage all the steps on their own. Why is that so? Cooking almost always involves an expectation of an edible result, which could create uncertainty in the teacher relating to the children's performance, and it can be assumed that this uncertainty primarily has to do with the teacher's own lack of didactic knowledge and food-related skills.

Educational theory assumes that children learn from and with each other, which no teacher in this study seems to have considered in relation to food before, but which became obvious during the project. This result surprised us. Is it because food and meals are an everyday activity, a routine situation, where teachers haven't really thought about food in relation to their profession? This implies a need for a holistic approach to understand and work with food in preschool.

Methodological considerations

A total of 20 interviews were conducted, either individually or in groups of 2–5 participants. Patton (41) states that group interviews generate high-quality and data-intense material, which also was observed in this study, as the individual interviews were less rich. Thus, to maintain rigor in the material, only group interviews were selected for the final analysis.

There is a shortage of educational material related to food in preschool, and therefore, Cook and learn step-by-step was chosen (33). The Sapere method (32) was chosen because it has proven to be a successful method (34–38). Because the books are self-explanatory, we assumed that there was no need for training in methods. Judging by the result, we can retrospectively see that we should have educated the teachers about the methods so they would feel secure. Moreover, even the kitchen staff should have been included, even though the study focused on the planned educational activities, since it became apparent that it was impossible for the preschool teachers to talk about food without bringing in the whole meal situation, which involves the kitchen staff very much.

For this study, we chose a social constructionist perspective for analysis of the material because the intention was to gain insight into the experiences of preschool teachers with a focus on food as part of their everyday activities, rather than on processes of learning and teaching or which pedagogic perspectives different preschools work with. Therefore, we believe that a social constructionist perspective was an adequate approach to process the results.

Implications for research and practice

To include food as an important part in everyday activities at preschool, a holistic understanding of food in preschool is required for long-term work. The lack of experienced individual and/or structural support makes it hard to integrate food as a tool for leaning as a natural part of everyday activities. There is no potential at all to work with food if the system is reluctant. However, if either individual or structural support is lacking, it may still be possible to work with food during a limited time, as was the case with the reported project. To enable long-term work, with food as a natural part of the everyday activities and with food as a way to work with the preschool curriculum for a sustainable lifestyle, an allowing system is needed. The preschool teachers need knowledge, skills, and tools, as well as the support of managers concerning both organisation and the allocation of resources. Otherwise, the success of implementing food as a tool for learning relies on enthusiasts who consider it important that food should be integrated as a natural part of preschool.

Acknowledgements

The first author (HS) thanks Gastronomiska Akademien [Academy of Gastronomy] for funding as well as Kristianstad University and the platform for research on work-integrated education and professional learning. The authors thank Susanne Thorén, project manager for 'The children's best table', who made the collection of data possible. The authors also want to thank the reviewers who helped to identify weaknesses.

Conflict of interest and funding

The authors declare that they have no conflict of interest.

References

1. EUFIC (2013). EUFIC's Cool Food Planet educational website: nutrition, food safety & physical activity for children! Available from: http://www.eufic.org/article/en/artid/Cool-Food-Planet-educational-website-nutrition-food-safety-physical-activity-children/ [cited 28 September 2016].
2. Craigie AM, Lake AA, Kelly SA, Adamson AJ, Mathers JC. Tracking of obesity-related behaviours from childhood to adulthood: a systematic review. Maturitas 2011; 70(3): 266–84.
3. Knai C, Pomerleau J, Lock K, McKee M. Getting children to eat more fruit and vegetables: a systematic review. Prev Med 2006; 42(2): 85–95.
4. Howerton MW, Bell BS, Dodd KW, Berrigan D, Stolzenberg-Solomon R, Nebeling L. School-based nutrition programs produced a moderate increase in fruit and vegetable consumption: meta and pooling analyses from 7 studies. J Nutr Educ Behav 2007; 39(4): 186–96.
5. Van Cauwenberghe E, Maes L, Spittaels H, van Lenthe FJ, Brug J, Oppert JM, et al. Effectiveness of school-based interventions in Europe to promote healthy nutrition in children and adolescents: systematic review of published and 'grey' literature. Br J Nutr 2010; 103(6): 781–97.
6. Delgado-Noguera M, Tort S, Martinez-Zapata MJ, Bonfill X. Primary school interventions to promote fruit and vegetable consumption: a systematic review and meta-analysis. Prev Med 2011; 53(1–2): 3–9.
7. Evans CE, Christian MS, Cleghorn CL, Greenwood DC, Cade JE. Systematic review and meta-analysis of school-based interventions to improve daily fruit and vegetable intake in children aged 5 to 12 y. Am J Clin Nutr 2012; 96(4): 889–901.
8. Mikkelsen MV, Husby S, Skov LR, Perez-Cueto FJ. A systematic review of types of healthy eating interventions in preschools. Nutr J 2014; 13: 56.
9. Birch LL, Ventura AK. Preventing childhood obesity: what works? Int J Obes (Lond) 2009; 33(Suppl 1): S74–81.
10. Waters E, de Silva-Sanigorski A, Hall BJ, Brown T, Campbell KJ, Gao Y, et al. Interventions for preventing obesity in children. Cochrane Database Syst Rev 2011; (12): CD001871.
11. Silveira JA, Taddei JA, Guerra PH, Nobre MR. Effectiveness of school-based nutrition education interventions to prevent and

reduce excessive weight gain in children and adolescents: a systematic review. J Pediatr (Rio J) 2011; 87(5): 382–92.
12. Payr A, Birnbaum J, Wildgruber A, Kreichauf S, Androutsos O, Lateva M, et al. Concepts and strategies on how to train and motivate teachers to implement a kindergarten-based, family-involved intervention to prevent obesity in early childhood. The ToyBox-study. Obes Rev 2014; 15(S3): 40–7.
13. Manios Y, Grammatikaki E, Androutsos O, Chinapaw MJM, Gibson EL, Buijs G, et al. A systematic approach for the development of a kindergarten-based intervention for the prevention of obesity in preschool age children: the ToyBox-study. Obes Rev 2012; 13: 3–12.
14. Manios Y, Androutsos O, Katsarou C, Iotova V, Socha P, Geyer C, et al. Designing and implementing a kindergarten-based, family-involved intervention to prevent obesity in early childhood: the ToyBox-study. Obes Rev 2014; 15(Suppl 3): 5–13.
15. Witt KE, Dunn C. Increasing fruit and vegetable consumption among preschoolers: evaluation of color me healthy. J Nutr Educ Behav 2012; 44(2): 107–13.
16. De Bock F, Breitenstein L, Fischer JE. Positive impact of a pre-school-based nutritional intervention on children's fruit and vegetable intake: results of a cluster-randomized trial. Public Health Nutr 2012; 15(3): 466–75.
17. Dev DA, McBride BA. Academy of Nutrition and Dietetics benchmarks for nutrition in child care 2011: are child-care providers across contexts meeting recommendations? J Acad Nutr Diet 2013; 113(10): 1346–53.
18. Benjamin Neelon SE, Briley ME. Position of the American Dietetic Association: benchmarks for nutrition in child care. J Am Diet Assoc 2011; 111(4): 607–15.
19. Mennella JA. Ontogeny of taste preferences: basic biology and implications for health. Am J Clin Nutr 2014; 99(3): 704S–11.
20. The Swedish National Agency for Education (2011). Curriculum for the preschool Lpfö 98 revised 2010. Stockholm: Skolverket.
21. National Education Agency. Statistik – Förskola – Barn och grupper – Riksnivå [Statistics – Pre-school – Children and groups – National level]. Available from: http://www.skolverket.se/statistik-och-utvardering/statistik-i-tabeller/forskola/barn-och-grupper/barn-och-grupper-i-forskolan-15-oktober-2015-1.248719 [cited 28 September 2016].
22. National Food Agency (2007). Bra mat i förskolan: råd för förskola och familjedaghem [Good food in preschool: advice for pre-school and family daycare]. Uppsala: Livsmedelsverket.
23. Sepp H, Abrahamsson L, Fjellström C. Pre-school staffs' attitudes toward foods in relation to the pedagogic meal. Int J Consum Stud 2006; 30(2): 224–32.
24. Eidevald C. Det finns inga tjejbestämmare: att förstå kön som position i förskolans vardagsrutiner och lek [There are no girl decision-makers – Understanding gender as a position in pre-school practices Language: Swedish, with a summary in English]. Jönköping: Högskolan för lärande och kommunikation; 2009.
25. Kultti A, Pramling N. Limes and lemons: teaching and learning in preschool as the coordination of perspectives and sensory modalities. Int J Early Child 2015; 47(1): 105–17.
26. Norman J. Språkspel i förskolan – uppfostran vid matbordet [Language in preschool – upbringing at the dinner table]. Malmö: Forskarutbildningen i pedagogik, Malmö högskola; 2003.
27. Kultti A. Mealtimes in Swedish preschools: pedagogical opportunities for toddlers learning a new language. Early Years 2014; 34(1): 18–31.
28. Munck Sundman U. Hur barn gör måltid [How children do meal]. Stockholm: Barn- och ungdomsvetenskapliga institutionen, Stockholms universitet; 2013.
29. Ødegaard EE. What's up on the teachers' agenda? Int J Early Child 2007; 39(2): 45–64.
30. Johansson E, Pramling Samulesson I. Omsorg- en cetral aspekt av förskolepedagogiken. Exemplet måltiden [Care – a central aspect of early childhood education. The example meal]. Pedagogisk forskning i Sverige 2001; 6(2): 81–101.
31. Swedish Board of Agriculture (2013). The Leader approach in Sweden. Swedish Board of Agriculture. The Children's Best Table. Available from: https://www.jordbruksverket.se/download/18.../Barnens+Bästa+Bord.pdf [cited 28 September 2016].
32. Algotson S, Öström Å, Alfredsson K. Sinnenas skafferi [The senses of the pantry]. Grythyttan: Måltidsakademiens förlag; 2011.
33. Andersson M. Laga mat och baka med förskolebarn [Cook and bake with preschool children]. Lund: Studentlitteratur; 1994.
34. Reverdy C, Chesnel F, Schlich P, Koster EP, Lange C. Effect of sensory education on willingness to taste novel food in children. Appetite 2008; 51(1): 156–65.
35. Jonsson IM, Ekström MP, Gustafsson I-B. Appetizing learning in Swedish comprehensive schools: an attempt to employ food and tasting in a new form of experimental education. Int J Consum Stud 2005; 29(1): 78–85.
36. Mustonen S, Rantanen R, Tuorila H. Effect of sensory education on school children's food perception: a 2-year follow-up study. Food Qual Prefer 2009; 20(3): 230–40.
37. Mustonen S, Tuorila H. Sensory education decreases food neophobia score and encourages trying unfamiliar foods in 8–12-year-old children. Food Qual Prefer 2010; 21(4): 353–60.
38. Dazeley P, Houston-Price C, Hill C. Should healthy eating programmes incorporate interaction with foods in different sensory modalities? A review of the evidence. Br J Nutr 2012; 108(5): 769–77.
39. Battjes-Fries M. Effectiveness of nutrition education in Dutch primary schools. Wageningen: Wageningen University; 2016.
40. Harms T. Learning from cooking experiences. A teacher's guide to accompany cook and learn. Chapel Hill, NC: Addison-Wesley Innovative Division; 1977.
41. Patton MQ. Qualitative research & evaluation methods. London: SAGE; 2002.
42. Wortham S, Jackson K. Educational constructionisms. In: Holstein JA, Gubrium JF, eds. Handbook of constructionist research. New York: Guilford Press; 2008.
43. Woo T, Lee KH. Effects of sensory education based on classroom activities for lower grade school children. Nutr Res Pract 2013; 7(4): 336–41.
44. Shon C, Park Y, Ryou H, Na W, Choi K. The development of a taste education program for preschoolers and evaluation of a program by parents and childcare personnel. Nutr Res Prac 2012; 6(5): 466–73.
45. Altin C, Lindholm SK, Wejdmark M, Lättman-Masch R, Boldemann C. Upgrading preschool environment in a Swedish municipality evaluation of an implementation process. Health Promot Pract 2015; 16(4): 583–91.
46. Brodin J, Renblad K. Reflections on the revised national curriculum for preschool in Sweden–interviews with the heads. Early Child Dev Care 2014; 184(2): 306–21.
47. Jonsson A. Att skapa läroplan för de yngsta barnen i förskolan: barns perspektiv och nuets didaktik [Creating curriculum for the youngest children in preschool. Children's perspective and didactics of the present moment]. Göteborg: Acta Universitatis Gothoburgensis; 2013.

*Hanna Sepp
Food and Meal Science
School of Education and Environment
Kristianstad University
SE-291 88 Kristianstad, Sweden
Email: hanna.sepp@hkr.se

14

Dietary supplementation with a specific melon concentrate reverses vascular dysfunction induced by cafeteria diet

Julie Carillon[1,2], Bernard Jover[3,4], Jean-Paul Cristol[4], Jean-Max Rouanet[1], Sylvain Richard[4] and Anne Virsolvy[4]*

[1]Nutrition & Metabolism, UMR 204 NutriPass, University of Montpellier, Montpellier, France; [2]Bionov Research, Montpellier, France; [3]EA7288, University of Montpellier, Montpellier, France; [4]PhyMedExp, INSERM U1046, UMR CNRS 9214, University of Montpellier, Montpellier, France

Abstract

Background: Obesity-related metabolic syndrome is associated with high incidence of cardiovascular diseases partially consecutive to vascular dysfunction. Therapeutic strategies consisting of multidisciplinary interventions include nutritional approaches. Benefits of supplementation with a specific melon concentrate, enriched in superoxide dismutase (SOD), have previously been shown on the development of insulin resistance and inflammation in a nutritional hamster model of obesity.

Objective: We further investigated arterial function in this animal model of metabolic syndrome and studied the effect of melon concentrate supplementation on arterial contractile activity.

Design and results: The study was performed on a hamster model of diet-induced obesity. After a 15-week period of cafeteria diet, animals were supplemented during 4 weeks with a specific melon concentrate (*Cucumis melo* L.) Contractile responses of isolated aorta to various agonists and antagonists were studied *ex vivo*. Cafeteria diet induced vascular contractile dysfunction associated with morphological remodeling. Melon concentrate supplementation partially corrected these dysfunctions; reduced morphological alterations; and improved contractile function, especially by increasing nitric oxide bioavailability and expression of endogenous SOD.

Conclusions: Supplementation with the specific melon concentrate improves vascular dysfunction associated with obesity. This beneficial effect may be accounted for by induction of endogenous antioxidant defense. Such an approach in line with nutritional interventions could be a useful strategy to manage metabolic syndrome–induced cardiovascular trouble.

Keywords: *vascular function*; *oxidative stress*; *antioxidant*; *superoxide dismutase*; *obesity*

Human obesity is not only consecutive to excessive saturated fat intake, but also results from a complex combination of multiple nutritional and lifestyle-related factors directly linked to the excessive consumption of industrial era foods (1). The modern Western lifestyle, merging stress, low-quality food (rich in fat and energy, but poor in micronutrients), and the disruption of chronobiological function/rhythms, contributes to the increase of metabolic syndrome incidence (2). Diets consisting of palatable industrially processed foods (named cafeteria diets) are suitable for modeling in animals the metabolic disorders of human obesity. Indeed, these cafeteria models lead to a phenotype of exaggerated obesity and related disorders similar to those responsible of metabolic syndrome (3).

The metabolic syndrome combines multifactorial health issues, such as glucose intolerance, central obesity, dyslipidemia, and insulin resistance (4), and it is frequently associated with hypertension. These conditions increase the risk of development of several pathologies, especially cardiovascular diseases and type 2 diabetes (5–7). Vascular disorders are central, involving morphological and functional remodeling of the arterial vasculature. Hemodynamic parameters are altered that imposes stress in the heart and other organs (8). Major changes are arterial stiffening (9), arterial wall thickening, and endothelial dysfunction (10). In the presence of physiological and pathological stimuli, the components of the arterial wall reorganize to maintain the integrity of the vessel wall, and these changes could increase the potential for vascular dysfunction (8).

Oxidative stress, associated with many components of metabolic syndrome, plays an important role in the pathogenesis of vascular dysfunction (11, 12). Oxidative stress results from an imbalance between production and inactivation of reactive oxygen species (ROS), which contributes to cellular dysfunction. An elevation in ROS production is associated with endothelial dysfunction, and vascular ROS may play a role in the development of obesity and metabolic syndrome (13).

Antioxidant dietary supplementations have beneficial effects on vascular dysfunction (14, 15). Supporting the efficiency of such nutritional approaches is the increasing emphasis on the positive effects of micronutrients found in natural products for controlling the pathogenesis of chronic disease such as metabolic syndrome (16).

Since 2000, a proprietary melon juice concentrate containing a high level of superoxide dismutase (SOD) has been developed. Its use as a dietary supplement has been a new subject of interest, and its antioxidant and anti-inflammatory properties have been demonstrated (17–21). Recently, it was reported that supplementation with this melon concentrate increases endogenous antioxidant defenses and thus reduces oxidative stress, insulin resistance, and corrected adipose tissue alterations in a hamster model of metabolic syndrome (18). Beneficial cardiac effects, correlated with induction of endogenous antioxidant defenses, were also observed in a rat model of cardiac hypertrophy (22, 23). Oxidative stress has been associated with the onset of cardiovascular complications in subjects with metabolic syndrome and especially with vascular dysfunction (24). In that context, information regarding the potential effects of this melon concentrate on vascular alterations was lacking.

Currently, the therapeutic strategy to specifically treat metabolic syndrome consists of multidisciplinary interventions including nutritional approaches. As many issues associated with obesity are mediated by oxidative stress, the use of a dietary antioxidant derived from a natural food source to antagonize such damage offers great potential.

In this work, we hypothesized that this specific melon concentrate can reverse vascular morphological and functional alterations associated with obesity through antioxidant properties. We investigated the effect of a 1-month oral supplementation with the melon concentrate on vascular function in a Golden Syrian hamster model of diet-induced metabolic syndrome. Supplementation was given to animals fed for 3 months with a diet consisting of high-fat, high-sugar, and high-salt supermarket products (Western diet). Endpoint direct arterial pressure was measured. Measurements of vascular reactivity and morphological analysis of thoracic aorta were performed to evaluate obesity-induced alterations. Oxidative status was also determined to understand the mechanism.

Materials and methods

Preparation and characterization of the melon concentrate

SODB (Bionov, Avignon, France) is a dried melon juice concentrate that is particularly rich in SOD, as a result of a patented process.

Approximately 625 kg of a specific proprietary and no–genetically modified organism melon variety *Cucumis melo* L. (equivalent to 15 kg of dried melon pulp) is needed to produce 1 kg of this dried melon juice concentrate. In brief, the melon pulp is separated from skin and seeds and crushed before centrifugation. Then, the melon juice undergoes filtration and concentration steps. Finally, the obtained melon juice concentrate is freeze-dried. For nutraceutical applications, this freeze-dried melon juice concentrate is coated with palm oil by spray drying method to preserve SOD activity from the digestive enzymes secreted above the small intestine. Detailed information about the antioxidant content of this dried melon juice concentrate has been published in a previous study (25).

Experimental design

The present animal experiments complied with European and French laws conformed to the *Guide for the Care and Use of Laboratory Animals, 8th ed.* (2011) published by the National Institutes of Health (National Academies Press, Washington, DC) and were approved by the Committee for Animal Care at the University of Montpellier (France) (permission no. C 34 249).

Eighteen 3-week-old male Golden Syrian hamsters (Janvier, Le Genest-St-Isle, France) were used. They were housed at 23 ± 1°C and subjected to a 12-h light/dark cycle, with free access to both food and water. After an 18-day adaptation period, the hamsters (75–80 g) were randomly divided into three groups. Two groups of hamsters ($n = 6$ per group) were assigned for 19 weeks to a cafeteria diet consisting of nine types of palatable industrially processed foods designed for human consumption (e.g. cake, potato crisps, sweets, cheese) and selected for their high-energy, -fat, -sugar and/or -salt content. The cafeteria items were weighed before being presented to the hamsters, and they were provided in excess, thereby inducing obesity. Detailed information about the nutritional value and ingredients of all foodstuffs used in this diet are presented in our previous study (17). After 15 weeks, one of the two groups of obese animals was orally supplemented with the melon concentrate (10 U SOD equivalent/day, corresponding to 10 mg/day, mixed with food) for the last 4 weeks (OB-treated group), whereas the other group was maintained on the cafeteria diet (OB group). The third group of hamsters ($n = 6$) received a standard pelleted diet (EF Hamster Control E21000-04, SSNIFF, Soest, Germany) and served as control (standard [STD] group). Food intake and body weight were recorded daily.

Direct arterial pressure measurement

At the end of the experimental protocol and the day of sacrifice, systolic arterial pressure was measured in the carotid artery. Hamsters were anesthetized (ketamine and xylazine, 75 and 25 mg/kg, respectively), and a polyethylene catheter (PE-50) was inserted into the right carotid artery for arterial pressure recordings.

Vascular reactivity

The thoracic aorta was used to study *ex vivo* the responses to agonists and antagonists of arterial contraction. Immediately after removal, arterial tissue was immersed in phosphate saline solution (PSS), pH 7.4, containing (in mM) 140 NaCl, 5 KCl, 1 $MgCl_2$, 0.5 KH_2PO_4, 0.5 Na_2HPO_4, 2.5 $CaCl_2$, 10 HEPES, and 10 glucose. Aortic tissue was cleaned of fat and connective tissue and cut into 2–3-mm-wide rings. Aortic rings were mounted in standard organ bath chambers (EMKA Technologies, Paris, France) maintained at 37°C and continuously bubbled with O_2. Then, changes in isometric tension were recorded as described previously (26). Each arterial segment was subjected to a 60-min equilibration period at the predetermined optimal basal tension of 1 g. The contractile function of each segment was assessed with 1 μM phenylephrine (PE), and the presence of endothelium was confirmed by the vasorelaxation induced by application of acetylcholine (Ach, 1 μM). After several washouts and a 20–30-min period of stabilization, dose responses were performed by cumulative increases in the concentration of the agonist PE (0.01–100 μM range) or the depolarizing agent KCl (1–80 mM). Endothelial function was assessed by studying the relaxing effects of cumulative increases of Ach between 1 nM and 10 μM on arteries contracted with a submaximally active concentration of PE (10 μM). The effects of the nitric oxide (NO)-synthase inhibitor N^{ω}-nitro-L-arginine methyl ester (L-NAME, 10 μM) and the ROS scavenger tempol (10 μM) were evaluated on the relaxing effect of Ach. Inhibitors were added for a 15-min period of incubation before PE addition. Endothelium-independent relaxations to sodium nitroprusside (SNP, 1 nM–200 μM) were studied in endothelium-denuded rings previously contracted with PE (10 μM). Each protocol was performed in triplicate for each aorta. All chemical compounds were purchased from Sigma-Aldrich (Saint Quentin Fallavier, France).

Aortic morphology

Thickness and internal diameter determinations were performed according to two methods. First, aortic rings were immersed in PSS, and optical images of the aortic cross-section were recorded to allow determination of basal internal diameter and thickness. Second, light microscope images were taken after hematoxylin-eosin staining realized on paraffin-embedded tissue sections. The mean internal aortic diameter and media thickness were determined from three measures realized on at least four arterial segments per animal by using ImageJ (National Institutes of Health, Bethesda, MD). Media cross-sectional area was calculated from these measures. Both methods gave similar results, and data represent means of all values obtained.

Determination of aortic SOD expression by real-time PCR

Total RNAs were extracted from frozen aorta using Trizol® (Sigma-Aldrich) according to manufacturer's instructions. DNase-treated (DNase I, Invitrogen, Saint Aubin, France) total RNA (1–2 μg) was transcribed into cDNA by using SuperScript II reverse transcriptase (Invitrogen) and random primer oligonucleotides (Invitrogen). Gene-specific primers for SOD3 and the housekeeping gene glyceraldehyde 3-phosphate dehydrogenase (GAPDH) were designed using the Universal Probe Library Assay Design center (Roche, Boulogne-Billancourt, France) and are as follows: SOD3-forward, 5′-tgtatgcaatctgccaggtg-3′; SOD3-reverse, 5′-tgacagctgcttgaagagga-3′; GAPDH-forward, 5′-tggcta cagcaacagagtgg-3′, and GAPDH-reverse, 5′-ggggttattgga cagggact-3′. Real-time quantitative polymerase chain reaction (PCR) was performed in a LightCycler System (Roche) in combination with the Absolute QPCR SYBR Green Capillary mix (Thermo Fisher Scientific, Illkirch, France). After a hot start (5 min at 95°C), the parameters for amplification were as follows: 10 sec at 95°C, 10 sec at 58°C, and 15 sec at 72°C for 50 cycles. Primers (Table 1) selected were of equal efficiency ($E_{ff} = 1.9$) across the range of template concentrations (1–10 ng of cDNA). Expression levels normalized with GAPDH were calculated relative to the less abundant isoform (Na_v1.6) by using the $E_{ff}^{-\Delta\Delta Ct}$ method.

Statistical analyses

Values are presented as mean ± standard error of the mean (SEM). Statistical analysis of the data was carried out using Prism® software (GraphPad, La Jolla, CA) by one-way analysis of variance (ANOVA) followed by a Mann–Whitney protected least significant difference test.

Table 1. Body weight and blood pressure of animals for various diets

	STD	OB	OB treated
Body weight at 15 weeks (g)	111 ± 2	195 ± 3*	195 ± 2*
Body weight at 19 weeks (g)	114 ± 2	200 ± 2*	188 ± 2*§
Systolic arterial pressure (mmHg)	136 ± 15	135 ± 8	134 ± 13

STD = standard diet, OB = cafeteria diet, OB treated = cafeteria diet plus melon concentrate supplementation. Values are presented as mean ± SEM. *$p < 0.05$, OB and OB-treated vs. STD animals; §$p < 0.05$, effect of the melon concentrate.

For dose–response curves, data were analyzed by two-way ANOVA followed by Bonferroni post-test. p values <0.05 were considered to be significant.

Results

Melon concentrate supplementation reduced body weight gain

Cafeteria diet induced a significant increase in body weight (OB group) compared with the standard diet (STD; Table 1). The melon concentrate supplementation slightly decreased body weight (5% lower than in the untreated OB group), although food intake was not affected. As shown in Table 1, systolic arterial pressure was similar in all groups.

Melon concentrate supplementation improved morphological alterations of aorta

In animals subjected to cafeteria diet (OB group), we observed increases in both internal diameter and media thickness of aorta (Fig. 1), corresponding to $7 \pm 1\%$ ($p = 0.0007$) and $19 \pm 2\%$ ($p < 0.0001$), respectively, compared with the same parameters measured in the reference STD group. Consequently, the cross-sectional area was $16 \pm 4\%$ higher in the OB group than in the STD group ($p = 0.0318$). The melon concentrate supplementation tended to reverse the increase in internal diameter (Fig. 1a; $p = 0.0581$) induced by the cafeteria diet in the OB-treated group; no difference was observed with STD group ($p = 0.2564$). In contrast, the melon concentrate supplementation had no effect on the media thickness in the OB group (Fig. 1b). As a result, the cross-sectional area in the OB-treated group was intermediate between that of the OB and that of the STD group (Fig. 1c). Thus, arterial remodeling induced by cafeteria diet reflected outward hypertrophic remodeling, partially reversed by the melon concentrate supplementation (Fig. 1d).

Melon concentrate supplementation corrected alterations of vascular contractility

PE and KCl induced robust dose-dependent vasoconstriction of hamster aorta (Fig. 2). PE promoted contractile response weaker in the OB group than in the STD group, irrespective of the concentration, and the EC_{50} value was increased (0.82 ± 0.16 μM in STD vs. 1.5 ± 0.16 μM in OB; $p = 0.0079$) (Fig. 2a). Maximal PE-induced contraction was decreased by $24 \pm 3\%$ ($p = 0.0102$). The melon concentrate supplementation fully corrected the loss of aortic contraction ($p = 0.004$, OB treated vs. OB) with a partial recovery of half maximal effective concentration (EC_{50}) value (1.21 ± 0.26 μM; $p = 0.0506$). The maximal responses to PE were identical in the OB-treated and STD groups (Fig. 2a; $p = 0.9661$). Cafeteria diet also induced modifications in the responses to KCl (Fig. 2b). We observed a rightward shift of the dose–response curve

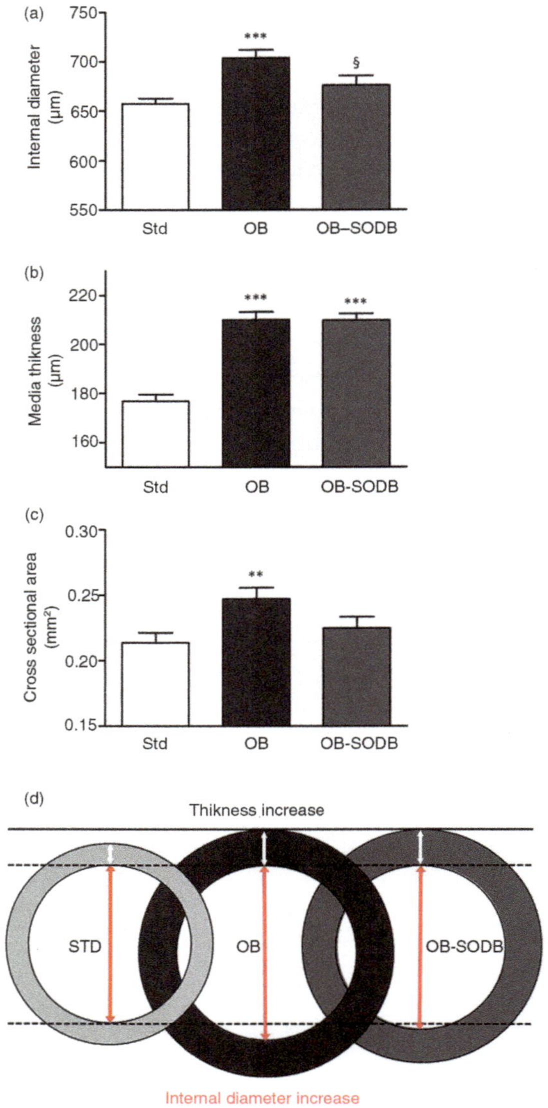

Fig. 1. Morphological changes in aorta isolated from STD, OB, and OB-treated animals. (a) Intraluminal diameters. (b) Mean thickness of aortic media. (c) Cross-sectional area calculated from values obtained for internal diameter and media thickness for each arterial segment. (d) Schematic representation of aorta cross-section illustrates changes for each group: STD, OB, and OB-treated animals. Data are presented as mean $\pm$ SEM ($n = 6$ hamsters in each group). At least four segments per animal were analyzed. $^{**}p < 0.01$, $^{***}p < 0.001$, OB and OB treated vs. STD animals; §§$p < 0.01$, effect of the melon concentrate.

for OB group. With no difference in the maximal KCl-induced contraction. The EC_{50} value was increased reflecting lower sensitivity to KCl depolarization (29.4 ± 1.7 for OB vs. 20.4 ± 1.1 mM for STD; $p < 0.0001$). The melon concentrate supplementation corrected this shift ($EC_{50} = 24.5 \pm 0.8$ mM; $p = 0.0495$, OB treated vs. OB). No significant difference in KCl sensitivity was detected compared to STD ($p = 0.0985$).

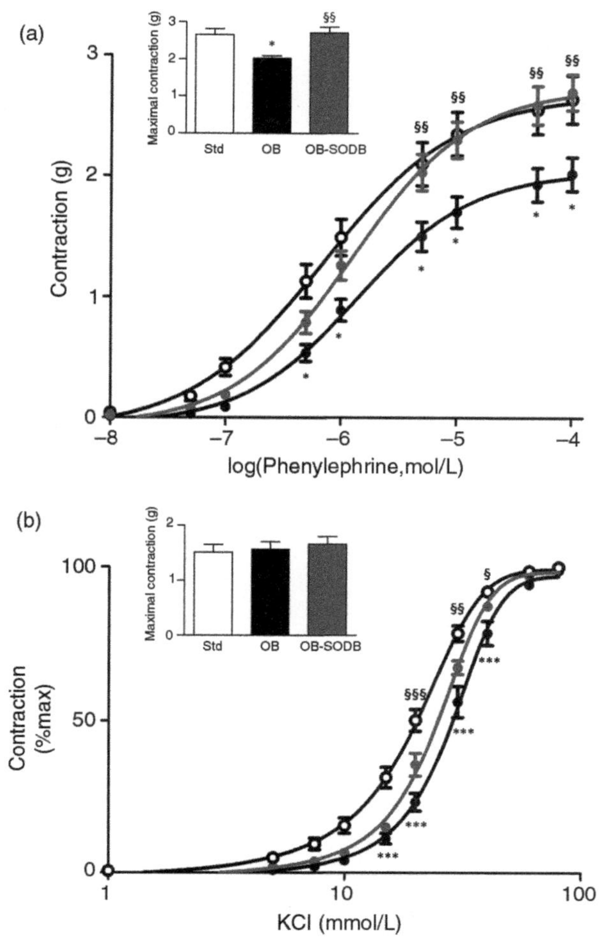

Fig. 2. Contractile responses of hamster aorta. Graphs represent cumulative response curves (a) to PE (0.01–100 μM) and (b) to KCl (1–80 mM) for aorta isolated from STD, OB, and OB-treated animals. Insets represent the maximal contraction induced by a maximally active concentration of PE (a) and KCl (b). Values are presented as mean ± SEM ($n = 6$). *$p < 0.05$, ***$p < 0.001$, OB and OB-treated vs. STD animals; §$p < 0.05$, §§$p < 0.01$, §§§$p < 0.001$ vs. effect of the melon concentrate.

Melon concentrate supplementation corrected alterations of vasorelaxation

Ach and SNP response were investigated to evaluate endothelium-dependent and -independent vasorelaxation, respectively. Both Ach and SNP induced vasorelaxation of hamster aorta pre-contracted with a submaximal dose of PE (Figs. 3 and 4). Ach-induced relaxation was higher in the OB compared to the STD group ($p = 0.0121$). The increase in maximal Ach response corresponded to 39 ± 2% of the response in the STD group (Fig. 3a). The melon concentrate supplementation tended to normalize the Ach-mediated relaxant properties. In the OB-treated group, Ach-induced relaxation was intermediate, with a trend to be different than in the OB group ($p = 0.0593$) and to be normalized as the STD ($p = 0.0691$). The presence of L-NAME suppressed the relaxant effect of Ach similarly whatever the diet.

The same experiments performed in the presence of tempol, a ROS scavenger, showed that Ach-induced relaxation was maintained in the STD and the OB-treated group, but it was potentiated in OB group (Fig. 3b) compared to Ach-induced relaxation in absence of tempol. Indeed, in the OB group, tempol amplified the maximal response to Ach, with a 40% increase (in absence vs. in presence of tempol; $p = 0.0209$). This potentiation was absent in the STD group ($p = 0.3198$) and was suppressed by the melon concentrate supplementation (OB treated, $p > 0.9999$). In the presence of tempol, PE response was also potentiated in OB group, whereas no potentiation was observed in STD as in OB treated (Fig. 3b, insets).

SNP dose dependently relaxed arteries previously contracted with a submaximally active concentration of PE (Fig. 4a). Cafeteria diet induced a potentiation of that relaxation (Fig. 4b). In the OB group, the maximal vasorelaxant capacity of aorta to SNP was increased by 30% compared to the STD group ($p = 0.0004$). The melon concentrate supplementation suppressed the potentiation of the SNP response ($p = 0.0125$) and in the OB-treated group, relaxation of aorta was identical to that of the STD group ($p = 0.3818$).

Melon concentrate supplementation modulated aortic oxidative status

Expression of antioxidant enzymes and especially SOD could be modified by cafeteria diet. In our model, we observed that SOD mRNA level was significantly lower in the OB group (Fig. 5). It was decreased by 34% compared to the STD group ($p = 0.0318$). The melon concentrate supplementation corrected this parameter. In OB-treated group, the endogenous SOD level, which was higher than that of the OB group ($p = 0.0439$), did not differ from that of the STD group.

Discussion

The beneficial effects of dietary supplementation with the melon concentrate reported in various animal and human models are currently presented as consecutive to a reduction of oxidative stress in relation with an increase in the endogenous antioxidant defenses, especially SOD (17, 18, 22). The present study extends this concept to the vascular level. In our hamster model, cafeteria diet induced vascular alterations mainly characterized by tissue remodeling, contractile dysfunction, and oxidative stress. A dietary supplementation with the particular melon concentrate corrected these disorders.

We have previously reported that, in the same animal model, cafeteria diet induces obesity and various related disorders such as dyslipidemia, insulin resistance, oxidative stress, or adipose tissue fibrosis that mimic metabolic syndrome disorders in humans (17, 18). Presently, we

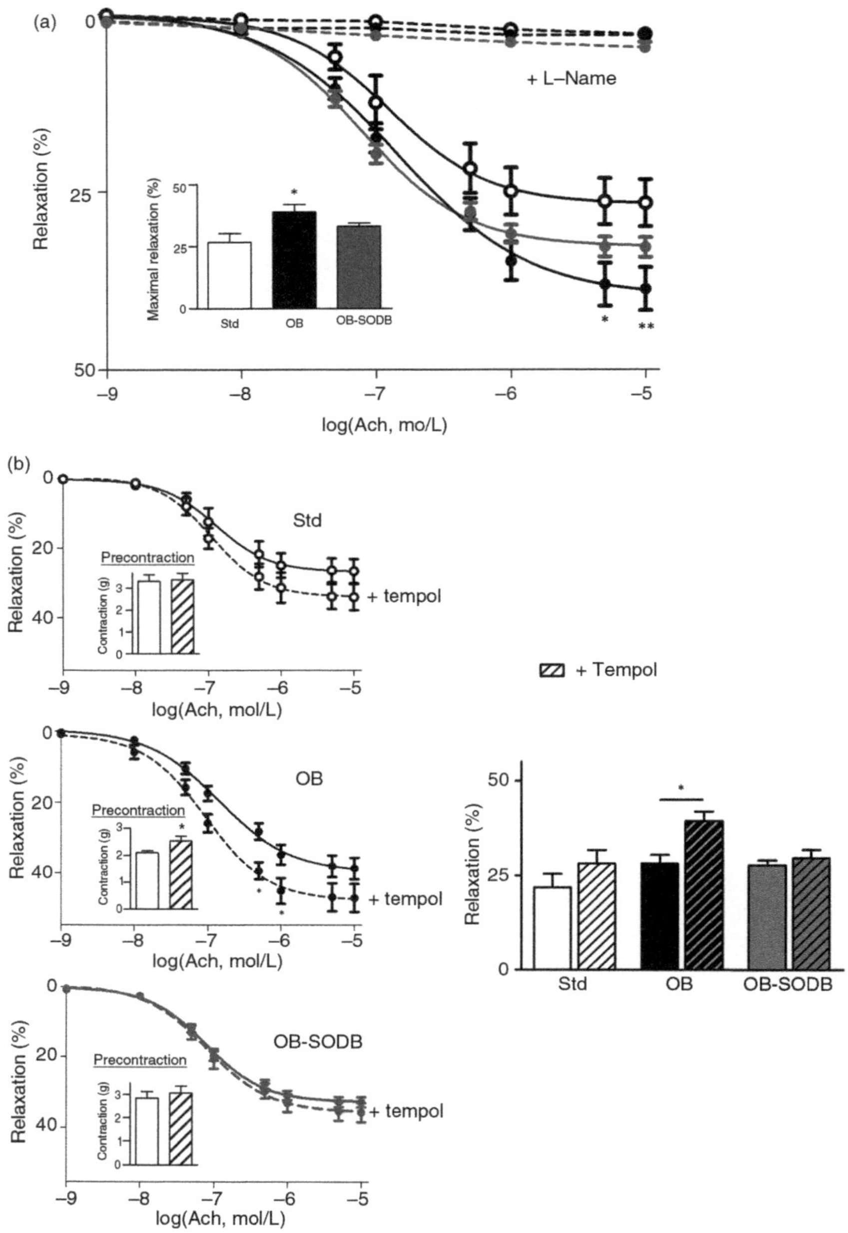

Fig. 3. Ach-mediated relaxation. Graphs represent cumulative dose–response curves to Ach, in the presence of endothelium, in aortic rings previously contracted with a submaximally active concentration of PE (10 μM). Data are expressed as percentage of relaxation relatively to the contraction induced by PE. (a) Relaxing effects of cumulative concentrations of Ach were studied in the absence (plain lines) and in the presence (dotted lines) of L-NAME (10 μM). The inset shows the maximal relaxing effect of Ach (10 μM) for each group (STD, OB, and OB treated). (b) Effect of PE and Ach was evaluated in the presence of tempol (10 μM). Dose–response curves for Ach are shown for each group; the insets represent the previous contractions obtained for PE before Ach addition and for both conditions absence and presence of tempol. The bar graph summarizes the relaxing effects of 1 μM Ach in the absence and in the presence of tempol for STD, OB, and OB-treated groups. Values are presented as mean ± SEM ($n = 6$). *$p < 0.05$, **$p < 0.01$, OB and OB-treated vs. STD animals.

observed that the cafeteria diet induced a morphological remodeling characterized by increases in both intraluminal diameter and media thickness of large arteries. These modifications reflect outward hypertrophic remodeling as shown in both human and animal models (9, 27). It is seen as an adaptive mechanism associated with metabolic syndrome and consecutive to flow-mediated shear stress (28, 29). At first, these adaptations are compensatory and aim to ensure adequate tissue perfusion in relation to higher metabolic requirement. However, in later stages, they become detrimental and contribute to accelerated risk for cardiovascular disorders (8). Increased blood

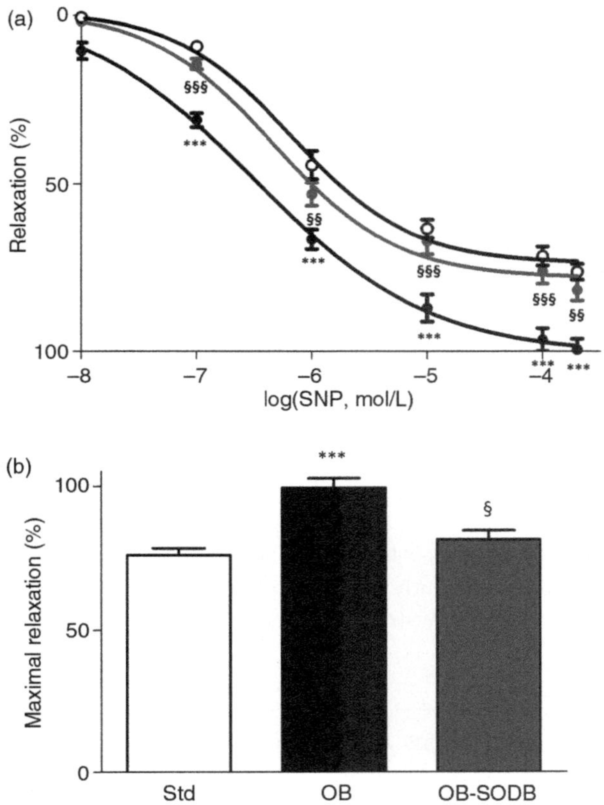

Fig. 4. SNP-induced endothelium-independent vasorelaxation. (a) Cumulative dose–response curves to SNP (0.01–200 μM) of aortic rings endothelium denuded and previously contracted with PE (10 μM) in STD, OB, and OB-treated groups. Data are expressed as percentage of relaxation relatively to the contraction induced by PE. (b) Bar graph represents the maximal relaxation obtained for each group. Values are presented as mean ± SEM. ***$p < 0.001$, OB and OB-treated vs. STD animals; §$p < 0.05$, §§$p < 0.01$, §§§$p < 0.001$ vs. effect of the melon concentrate.

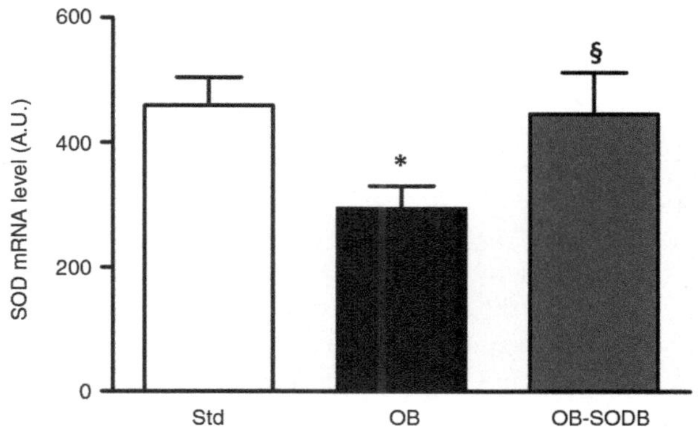

Fig. 5. Expression of aortic SOD. SOD3 mRNA levels were quantified by real-time PCR in aorta. GAPDH was used to normalize total RNA amount. Relative levels were presented in arbitrary units as mean ± SEM of two determinations in all animals in each group ($n = 6$). *$p < 0.05$, OB and OB-treated vs. STD animals; §$p < 0.05$ vs. effect of the melon concentrate.

flow and hypertension, usually associated with obesity, are correlated to arterial stiffness (8, 30). At high blood pressure, vascular-wall stress is prominent and in arteries, less compliant collagen fibers predominate. Abnormalities of arterial function described in humans include both endothelium-dependent and -independent vasodilatation (31). In animal models, vascular reactivity abnormalities mainly consisted of increased contractility and reduced vasodilation (32). Here, in our hamster model of diet-induced obesity, arterial dysfunction was characterized by decreased contractile and increased vasodilatory responses. Such alterations and absence of arterial pressure elevation after high-fat diet have been otherwise reported in another kind of muscular arteries, coronary arteries (33–36). These discrepancies remain unexplained, but they could be due to differences in the disease state studied, or related to diet and different models. Nevertheless, the vascular dysfunction observed in OB group is consistent with the absence of hypertension and revealed an adaptive response resulting in an enhancement of vasorelaxation and a decrease in contractility to maintain adequate tissue perfusion. As a major result of this work, we showed that the melon concentrate supplementation partially reversed the vascular remodeling and improved arterial function. The improvement of arterial function was illustrated by the contractile and vasorelaxant responses in OB-treated group compared to the OB group.

Vasomotor responses are the result of smooth muscle activity regulated by the endothelium. Impaired vascular function can involve endothelial and smooth muscle dysfunction. A high-fat diet is usually related to endothelium dysfunction and reduced NO bioactivity (37). In our model, we observed that both Ach- and SNP-induced relaxations were enhanced in the OB group. This suggests that increased sensitivity to NO, rather than endothelium dysfunction, occurred. Indeed, SNP-induced relaxation is NO dependent, but endothelium independent, whereas Ach induced an NO- and endothelium-dependent relaxation. Enhanced vasodilator capacity of vessels in response to NO and SNP has been previously reported in some models of obesity (33, 36). This phenomenon, thought to be an adaptive mechanism providing adequate tissue perfusion, has been shown to involve increased NO sensitivity that is probably associated with impaired NO bioavailability (34, 38). We observed that the ROS scavenger tempol potentiated Ach-induced relaxation and PE-induced contraction in the OB group. Thus, in the presence of tempol, PE-induced contraction otherwise decreased in the OB group tended to be normalized and identical to STD animals. Tempol is known to prevent NO degradation and thus increases NO bioavailability (39) and mimics the effect of endogenous cellular defense.

The effect of tempol on vasomotor responses in the OB group unmasked an increased NO degradation that was probably related to high level of cellular ROS and oxidative stress, as observed previously (18). One major cellular defense against oxidative stress is a group of oxidoreductases known as SODs. SODs catalyze the dismutation of $O_2^{\bullet -}$ into H_2O_2 and oxygen and thus prevent the inactivation of NO. In blood vessel walls and particularly in the arteries, extracellular SOD (or SOD3) is the main antioxidant defense enzyme (39). Interestingly, the SOD3 mRNA level was decreased in the OB group compared to the STD group. Thus, cafeteria diet triggered vascular disorders related to increased oxidative stress and decreased antioxidant defenses.

The potentiating effect of tempol on Ach-induced relaxation was not observed in the OB-treated group like in the STD group, consistently with a low level of oxidative stress. Thus, the melon concentrate supplementation seemed to correct the decrease in antioxidant defense. This was corroborated by an SOD3 mRNA level that was higher in the OB-treated group than in the OB group and not different from that of the STD group. Vascular SOD3 is localized in a high concentration between the endothelium and the smooth muscle. This localization, at the extracellular matrix level and endothelial cell surfaces, confers a critical role for SOD3 in preventing oxidation of NO released by the endothelium, which is of importance in the regulation of NO bioavailability (40). The beneficial effect of the melon concentrate supplementation on vascular function could be accounted for by an increase in NO bioavailability through SOD3 up-regulation. Consequently, this is associated with a reduction in ROS production that is probably related to a reduced inflammatory status and is consistent with our previous observations (17, 22).

We observed in our model that the melon concentrate supplementation triggers endogenous SOD3 expression. This is in line with previous studies reporting increased levels of antioxidant enzymes in various animal models after melon concentrate supplementation (17, 22, 41). The precise mechanism of the induction remains to be clarified and warrants further investigation. Although the melon concentrate contains a high level of SOD, a direct effect of the enzyme is not considered because its high molecular weight excludes intestinal absorption. Currently, this particular melon concentrate is thought to trigger a cascade of events that initiates the induction of antioxidant defense in various tissues from the intestine through a local stimulation of the immune system (42). The natural product contains active ingredients that will activate antioxidant defense of the host, with a systemic effect at multiple organ levels.

Our results suggest an impact in cardiovascular protection and illustrate that this specific melon concentrate could be used to prevent or attenuate Western diet–related vascular dysfunction. More generally, the induction of endogenous defense implies that this melon concentrate could prevent alterations induced by different pathological situations in which oxidative stress is enhanced. Such a nutritional strategy is in line with the therapeutic guidelines and with the current concept that bioactive phytochemicals play a significant therapeutic role in attenuating oxidative damage induced by metabolic syndrome. However, the beneficial influence of this specific melon concentrate as a dietary supplementation has to be validated in humans.

Acknowledgements

JC was financially supported by Bionov Company with a CIFRE fellowship (Industrial Agreement of Training Through Research).

Conflict of interest and funding

Except JC, the authors have not received any funding or benefits from industry or elsewhere to conduct this study.

References

1. Cordain L, Eaton SB, Sebastian A, Mann N, Lindeberg S, Watkins BA, et al. Origins and evolution of the Western diet: health implications for the 21st century. Am J Clin Nutr 2005; 81: 341–54.
2. Wilsgaard T, Jacobsen BK. Lifestyle factors and incident metabolic syndrome. The Tromsø Study 1979–2001. Diabetes Res Clin Pract 2007; 78: 217–24.
3. Sampey BP, Vanhoose AM, Winfield HM, Freemerman AJ, Muehlbauer MJ, Fueger PT, et al. Cafeteria diet is a robust model of human metabolic syndrome with liver and adipose inflammation: comparison to high-fat diet. Obes Silver Spring Md 2011; 19: 1109–17.
4. Azevedo A, Santos AC, Ribeiro L, Azevehdo I. The Metabolic Syndrome. In: Soares R, Costa C, eds. Oxidative stress, inflammation and angiogenesis in the metabolic syndrome. New York: Springer Science; 2009, pp. 1–19.
5. Caterson ID, Hubbard V, Bray GA, Grunstein R, Hansen BC, Hong Y, et al. Prevention Conference VII: obesity, a worldwide epidemic related to heart disease and stroke: Group III: worldwide comorbidities of obesity. Circulation 2004; 110: e476–83.
6. Eckel RH, Alberti KGMM, Grundy SM, Zimmet PZ. The metabolic syndrome. Lancet Lond Engl 2010; 375: 181–3.
7. Galassi A, Reynolds K, He J. Metabolic syndrome and risk of cardiovascular disease: a meta-analysis. Am J Med 2006; 119: 812–19.
8. Chantler PD, Frisbee JC. Arterial function in cardio-metabolic diseases: from the microcirculation to the large conduits. Prog Cardiovasc Dis 2015; 57: 489–96.
9. Scuteri A, Najjar SS, Muller DC, Andres R, Hougaku H, Metter EJ, et al. Metabolic syndrome amplifies the age-associated increases in vascular thickness and stiffness. J Am Coll Cardiol 2004; 43: 1388–95.
10. Brook RD, Bard RL, Rubenfire M, Ridker PM, Rajagopalan S. Usefulness of visceral obesity (waist/hip ratio) in predicting vascular endothelial function in healthy overweight adults. Am J Cardiol 2001; 88: 1264–9.

11. Griendling KK, Sorescu D, Ushio-Fukai M. NAD(P)H oxidase: role in cardiovascular biology and disease. Circ Res 2000; 86: 494–501.
12. Guzik TJ, West NE, Black E, McDonald D, Ratnatunga C, Pillai R, et al. Vascular superoxide production by NAD(P)H oxidase: association with endothelial dysfunction and clinical risk factors. Circ Res 2000; 86: E85–90.
13. Youn JY, Siu KL, Lob HE, Itani H, Harrison DG, Cai H. Role of vascular oxidative stress in obesity and metabolic syndrome. Diabetes 2014; 63: 2344–55.
14. Böger RH, Bode-Böger SM, Phivthong-ngam L, Brandes RP, Schwedhelm E, Mügge A, et al. Dietary l-arginine and α-tocopherol reduce vascular oxidative stress and preserve endothelial function in hypercholesterolemic rabbits via different mechanisms. Atherosclerosis 1998; 141: 31–43.
15. Jiang F, Guo Y, Salvemini D, Dusting GJ. Superoxide dismutase mimetic M40403 improves endothelial function in apolipoprotein(E)-deficient mice. Br J Pharmacol 2003; 139: 1127–34.
16. Soory M. Relevance of nutritional antioxidants in metabolic syndrome, ageing and cancer: potential for therapeutic targeting. Infect Disord Drug Targets 2009; 9: 400–14.
17. Carillon J, Romain C, Bardy G, Fouret G, Feillet-Coudray C, Gaillet S, et al. Cafeteria diet induces obesity and insulin resistance associated with oxidative stress but not with inflammation: improvement by dietary supplementation with a melon superoxide dismutase. Free Radic Biol Med 2013; 65: 254–61.
18. Carillon J, Knabe L, Montalban A, Stévant M, Keophiphath M, Lacan D, et al. Curative diet supplementation with a melon superoxide dismutase reduces adipose tissue in obese hamsters by improving insulin sensitivity. Mol Nutr Food Res 2014; 58: 842–50.
19. Décordé K, Agne A, Lacan D, Ramos J, Fouret G, Ventura E, et al. Preventive effect of a melon extract rich in superoxide scavenging activity on abdominal and liver fat and adipokine imbalance in high-fat-fed hamsters. J Agric Food Chem 2009; 57: 6461–7.
20. Décordé K, Ventura E, Lacan D, Ramos J, Cristol JP, Rouanet JM. An SOD rich melon extract Extramel prevents aortic lipids and liver steatosis in diet-induced model of atherosclerosis. Nutr Metab Cardiovasc Dis NMCD 2010; 20: 301–7.
21. Vouldoukis I, Lacan D, Kamate C, Coste P, Calenda A, Mazier D, et al. Antioxidant and anti-inflammatory properties of a *Cucumis melo* LC. extract rich in superoxide dismutase activity. J Ethnopharmacol 2004; 94: 67–75.
22. Carillon J, Rugale C, Rouanet JM, Cristol JP, Lacan D, Jover B. Endogenous antioxidant defense induction by melon superoxide dismutase reduces cardiac hypertrophy in spontaneously hypertensive rats. Int J Food Sci Nutr 2014; 65: 602–9.
23. Carillon J, Gauthier A, Barial S, Tournier M, Gayrard N, Lajoix AD, et al. Relaxin and atrial natriuretic peptide pathways participate in the anti-fibrotic effect of a melon concentrate in spontaneously hypertensive rats. Food Nutr Res 2016; 60: 30985, doi: http://dx.doi.org/10.3402/fnr.v60.30985
24. Roberts CK, Sindhu KK. Oxidative stress and metabolic syndrome. Life Sci 2009; 84: 705–12.
25. Carillon J, Del Rio D, Teissèdre PL, Cristol JP, Lacan D, Rouanet JM. Antioxidant capacity and angiotensin I converting enzyme inhibitory activity of a melon concentrate rich in superoxide dismutase. Food Chem 2012; 135: 1298–302.
26. Suh JH, Virsolvy A, Goux A, Cassan C, Richard S, Cristol JP, et al. Polyphenols prevent lipid abnormalities and arterial dysfunction in hamsters on a high-fat diet: a comparative study of red grape and white persimmon wines. Food Funct 2011; 2: 555–61.
27. Ferreira I, Beijers HJ, Schouten F, Smulders YM, Twisk JW, Stehouwer CD. Clustering of metabolic syndrome traits is associated with maladaptive carotid remodeling and stiffening: a 6-year longitudinal study. Hypertension 2012; 60: 542–9.
28. Belin de Chantemèle EJ, Vessières E, Dumont O, Guihot AL, Toutain B, Loufrani L, et al. Reactive oxygen species are necessary for high flow (shear stress)-induced diameter enlargement of rat resistance arteries. Microcirculation 2009; 16: 391–402.
29. Glagov S, Vito R, Giddens DP, Zarins CK. Micro-architecture and composition of artery walls: relationship to location, diameter and the distribution of mechanical stress. J Hypertens Suppl 1992; 10: S101–4.
30. Jia G, Aroor AR, DeMarco VG, Martinez-Lemus L, Meininger GA, Sowers JR. Vascular stiffness in insulin resistance and obesity. Front Physiol 2015; 6: 231.
31. Walther G, Obert P, Dutheil F, Chapier R, Lesourd B, Naughton G, et al. Metabolic syndrome individuals with and without type 2 diabetes mellitus present generalized vascular dysfunction: cross-sectional study. Arterioscler Thromb Vasc Biol 2015; 35: 1022–9.
32. Frisbee JC, Delp MD. Vascular function in the metabolic syndrome and the effects on skeletal muscle perfusion: lessons from the obese Zucker rat. Essays Biochem 2006; 42: 145–61.
33. Prakash R, Mintz JD, Stepp DW. Impact of obesity on coronary microvascular function in the Zucker rat. Microcirculation 2006; 13: 389–96.
34. Jebelovszki E, Kiraly C, Erdei N, Feher A, Pasztor ET, Rutkai I, et al. High-fat diet-induced obesity leads to increased NO sensitivity of rat coronary arterioles: role of soluble guanylate cyclase activation. Am J Physiol Heart Circ Physiol 2008; 294: H2558–64.
35. Lehnen AM, Rodrigues B, Irigoyen MC, De Angelis K, Schaan BD. Cardiovascular changes in animal models of metabolic syndrome. J Diabetes Res 2013; 2013: 761314.
36. Mourmoura E, Chaté V, Couturier K, Laillet B, Vial G, Rigaudiere JP, et al. Body adiposity dictates different mechanisms of increased coronary reactivity related to improved in vivo cardiac function. Cardiovasc Diabetol 2014; 13: 54.
37. Damjanovic M, Barton M. Fat intake and cardiovascular response. Curr Hypertens Rep 2008; 10: 25–31.
38. Brandes RP, Kim D, Schmitz-Winnenthal FH, Amidi M, Gödecke A, Mülsch A, et al. Increased nitrovasodilator sensitivity in endothelial nitric oxide synthase knockout mice: role of soluble guanylyl cyclase. Hypertension 2000; 35: 231–6.
39. Simonsen U, Christensen FH, Buus NH. The effect of tempol on endothelium-dependent vasodilatation and blood pressure. Pharmacol Ther 2009; 122: 109–24.
40. Fukai T, Ushio-Fukai M. Superoxide dismutases: role in redox signaling, vascular function, and diseases. Antioxid Redox Signal 2011; 15: 1583–606.
41. Vouldoukis I, Conti M, Krauss P, Kamaté C, Blazquez S, Tefit M, et al. Supplementation with gliadin-combined plant superoxide dismutase extract promotes antioxidant defences and protects against oxidative stress. Phytother Res 2004; 18: 957–62.
42. Carillon J, Rouanet JM, Cristol JP, Brion R. Superoxide dismutase administration, a potential therapy against oxidative stress related diseases: several routes of supplementation and proposal of an original mechanism of action. Pharm Res 2013; 30: 2718–28.

***Anne Virsolvy**
INSERM U1046, UMR CNRS 9214
CHU Arnaud de Villeneuve
FR-34495 Montpellier, France
Email: anne.virsolvy@inserm.fr

15

Microalgae as a safe food source for animals: nutritional characteristics of the acidophilic microalga *Coccomyxa onubensis*

Francisco Navarro[1,2], Eduardo Forján[2], María Vázquez[2], Zaida Montero[1,2], Elisabeth Bermejo[2], Miguel Ángel Castaño[3], Alberto Toimil[1], Enrique Chagüaceda[4], Miguel Ángel García-Sevillano[5], Marisa Sánchez[6], María José Domínguez[2], Rosario Pásaro[7], Inés Garbayo[2], Carlos Vílchez[2]* and José María Vega[8]

[1]Department of Environmental Biology and Public Health, Cell Biology, Faculty of Experimental Sciences, University of Huelva, Huelva, Spain; [2]Algal Biotechnology Group, CIDERTA and Faculty of Sciences, University of Huelva and Marine International Campus of Excellence (CEIMAR), Huelva, Spain; [3]University Hospital Complex of Huelva Juan Ramón Jiménez, Huelva, Spain; [4]CIDERTA Investigation Center, University of Huelva, Huelva, Spain; [5]Department of Chemistry and Materials Science, Faculty of Experimental Sciences, University of Huelva, Huelva, Spain; [6]Riotinto Hospital, Huelva, Spain; [7]Department of Physiology, Faculty of Biology, University of Seville, Seville, Spain; [8]Department of Plant Biochemistry and Molecular Biology, Faculty of Chemistry, University of Seville, Seville, Spain

Abstract

Background: Edible microalgae are marine or fresh water mesophilic species. Although the harvesting of microalgae offers an abundance of opportunities to the food and pharmaceutical industries, the possibility to use extremophilic microalgae as a food source for animals is not well-documented.
Objective: We studied the effects of dietary supplementation of a powdered form of the acidophilic microalga *Coccomyxa onubensis* on growth and health parameters of laboratory rats.
Method: Four randomly organized groups of rats ($n = 6$) were fed a standard diet (Diet 1, control) or with a diet in which 0.4% (Diet 2), 1.25% (Diet 3), or 6.25% (Diet 4) (w/w) of the standard diet weight was substituted with dried microalgae powder, respectively. The four groups of animals were provided *ad libitum* access to feed for 45 days.
Results: *C. onubensis* biomass is rich in protein (44.60% of dry weight) and dietary fiber (15.73%), and has a moderate carbohydrate content (24.8%) and a low lipid content (5.4%) in which polyunsaturated fatty acids represent 65% of the total fatty acid. Nucleic acids are present at 4.8%. No significant difference was found in growth rates or feed efficiency ratios of the four groups of rats. Histological studies of liver and kidney tissue revealed healthy organs in control and *C. onubensis*-fed animals, while plasma hematological and biochemical parameters were within healthy ranges for all animals. Furthermore, animals fed a microalgae-enriched diet exhibited a statistically significant decrease in both blood cholesterol and triglyceride levels. The blood triglyceride content and very low density lipoprotein-cholesterol levels decreased by about 50% in rats fed Diet 4.
Conclusions: These data suggest that *C. onubensis* may be useful as a food supplement for laboratory animals and may also serve as a nutraceutical in functional foods. In addition, microalgae powder-supplemented diets exerted a significant hypocholesterolemic and hypotriglyceridemic effect in animals.

Keywords: Coccomyxa onubensis; *rats*; *safe food*; *nutraceuticals*; *hypolipidemic induction*

The health of people is linked directly to lifestyle, of which a balanced diet plays a fundamental role. Within the concept of what is meant by such a diet, nutraceuticals and functional foods have become progressively relevant. From the middle of the 20th century, large-scale microalgae cultivation has been carried out in regions with harsh climatic conditions where other crops cannot be grown, such as desert and coastal areas, and the obtained biomass used for biotechnological applications (1).

Microalgae such as *Chlorella* spp., *Dunaliella* spp., *Scenedesmus* spp., *Nannochloropsis* spp., *Tetraselmis* spp., *Spirulina* spp., and *Aphanizomenon flos-aquae* have been used as nutrient-dense foods and sources of nutraceuticals for functional foods (2–4). The use of microalgae for animal feed and aquaculture is of particular interest (5). While edible microalgae have been obtained from marine or freshwater mesophilic species, just a few attempts have been made to the present time to introduce the production of extremophilic microalgae, including *Dunaliella*, *Spirulina*, and *Galdieria* species (6, 7), to be used as a feed or food source, probably due to low growth rates and poor biomass productivity. However, recent studies have shown that acidophilic *Coccomyxa onubensis* can be phototrophically cultivated at pH 2.5 in minimum mineral medium, thereby reaching a moderate growth rate (8).

Issues associated with the use of microalgal biomass as a direct food source for animals include its high nucleic acid content and possible contamination, which raise concerns regarding potential toxicity and long-term effects on human health (3). Some authors indicate that the future use of microalgae biomass in the food industry will be as a source of nutraceuticals for functional foods rather than the direct use of such biomass. Microalgal biomass contains variable amounts of biological compounds that are beneficial to human and animal health, including lipids, polysaccharides, antioxidants, vitamins, minerals, and biomolecules with pharmaceutical activities (9–11). Some of these compounds are considered as functional ingredients in traditional foods, such as breakfast cereals, spreads, breads, cookies, brownies, energy bars, mayonnaises, gelled dessert, pastas, emulsions, ice creams, and beverages (12).

Several polyhydroxysterols from microalgae have also been found to display cytotoxic and anticancer activities (13). Polysaccharides belong to a large family of highly diverse chemical compounds, some of which have been described to stimulate the human immune system and/or have potential biomedical applications (14). Therefore, there is no doubt concerning the high potential value of microalgal biomass as a possible source of nutraceuticals for functional foods.

Because the natural habitat of *C. onubensis* supports high irradiation and oxidative conditions, physicochemical and nutritional parameters can be adequately fixed to produce biomass with a high carotenoid (mainly lutein) and polyunsaturated fatty acid (PUFA) content (15). As such, *C. onubensis* might be a good model to investigate the potential role of an acidophilic photosynthetic microalga to be used in animal feed. This study was undertaken to elucidate the effects of microalgae-supplemented diets on the health of laboratory rats. Hematological and biochemical parameters were analyzed in parallel with histological studies, with results demonstrating no adverse effects on rat health. In addition, *C. onubensis*–supplemented diets exhibited a potent hypocholesterolemic and hypotriglyceridemic effect in experimental animals.

Materials and methods

Microalgal biomass production

The microalga *C. onubensis* (SAG 2510) (16), deposited at the Culture Collection of Algae at Goettingen University, was bulk produced in 400 L transparent plastic bags of 60 cm diameter and 2.1 m height. The bags were maintained indoors at 20°C, filled with K9 culture medium (adjusted to pH 2.5), and bubbled with CO_2-enriched air (5% v/v) *via* air diffusers placed at the bottom of the bags. The cultures were illuminated with white fluorescent light at 200-μmol photons/m^2s at the bag surface. The cells were harvested by continuous flow centrifugation at 8,400 rpm using an industrial centrifuge (GEA Westfalia Separator model KA-6, Oelde, Germany), and the collected pellet was washed twice with deionized water. The biomass was dried in an oven with fan-assisted circulation (JP Selecta DRY-BIG 2002972, Barcelona, Spain) and converted into a powder of grain size <100 μm using a vibratory disc mill (Retsch GmbH RS100, Haan, Germany). The powder was then vacuum packed and stored at −80°C until use.

Chemical analysis of the C. onubensis *biomass*

The main components of the algal biomass were analyzed by the Central Services Unit of the University Pablo de Olavide (Seville, Spain). To determine the fatty acid composition of the biomass, the acid catalyzed transesterification of extracted glycerides was carried out in flasks according to the following procedure: the standard reaction mixture containing glycerides, methanol, and concentrated sulfuric acid (5% v/v) was heated at 70°C for 3 h, then cooled and treated with hexane and water. The mixture was separated by centrifugation (2,000 rpm, 10 min) into two layers, the upper lipidic layer of which was washed with water until the washing water was pH neutral. Analysis of the resulting fatty acid monoester (FAME) composition of this hexane layer was carried out using an Agilent 7890A gas chromatography unit (Agilent Technologies, Wilmington, DE, USA) equipped with flame ionization detector. Samples (1 μL) were injected into an OMEGAWax-fused silica capillary column (30 m, 0.32 mm id, and 0.25 μm film thickness) in which the flow rate of the carrier gas helium was constant at 1.5 mL/min and a split ratio of 20:1 was used. A solvent delay period of 1.5 min was assigned. The injector temperature was 100°C, and the detector temperature was maintained at 200°C. The oven temperature was raised from 80 to 140°C at 5°C/min, then increased up to 170°C at 4°C/min, and maintained for 2 min at that temperature. It was then raised to 190°C at 1°C/min and maintained for 2 min, and finally, the oven temperature program was increased to 200°C. Individual FAMEs were identified by comparing their retention times with those of a mixed FAME standard (FAMEs MIX C4-C24 SUPELCO

Analytical, Bellefonte, PA, USA). Concentrations of FAMEs in the injected hexane solution were quantified by comparing their peak areas with those obtained from the standards of known concentration. Fatty acid composition was calculated as the percentage of total fatty acids in the volume of hexane.

Experimental diet preparation
The experimental diets used in this work were based on conventional rodent chow pellets from Harlan Laboratories, Inc. (Indianapolis, IN, USA), which were grounded into powder using a jaw crusher (Retsch GmbH BB200) and a vibratory disc mill until the grain size was < 100 μm. The four diets were prepared as follows: Diet 1, control: composed of standard diet powder only; Diet 2: 4 mg of microalgae powder were mixed with 996 mg of standard diet powder; Diet 3: composed of 12.5 mg microalgae powder plus 987.5 mg standard diet powder; and Diet 4: 62.5 mg microalgae powder plus 937 mg standard diet powder. In all cases, the powders were mixed homogeneously, reconstituted with distilled water in a kneader (Fimar AM1, Rimini, Italy), and then made into pellets again with an extruder (Fimar MPF4). The four reconstituted pellet diets were dried in an oven with fan-assisted circulation to obtain the same degree of humidity as the original standard rodent diet. Dried pellets were stored at 4°C under vacuum until used.

According to equivalences shown in Table 1, the amount of microalga used in these experimental diets was comparable to a human consumption of 20.4–255 g/day microalgae powder, which would be sufficient quantities to enable information about toxicity to be obtained.

Animal handling
Experiments were performed on 4-week-old Long Evans male rats ($n = 24$) weighing 130–140 g, obtained from the Charles River Laboratories (St. Germain-Nuelles, France). Animals were handled in accordance with Directive 8609/CEE of the European Community Council and Spanish Legislation (R.D. 53/2013). The protocols used in this work were approved by the Ethics Committee of the University of Huelva (Spain). Animals were allowed to acclimatize for 5 days with free access to food (Diet 1) and water under controlled conditions of temperature (22.0 ± 1.3°C) and a 12 h light–dark cycle prior to the start of experiments. They were then randomly distributed into four groups of six rats each, with similar mean weights, housed individually, and fed with one of the described diets (Diet 1, Diet 2, Diet 3, and Diet 4). They were weighed every second day, and biochemical and histological analyses were performed on all animals after a period of 45 days of *ad libitum* feeding.

Table 1. Relationship of microalga powder in rat diets and its corresponding equivalence in human diets

Diet	Alga amount in rat diet (%)	Alga consumption by rats (mg/day)	Equivalent alga consumption by 68 kg person (g/day)
1	0	0	0
2	0.4	60	20.4
3	1.25	187.5	63.8
4	6	750	255

Calculations were made for an average size (200 g) rat consuming 15 g/day of feed (26).

Hematological and biochemical analyses
Rats were fasted for 8 h and anesthetized with inhaled isoflurane prior to sacrifice. Following a cardiac puncture, blood was collected from the left ventricle in a 2 mL glass BD Vacutainer K3 EDTA tube (Becton, Dickinson and Company, Franklin Lakes, NJ, USA) and processed immediately according to the manufacturer's instructions for hematological studies. The hematological analysis was carried out on a Sysmex XT-4000i automated hematology analyzer (Sysmex America, Inc., Lincolnshire, IL, USA). To study the erythrocyte morphology, blood smears were prepared following the procedure of Bain et al. (17), stained with Hemacolor® staining kit (Merck Millipore, Darmstadt, Germany), and examined under a Nikon Eclipse E400 microscope (Nikon, Tokyo, Japan).

Samples for serum biochemistry determinations were collected in 2 mL tubes with the Advanced BD Vacutainer SST II gel separator and suction system. Blood samples were first cooled in a refrigerator and protected from light for 60 min to allow clot retraction, and serum obtained after centrifugation at 4,000 rpm for 30 min at 4°C. Parameter determinations were carried out on a Sysmex XT-4000i automated hematology analyzer (Sysmex America, Inc.). Enzyme activities were determined on a Cobas 8000 modular analyzer (Roche Diagnostics, Basel, Switzerland) according to the manufacturer's instructions. Plasma total cholesterol (TC) and triglyceride concentrations were determined enzymatically on the Cobas 8000 modular analyzer according to the manufacturer's instructions. The same instrument was also used to analyze high density lipoprotein (HDL)- and very low density lipoprotein (VLDL)-cholesterol contents following the manufacturer's instructions in each case.

Histological analysis
Liver and kidney tissues from animals in the different group were extracted, weighed, cleaned with 0.9% (w/v) NaCl solution, and fixed in 4% neutral buffered formalin. This was followed by dehydration in ascending grades of alcohol for 51 h, xylene for 1 h, and finally embedding in paraffin wax. Liver and kidney sections (4 mm thickness) were obtained with a Leica Leitz 1512 precision rotary microtome (Leitz, Wetzlar, Germany) and stained with hematoxylin and eosin for histological examination.

Slide-mounted sections were observed under light microscope (Nikon Eclipse E400 microscope) for the evaluation of tissue integrity.

Statistical analyses

Statistical analyses were conducted by using the SPSS version 19 statistical analysis package. The data of the four dietary groups were analyzed by a non-parametric test (Kruskal–Wallis). Differences were accepted as significant for values of $p < 0.05$.

Results

Effect of C. onubensis *biomass on rat body weights*

The composition of *C. onubensis* biomass is indicated in Table 2. Of particular interest from a nutritional point of view was the high protein (44.60% of dry weight) and dietary fiber (15.73%) content of the material, together with a moderate carbohydrate content (24.80%), and a low lipid (5.40%) and nucleic acids (4.8%) content. An additional dietary advantage of this biomass is its low monosaccharide and disaccharide content (0.1%), and high PUFA content (65% of total fatty acid content).

The four groups of rats exhibited constant weekly weight gain, which at the end of the experiment ranged from 210±8.08 g for control animals (Diet 1) to 205±8.46 g for the Diet 4 group. Rats did not show any visible physiological or behavioral alterations over the experimental period. The ratio of food consumed (g)/weight gained (g) (feeding efficiency) was between 5.04±0.20 (Diet 1, control) and 4.40±0.11 (Diet 4) (Table 3), which is within the normal range for rats.

Table 2. Chemical composition of dry biomass from *C. onubensis*

Parameter	Fraction composition (%)	Sub-fraction composition (%)
Proteins	44.60	–
Carbohydrates	24.80	–
Soluble sugars	–	4.11
Dietary fiber	15.73	–
Triglycerides	5.40	–
Saturated FA	–	17.55
Monounsaturated FA	–	17.45
Polyunsaturated FA	–	65.00
Nucleic acids	4.8	–

The dry weight represents 24.35% of the biomass. Numbers are per cent of dry weight. Parameters were determined as indicated in Materials and Methods. FA, fatty acids.

Histological studies of liver and kidney

At the end of the experiment, each rat was sacrificed, and its liver and kidneys extracted and studied. Freshly excised organs showed a normal aspect in all groups and weighed 10.48±0.55 g for liver and 2.13±0.28 g for kidneys (Table 3). The relative weights of the liver and kidney tissues (g/100 g body weight) were similar for all groups of animals; at around 3.00 for liver and 0.60 for kidney in the control and Diet 4 groups (Table 3).

The thickness and configuration of the trabeculae, the presence of regenerative changes, and an initial assessment of fibrosis in the liver were carried out, with no pathogenic changes observed for any groups (Fig. 1a–d). In addition, parameters indicative of degeneration and substance deposition, such as ballooning degeneration (swelling), presence of cholestasis, and of macro and micro vesicular steatosis, were found to be normal in all groups. All of the sections studied showed a healthy hepatocyte architecture in the parenchyma and central vein, with similar degrees of steatosis in the different groups of rats. However, striking alterations were identified in the chromatin pattern of hepatocyte nuclei from the Diet 4 group (Fig. 1d), which did not affect the health of animals. Likewise, the cytoplasm presented an

Table 3. Anthropometric data for control rats and rats fed powdered *C. onubensis* in the diet

Anthropometric data	Diet 1	Diet 2	Diet 3	Diet 4
Initial weight (g)	134±4.64	137±2.38	125±4.64	123±3.35
Final weight (g)	344±6.62	338±7.72	336±8.76	328±7.77
Weight gain (g)	210±8.08	201±8.07	211±9.91	205±8.46
Feed consumption (g)	1,058±43.38	1,016±40.65	939.5±43.22	902±37.88
Feed efficiency ratio	5.04±0.20	5.06±0.22	4.45±0.17	4.40±0.11
Liver weight (g)	10.48±0.55	9.68±0.36	9.78±0.24	9.85±0.64
Relative weight (g/100 g bw)	3.00	2.86	2.90	3.00
Kidney weight (g)	2.13±0.28	2.04±0.35	1.97±0.42	2.01±0.38
Relative weight (g/100 g bw)	0.60	0.60	0.50	0.60

Each value is expressed as the mean±SE ($n = 6$) in all groups. Results were statistically analyzed with Kruskal–Wallis test. No significant differences were observed at the $p < 0.05$ level among the different diets. bw, body weight.

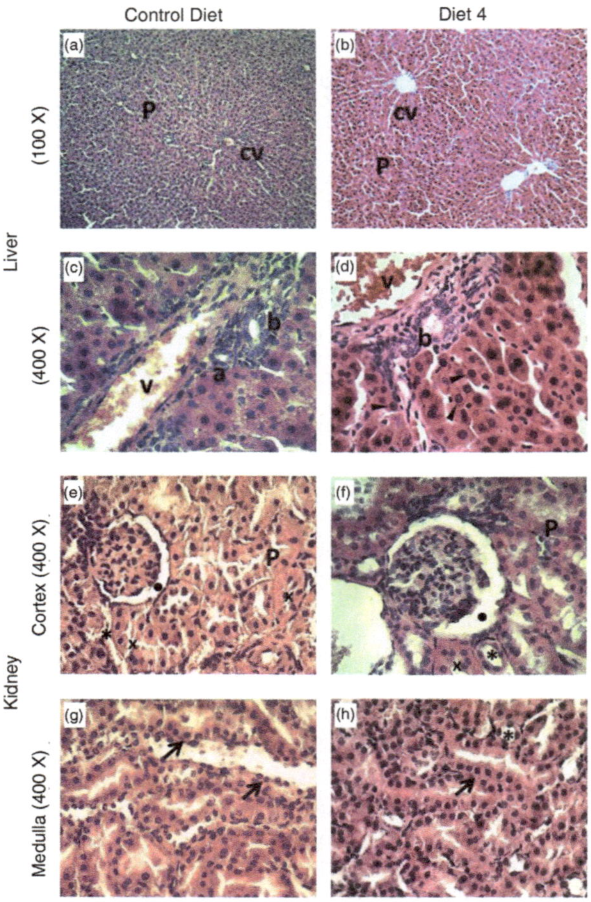

Fig. 1. Hematoxylin and eosin stained sections of rat liver and kidney from experimental rats. Liver: a,b. Hepatocyte architecture in parenchyma (P) and central vein (cv). c,d: Higher magnification of hepatic sections where the portal triad it can be observed: normal portal vein (v), artery (a), and bile duct (b) without occlusions. d. Black arrow heads indicate hepatocyte nuclei. Kidney: e-h. Sections of the cortex (black dot) and convoluted proximal (x) and distal (asterisks) tubules are shown in e,f. g,h: Medulla. Longitudinal section of tubule epithelium (black arrows).

increased uptake of hematoxylin in some areas without signs of cell swelling. No hepatocellular damage such as tissue necrosis or apoptosis was found. Predominant cell types and inflammation parameter levels were also found to be normal (Fig. 1a and b) (18).

With respect to kidney tissue, attention was focused on the glomerulus, where we looked for the possible presence of sclerosis, inflammatory infiltrates, thrombi, and/or deposits. We also examined the interstitium and tubules, where we looked for the presence of atrophy, inflammatory infiltrates, necrosis, and deposits. All of studied sections in the different groups of animals presented a normal histology, with no signs of degeneration (Fig. 1e–h) (18). In cortical regions of the kidney, where the Bowman's capsule is located, the capsular space and podocytes were distributed in a normal fashion, independently of the diet received by the rat (Fig. 1e and f). The proximal convoluted and distal tubules also showed a normal epithelial cell distribution. Most of the tubules in the medulla (Fig. 1g and h) presented a longitudinal section and an intact collecting tubule epithelium. Attention was paid to the structure of blood vessels to identify the possible presence of vasculitis, thrombi, hyalinization, or sclerosis, but all of the studied histological sections appeared normal (18), thereby indicating a lack of toxicity of the microalgae powder-containing diets.

Blood and biochemical parameters

Table 4 shows hematological parameters for the four experimental animal groups. No significant differences were identified, and the blood profiles were typical of healthy animals. In relation to biochemical parameters, the plasma total protein content was significantly lower for the Diet 3 and Diet 4 groups, whose diet had a higher percentage enrichment of algae. The plasma glucose concentration, 115.50 mg/dL, in rats fed with the Diet 4 was higher than the control group (70.18 mg/dL, Diet 1) (Table 5). However, values did not exceed 135 mg/dL, which is considered the upper limit for healthy rats. Levels of other plasma parameters such as albumin, creatinine, ferritin, bilirubin, and the Ca^{2+}, Na^{+}, K^{+}, Cl^{-}, and Fe^{2+} ions were similar across the different groups of rats, and within normal ranges (Table 5).

Diets supplemented with *C. onubensis* powder did not influence blood transaminase or alkaline phosphatase activity levels in rats. Glutamate-oxaloacetate transaminase (GOT) and glutamate-pyruvate transaminase activities in plasma were unchanged in rats fed supplemented diets compared with controls (Fig. 2). Finally, only a small decrease was observed in the plasma lipase activity level from rats fed the algae-supplemented feed with respect to control (Fig. 2).

Importantly, *C. onubensis* powder-supplemented diets induced a significant decrease in plasma triglyceride contents, which reached 50% in Diet 4-fed rats compared to control rats (Diet 1). A similar decrease was observed in the plasma VLDL-cholesterol content, while TC content decreased by around 20% (Fig. 3). On contrary, HDL-cholesterol content decreased significantly by 25%, while the low density lipoprotein (LDL) cholesterol content increased by 30% (not shown).

Discussion

The composition of *C. onubensis* biomass (Table 2) suggests that it has nutritional properties that may be more beneficial than other microalgae used in animal foods, where protein contents range from 1 to 65%, carbohydrate from 15 to 50%, and fat from 3 to 48% (4, 19). Biomass from *Chlorella vulgaris*, one of the most used species of microalgae, employed as a food supplement contains

Table 4. Hematological parameters of rats fed control or *C. onubensis*–supplemented diets

Parameter	Diet 1	Diet 2	Diet 3	Diet 4
Hemoglobin (g/dL)	14.58 ± 0.99	14.78 ± 1.1	15.88 ± 0.11	16.08 ± 0.05
Hematocrit (%)	44.43 ± 2.93	44.25 ± 3.12	47.38 ± 0.46	48.00 ± 0.36
Erythrocytes (cells × 10^{-6}/μL)	8.66 ± 0.60	8.24 ± 0.57	8.76 ± 0.13	8.61 ± 0.03
Leucocytes (cells × 10^{-3}/μL)	5.57 ± 0.89	5.35 ± 1.04	8.23 ± 1.89	6.65 ± 1.02
Lymphocytes (%)	84.75 ± 1.89	90.00 ± 2.64	85.75 ± 2.06	89.75 ± 0.63
Platelets (cells × 10^{-3}/μL)	584.67 ± 18.46	618.33 ± 29.80	665.00 ± 10.13	779.00 ± 14.12

Data obtained at the end of the experiment (45 days). Each value is expressed as the mean ± SD ($n = 6$ per group). Results were statistically analyzed with Kruskal–Wallis test. No significant differences were observed at the $p < 0.05$ level among the different diets. More details in Materials and Methods section.

28.0% protein, 49.5% carbohydrate, 17.5% lipid and 4.5% nucleic acids (20). Microalgal lipids are particularly interesting because they contain high levels of PUFAs such as docosahexaenoic (DHA) and eicosapentaenoic (EPA) acids, as well as carotenoids, such as astaxanthin and lutein, and other antioxidants (21). *C. onubensis* biomass is particularly rich in lutein and β-carotene, which have high antioxidant activities and are considered very useful as a source of nutraceuticals (8). Antioxidant phenolic compounds and vitamins (A precursor, E, and B group) are also produced by microalgae and accumulate at different levels depending on the cultivation conditions (4, 9). Further studies are necessary to examine ways to increase the antioxidant phenolic compounds and vitamin contents in *C. onubensis* biomass, and thereby to improve the properties of this material. The content in nucleic acids of *C. onubensis* is 4.8%, which is within the average nucleic acid content for most of microalgae, including those which are used as food for humans (22). This value should be compared with 1.5 and 2.2% of nucleic acids content found in beef and beef liver, respectively. It is generally considered that the long-term maximum acceptable daily intake of nucleic acid is about 4.0 g/day for an adult (23).

In general, the use of powdered microalgae in diets here was well tolerated by rats, as indicated by the similar weight gains in the four experimental groups over the course of the experiment (Table 3). In this context, a decrease in the body weight of animals has been observed with other microalgae-supplemented diets such as *Isochrysis galbana* and *Nannocholopsis oculata* (24), and the red microalga *Porphyridium* sp. (25). In contrast, rats fed a powdered form of the cyanobacteria *A. flos-aquae* showed a body weight increase of around 10% with respect to the control group (26).

Histological studies, along with hematological and biochemical analyses demonstrated that the *C. onubensis* powder-supplemented diets were not associated with any toxic side-effects to animals. The observed plasma levels of albumin and creatinine suggested that the four groups of animals had a good nutritional status and good renal

Table 5. Biochemical parameters of rats fed control or *C. onubensis*–supplemented diets

Parameter	Diet 1	Diet 2	Diet 3	Diet 4
Total protein (g/dL)	6.05 ± 0.05	6.18 ± 0.02	5.45 ± 0.31*#	5.65 ± 0.35*#
Albumin (g/dL)	4.40 ± 0.11	4.48 ± 0.11	4.23 ± 0.25	4.28 ± 0.23
Ca^{2+} (mg/dL)	10.40 ± 0.50	10.40 ± 0.5	10.19 ± 0.19	10.40 ± 0.32
Na^{2+} (mEq/L)	145.00 ± 0.82	146.00 ± 1.78	144.25 ± 1.65	147.00 ± 0.91
K^{+} (mEq/L)	4.43 ± 0.19	4.43 ± 0.19	5.26 ± 0.69	4.22 ± 0.38
Cl^{-} (mEq/L)	90.13 ± 1.07	98.13 ± 1.07	99.15 ± 0.65	99.88 ± 1.62
Glucose (mg/dL)	70.18 ± 4.97	99.68 ± 7.63	115.50 ± 14.47	103.03 ± 15.44
Creatinine (mg/dL)	0.32 ± 0.02	0.32 ± 0.02	0.32 ± 0.02	0.27 ± 0.03
Fe^{2+} (μg/dL)	128.90 ± 6.44	136.33 ± 7.16	137.45 ± 7.89	139.58 ± 11.89
Ferritin (ng/mL)	185.30 ± 5.52	177.93 ± 2.81	174.38 ± 9.97	152.70 ± 25.70
Bilirubin (mg/dL)	0.04 ± 0.01	0.07 ± 0.01	0.10 ± 0.02	0.08 ± 0.03

Data obtained at the end of the experiment (45 days). Each value is expressed as the mean ± SD ($n = 6$ per group). Results were statistically analyzed with Kruskal–Wallis test. The only significant difference observed was for total protein. *$p < 0.05$ compared with the control group. #$p < 0.05$ compared with other groups. No significant difference was observed at the $p < 0.05$ for other parameters. More details in Materials and Methods section.

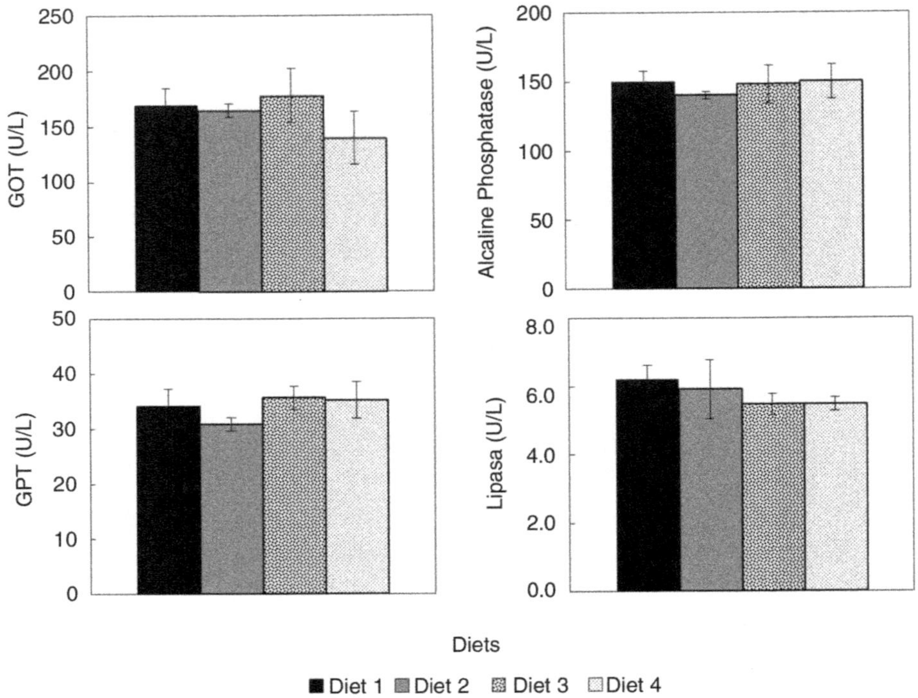

Fig. 2. Enzyme activities in plasma from rats fed diets supplemented with *C. onubensis* biomass. Experimental conditions are described in the Materials and Methods. GOT, glutamate-oxaloacetate transaminase; GPT, glutamate-pyruvate transaminase. Each value is expressed as the mean $\pm$ SD ($n = 6$ per group). Results were statistically analyzed with Kruskal–Wallis test. None of the diets (Diet 2, Diet 3, and Diet 4) showed significant differences at the $p < 0.05$ level with respect to each other, or relative to the control (Diet 1).

function, while plasma transaminase activity levels demonstrated that the liver status of animals was good. In line with these observations, Ekmay et al. (27) observed a lack of toxicity in laying hens fed diets supplemented with biomass from the green microalga *Desmodesmus* spp. or the diatom *Staurospira* spp. The high phenolic compound content in *Spirulina platensis* biomass seems to exert a hepatoprotective effect in rats (28).

Previous findings concerning the plasma glucose concentration in animals fed on microalgal biomass are contentious. For example, *I. galbana* induced a decrease in plasma glucose and cholesterol values, whereas consumption of the microalga *N. oculata* showed no benefit for normal and diabetic rats (24). The moderate hyperglycemic effect induced by *C. onubensis* powder in rats in this study (Table 5) had no apparent consequences on animal health status. This effect cannot be directly attributed to the microalgae powder because soluble carbohydrates found in this biomass were very low (Table 2).

The *C. onubensis* biomass induced a potent hypolipidemic activity in rats, which suggests that this material may have been used as a source of nutraceuticals in functional foods and/or have pharmacologic applications. It is important to note that, in humans and rodents, the liver is the primary site for *de novo* lipogenesis, where glucose is the main carbon precursor for this process. However, a principle difference between these species is that carry out the majority of cholesterol in the plasma of rodents is bound to HDL-lipoproteins, whereas in humans it is bound to LDL-lipoproteins (29). In animals, ProAlgaZyme, an infusion of fermented algae biomass, induces a significant reduction in body weight, body fat, TC, LDL-cholesterol, and triglycerides and is accompanied by a significant increase in HDL-cholesterol levels. This infusion is well tolerated by animals and does not cause significant side effects (30). Results obtained with *C. pyrenoidosa* are particularly interesting, as this microalga was shown to prevent hyperlipidemia and atherosclerosis in rats and hamsters fed chronically with a high-fat diet (31). A study performed on chickens demonstrated that both 5 and 10% levels of *Porphyridium* sp. biomass supplemented in the diet were effective in lowering cholesterol levels, while a trend toward lower cholesterol in eggs was also observed (32). The next step in our research will be to examine the hypolipidemic effects of *C. onubensis* on rats fed a cholesterol-rich diet.

Identification of the active constituents that give rise to the hypolipidemic activity of *C. onubensis* must be further investigated. In this context, PUFAs have been reported to reduce blood LDL-cholesterol and HDL-cholesterol levels (33). Van Beelen et al. (34) suggested that omega-3 fatty acids lowered blood LDL-cholesterol levels, producing

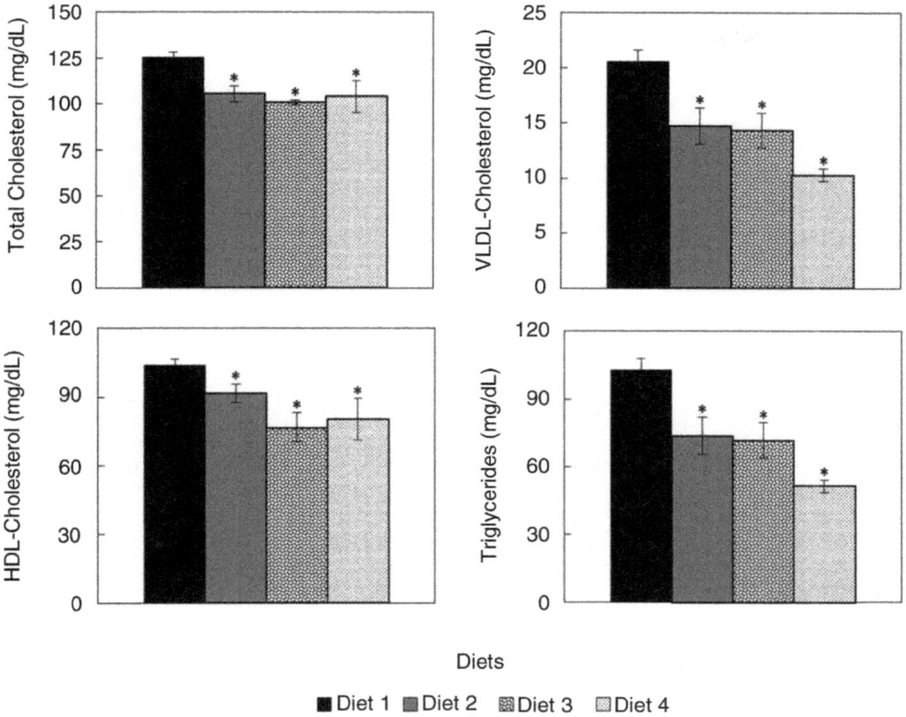

Fig. 3. Lipid profiles of rats fed with diets supplemented with *C. onubensis* biomass. Experimental conditions are described in the Materials and Methods section. Each value is expressed as the mean ± SD ($n = 6$ per group). Results were statistically analyzed with Kruskal–Wallis test. *$p < 0.05$ compared with the control group. None of the diets (Diet 2, Diet 3, and Diet 4) showed significant differences at the $p < 0.05$ level with respect to each other. HDL = High density lipoprotein. VLDL = Very low density lipoprotein.

similar protective effects to those of fish oil against heart disease, atherosclerosis, cancer, and diabetes. The fatty acid content of *C. onubensis* is rich in PUFAs (see Table 2), which could be responsible for the observed lipoprotein profile in rats, although it is possible that the presence of other components could also be involved. Chen et al. (35) concluded that microalgal lipids are the active compounds responsible for the triglyceride- and cholesterol-lowering activity induced in hamsters. Algal-DHA acid induced a significant dose-related decrease of triglycerides and cholesterol in rats fed a high fructose diet (36). In this context, it is important to note that algae rich in n-3 fatty acids have been used in feed supplements for dairy cattle (37).

Our study shows that the acidophilic microalga *C. onubensis* provides a good source of dietary fiber, which may help to promote hypocholesterolemic and hypotriglyceridemic outcomes in rats due to its high PUFA content. Polysaccharides and dietary fiber have also been demonstrated to be involved in the hypolipidemic effect of *Porphyridium* (25). Animal studies have shown that the consumption of dietary fiber is associated with changes in lipid metabolism (9). In addition, soluble polysaccharides and biomass obtained from the red microalga *Porphyridium* sp. altered the intestinal morphology and reduced serum cholesterol in rats (25). Several health benefits derived from the presence of algal polysaccharides in the diet have also been reported in humans (38, 39). On contrary, sterol extracts from the alga *Schizochytrium* sp. were as effective as β-sitosterol in reducing plasma cholesterol concentrations (40).

Conclusions

Based on histological, hematological, and biochemical analyses, this study shows that a diet enriched with *C. onubensis* biomass is non-toxic to rats. No negative effects were observed on body weight, physiological or morphological parameters over the course of the experimental period. *C. onubensis* biomass also had significant hypocholesterolemic and hypotriglyceridemic effects in rats. As such, *C. onubensis* biomass may serve directly as a functional food for animals or as source of nutraceutical and pharmacological compounds.

Acknowledgements

The authors acknowledge the financial support received from the University of Huelva and Andalusian Government (Research project. BIO-214).

Conflict of interest and funding

The authors declare no conflict of interest.

References

1. Forján E, Navarro F, Cuaresma M, Vaquero I, Ruiz-Domínguez MC, Gojkovic Z, et al. Microalgae: fast-growth sustainable green factories. Crit Rev Environ Sci Technol 2015; 45: 1705–55.
2. Kay RA. Microalgae as food and supplement. Crit Rev Food Sci Nutr 1991; 30: 555–73.
3. Gantar M, Svircev Z. Microalgae and cyanobacteria: food for thought. J Phycol 2008; 44: 60–8.
4. Bishop WM, Zubeck HM. Evaluation of microalgae for use as nutraceuticals and nutritional supplements. J Nutr Food Sci 2012; 2: 147–52.
5. Yaajob Z, Ali E, Zainai A, Mohamad M, Takriff MS. An overview: biomolecules from microalgae for animal feed and aquaculture. J Biol Res 2014; 21: 6.
6. Varshney P, Mikulic P, Vonshak A, Beardall J, Wangikar PP. Extremophilic micro-algae and their potential contribution in biotechnology. Bioresour Technol 2015; 184: 363–72.
7. Graziani G, Schiavo S, Nicolai MA, Buono S, Fogliano V, Pinto G, et al. Microalgae as human food: chemical and nutritional characteristics of the thermo-acidophilic microalga *Galdieria sulphuraria*. Food Funct 2013; 4: 144–52.
8. Vaquero I, Mogedas B, Ruiz-Domínguez MC, Vega JM, Vílchez C. Light-mediated lutein enrichment of an acid environment microalga. Algal Res 2014; 6: 70–7.
9. Spolaore P, Joannis-Cassan C, Duran E, Isambert A. Commercial applications of Microalgae. J Bios Bioeng 2006; 101: 87–96.
10. Vílchez C, Forján E, Cuaresma M, Bédmar F, Garbayo I, Vega JM. Marine carotenoids: biological functions and commercial applications. Mar Drugs 2011; 9: 319–33.
11. Plaza M, Santoyo S, Jaime L, García-Blairsy G, Herrero M, Señorans FJ, et al. Screening for bioactive compounds from algae. J Pharm Biomed Anal 2010; 51: 450–5.
12. Buono S, Langellotti AL, Martello A, Rinna F, Fogliano V. Functional ingredients from microalgae. Food Funct 2014; 5: 1669–85.
13. Gouveia L, Marques AE, Sousa JM, Moura P, Bandarra NM. Microalgae-source of natural bioactive molecules as functional ingredients. Food Sci Technol Bull Funct Foods 2010; 7: 21–37.
14. De Jesus-Raposo MF, de Morais AM, de Morais RM. Marine polysaccharides from algae with potential biomedical applications. Mar Drugs 2015; 13: 2967–3028.
15. Ruiz-Domínguez MC, Vaquero I, Obregón V, de la Morena B, Vílchez C, Vega JM. Lipid accumulation and antioxidant activity in the eukaryotic acidophilic microalga *Coccomyxa* sp. (strain *onubensis*) under nutrient starvation. J Appl Phycol 2015; 27: 1099–108.
16. Fuentes JL, Huss VAR, Montero Z, Torronteras R, Cuaresma M, Garbayo I, et al. Phylogenetic characterization and morphological and physiological aspects of a novel acidotolerant and halotolerant microalga *Coccomyxa onubensis* sp. nov. (Chlorophyta, Trebouxiophyceae). J Appl Phycol 2016; doi: http://dx.doi.org/10.1007/s10811-016-0887-3
17. Bain BJ, Lewis SM. Preparation and staining methods for blood and bone marrow film. In: Lewis SM, Bain B, Bates I, eds. Dacie and Lewis Practical Haematology, 10th ed. Philadelphia: Churchill Livingston; 2006, pp. 59–78.
18. Kierszenbaum AL. Histología y Biología Celular. Barcelona: Elsevier España; 2008.
19. Tibetts SM, Milley JE, Lall SP. Chemical composition and nutritional properties of fresh water and marine microalgal biomass cultured in photobioreactors. J Appl Phycol 2015; 27: 1109–19.
20. Lardon L, Hélias A, Sialve B, Steyer J-P, Bernard O. Life-cycle assessment of biodiesel production from microalgae. Environ Sci Technol 2015; 3: 386–95.
21. Christaki E, Florou-Paneri P, Bonos E. Microalgae: a novel ingredient in nutrition. Int J Food Sci Nutr 2011; 62: 794–9.
22. Becker EW. Microalgae: biotechnology and microbiology. Cambridge: Cambridge University Press; 1994.
23. Zepka LQ, Jacob-Lopes E, Goldbeck R, Souza-Soares LA, Queiroz MI. Nutritonal evaluation of single-cell protein produced by *Aphanothece microscopica* Nägeli. Bioresourc Technol 2010; 101: 7107–11.
24. Nuño K, Villarruel-López A, Puebla-Pérez AM, Romero-Velarde E, Puebla-Mora AG, Ascencio F. Effects of the marine microalgae *Isochrysis galbana* and *Nanochloropsis oculata* in diabetic rats. J Funct Foods 2013; 5: 106–15.
25. Dvir I, Chayoth R, Sod-Moriah U, Shany S, Nyska A, Stark A, et al. Soluble polysaccharide and biomass of red microalga *Pophyridium* sp. alter intestinal morphology and reduce serum cholesterol in rats. Br J Nutr 2000; 84: 469–76.
26. Kushak RI, Drapeau C, Winter HS. The effect of blue-green algae *Aphanizomenon flos-aquae* on nutrient assimilation in rats. J Nutrac Nutr 2001; 3: 35–9.
27. Ekmay RD, Chou K, Lei XG. Continual feeding of two types of microalgal biomass affected protein digestion and metabolism in laying hens. J Anim Sci 2015; 93: 287–97.
28. Kepekçi RA, Polat S, Çelik A, Bayat N, Saygideger SD. Protective effect of *Spirulina platensis* enriched in phenolic compounds against hepatotoxicity induced by CCl_4. Food Chem 2013; 141: 1972–9.
29. Bergen WG, Mersmann HJ. Comparative aspects of lipid metabolism: impact on contemporary research and use of animal models. J Nutr 2005; 135: 2499–502.
30. Geamanu A, Goja A, Saadat N, Khosla P, Gupta SV. ProAlgaZyme subfraction improves the lipoprotein profile of hypercholesterolemic hamsters, while inhibiting production of betaine, carnitine, and choline metabolites. Nutr Metabol 2013; 10: 55–64.
31. Cherng J-Y, Shih M-F. Preventing dyslipidemia by *Chlorella pyrenoidosa* in rats and hamsters after chronic high fat diet treatment. Life Sci 2005; 76: 3001–13.
32. Ginzberg A, Cohen M, Sod-Moriah UA, Shany S, Rosenshtrauch A, Arad S. Chickens fed with biomass of the red microalga *Porphyridium* sp. have reduced blood cholesterol level and modified fatty acid composition in egg yolk. J Appl Phycol 2000; 12: 325–30.
33. Komprda T, Zornikova G, Knoll A, Vykoukalova Z, Rozikova V, Skultety O, et al. Effect of dietary eicosapentaenoic and docosahexaenoic acid on expression of rat liver genes controlling cholesterol homeostasis and on plasma cholesterol level. Czech J Anim Sci 2014; 59: 391–8.
34. Van Beelen VA, Spenkelink B, Mooibroek H, Sijtsma L, Bosch D, Rietjens IM, et al. An n-3 PUFA-rich microalgal oil diet protects to a similar extent as a fish oil-rich diet against AOM-induced colonic aberrant *cryp foci* in F344 rats. Food Chem Toxicol 2009; 47: 316–20.
35. Chen J, Jiang Y, Ma K-Y, Chen F, Chen Z-Y. Microalga decreases plasma cholesterol by down-regulation of intestinal NPC1L1, hepatic LDL receptor, and HMG-CoA reductase. J Agric Food Chem 2011; 59: 6790–7.

36. Ryan AS, Bailey-Hall E, Nelson EB, Salem N Jr. The hypolipidemic effect of an ethyl ester of algal-docosahexaenoic acid in rats fed a high-fructose diet. Lipids 2009; 44: 817–26.
37. Stamey JA, Shepherd DM, de Veth MJ, Corl BA. Use of alga or algal oil rich in n-3 fatty acids as a feed supplement for dairy cattle. J Dairy Sci 2012; 95: 5269–412.
38. Werman MJ, Sukenik A, Mokady S. Effect of the marine unicellular alga *Nanochloropsis* sp. to reduce the plasma and liver cholesterol levels in male rats fed on diets with cholesterol. Biosci Biotechnol Biochem 2003; 67: 2266–8.
39. Misurcová L, Skrovanková S, Samek D, Ambrozová J, Machú L. Health benefits of algal polysaccharides in human nutrition. Adv Food Nutr Res 2012; 66: 75–145.
40. Chen J, Jiao R, Jiang Y, Bi Y, Chen Z-Y. Algal sterols are as effective as β-sitosterol in reducing plasma cholesterol concentration. J Agric Food Chem 2014; 62: 675–81.

***Carlos Vílchez**
Algal Biotechnology Group
CIDERTA and Faculty of Sciences
University of Huelva and
Marine International Campus of Excellence (CEIMAR)
ES-21007 Huelva, Spain
Email: cvilchez@uhu.es

16

Effect of a cheese rich in angiotensin-converting enzyme-inhibiting peptides (Gamalost®) and a Gouda-type cheese on blood pressure: results of a randomised trial

Rita Nilsen[1]*, Are H. Pripp[2], Arne T. Høstmark[3], Anna Haug[4] and Siv Skeie[1]

[1]Department of Chemistry, Biotechnology and Food Science, Norwegian University of Life Sciences, Ås, Norway; [2]Oslo Centre of Biostatistics and Epidemiology, Research Support Services, Oslo University Hospital, Oslo, Norway; [3]Institute of Health and Society, University of Oslo, Oslo, Norway; [4]Department of Animal and Aquacultural Sciences, Norwegian University of Life Sciences, Ås, Norway

Abstract

Background: High blood pressure (BP) is the leading risk factor for global disease burden, contributing to 7% of global disability adjusted life years. Angiotensin converting enzyme (ACE)-inhibiting bioactive peptides have the potential to reduce BP in humans. These peptides have been identified in many dairy products and have been associated with significant reductions in BP.
Objective: The objective of this trial was to examine whether a cheese rich in ACE-inhibiting peptides (Gamalost®), or a standard Gouda-type cheese could lower BP.
Design: A total of 153 healthy participants were randomised to one of three parallel arms: Gamalost® ($n = 53$, 50 g/day for 8 weeks), Gouda-type cheese ($n = 50$, 80 g/day for 8 weeks), and control ($n = 50$). BP and anthropometric measurements were taken at the baseline and at the end, with an additional BP measurement midway. Based on BP at baseline, participants were categorised as having optimal BP ($<$120/ $<$80 mmHg), normal-high BP (120–139/80–89 mmHg), or being hypertensive ($>$140/ $>$90 mmHg). Questionnaires about lifestyle, health, and dietary habits were completed at baseline, midway and end.
Results: In total, 148 participants (mean age 43, 52% female) completed the intervention. There were no differences among the three groups in relevant baseline characteristics. BP was reduced in the entire study population, but the cheese groups did not differ from control. However, in a subgroup of participants with slightly elevated BP, BP at 4 weeks of intervention seemed to be borderline significantly more reduced in the Gamalost® group compared with the control group (Dunnett test: diastolic BP −3.5 mmHg, 95% confidence interval (CI) −7.3, 0.4, systolic BP: −4.3 mmHg, 95% CI −9.8, 1.1).
Conclusion: An intention-to-treat analysis of the data showed no cheese effect upon BP compared to control, but Gamalost® seemed to have a small, non-significant lowering effect on diastolic BP after 4 weeks in people with a normal-high BP.

Keywords: *bioactive peptides*; *intervention*; *dairy*; *Gamalost*; *Gouda*; *cardiovascular diseases*

Cardiovascular diseases (CVD) are the most common contributors to worldwide morbidity and mortality (1), and ischemic heart disease is the leading cause of death in the world (2). Hypertension is a major risk factor for CVD, and it has been estimated from prospective observational studies that just a 5 mmHg reduction in diastolic blood pressure (BP) would reduce the risk of stroke by 34% (3). BP was identified as the leading risk factor contributing to global disease burden in 'the Global Burden of Disease Study 2010', and it was estimated that 16.5% of all deaths can be attributed to high BP (4).

Hypertension is mostly treated pharmacologically, but lifestyle and dietary changes, such as weight loss and reduced salt intake, have been effective in preventing hypertension (5). The dietary approach to stop hypertension (DASH diet), which emphasises a high intake of dairy and fruits and vegetables, is one of the trials showing that diet is a successful tool to reduce hypertension (6). Dairy products are rich sources of protein, calcium, and potassium, which have all been shown to independently reduce BP (7–9). Dairy proteins are also one of the main sources of bioactive peptides in the human diet (10), which are present in varying amounts in different cheeses. These bioactive peptides have several known activities, including angiotensin-converting enzyme (ACE) inhibition. The function of ACE is to activate angiotensin II, a vasoconstrictor, as well as inactivating bradykinin, a vasodilator (11), resulting in increased BP. ACE-inhibiting peptides have been identified in several cheeses and other fermented milk products, including cheddar (12), manchego (13), asiago (14), and the traditional Norwegian cheese Gamalost® (15). Some randomised, controlled trials have shown that fermented milks and extracts of ACE-inhibiting peptides from milk products can reduce BP in humans. A meta-analysis showed that food-derived peptides, such as the two lactotripeptdies valine-proline-proline (VPP) and isoleucine-proline-proline (IPP), had the potential to lower systolic BP by 5 mmHg (16).

Gamalost® is a cheese made from skimmed milk that does not contain salt and is naturally low in fat ($<1\%$) and very rich in protein (50%). A detailed account of the production of Gamalost® has been described previously (15). The cheese is rich in bioactive peptides and was found to have a better ACE-inhibitory activity, in terms of the concentration of cheese peptides needed to inhibit 50% of ACE, than other cheeses (15, 17, 18). Compared to cheeses from other studies, Gamalost was one of the cheeses with the highest ACE-inhibitory potential (19). A cross-sectional study on Gamalost® and BP was carried out in 2012 and showed that Gamalost® intake frequency was associated with slightly lower systolic BP (20). Given its bitter taste and crumbly texture, Gamalost® is not widely consumed, while mild and versatile Gouda-type cheeses have the highest consumption in Norway. A simulated human gastrointestinal digestion trial showed that the moderate ACE-inhibitory activity of Gouda-type cheeses increased greatly after digestion (18), making the cheese an interesting addition to this trial. We are not aware of any previously published randomised, controlled trials specifically investigating the effect of cheese on BP.

The aim of this work was to investigate whether the consumption of cheese might lower BP during 8 weeks of intervention.

Materials and methods

Subjects

Participants were recruited through local newspapers, radio, and television, from the general population. The target population was persons with moderately high blood BP, who were not medicated. Males and females over 18 years of age who spoke Norwegian fluently were included. Exclusion criteria included pregnancy and the use of BP-lowering medications.

Design

The study performed was a randomised, single-blinded controlled trial with three parallel arms, as illustrated in Fig. 1. The intervention period lasted for 8 weeks with measurements taken at baseline, midway, and at the end of the trial. An independent person not involved in the study prepared the randomisation envelopes containing information on which intervention the participants would follow. Independent of baseline BP, the participants were handed envelopes by two independent persons not involved in the conduct of the study. The sample size estimate for a one-way analysis of variance with three groups, with a power of 0.80 and criterion for significance set at 0.05, yielded a sample size of 53 cases per group and a total of 159. We initially aimed for a larger sample of about 300 participants, but recruitment yielded a total sample size of 153.

This study was carried out at the Department of Chemistry, Biotechnology and Food Science, Norwegian University of Life Sciences, Aas, Norway, from April 2013 to July 2013 and was approved by the Regional Committees for Medical and Health Research Ethics (Oslo, Norway) on 7 March 2013 (2013/166) (registered at www.clinicaltrials.gov; NCT01913756). The study was conducted according to the guidelines laid down in the Declaration of Helsinki and written informed consent was obtained from all subjects.

Interventions

Participants were randomised to one of three arms: Gamalost®, Gouda-type cheese, or control. All participants in the cheese groups were asked to maintain their habitual diet and not make any other major lifestyle changes. Subjects in the control group were asked to maintain their habitual diet, but to avoid the two intervention cheeses as well as similar cheeses. They were given lists of suggestions of other cheeses they could freely consume, such as blue cheese, mozzarella cheese, or cream cheese.

Participants in the Gamalost® group were instructed to consume 50 g/day of the cheese, whereas participants in the Gouda-type cheese group were instructed to consume 80 g/day of the cheese. These amounts were chosen because they were judged to be higher than the average intake of each cheese, but not so high that the participants were unable to consume the designated amount. In order to have similar cheese protein intakes in the two cheese groups, the Gouda-type intervention was larger than the Gamalost® intervention. The cheeses were not portioned, but the participants were provided with digital scales to accurately weigh out the daily intake. All the Gamalost® cheeses were from the same batch and were ripened for 10 days. All the Gouda-type cheeses were from the

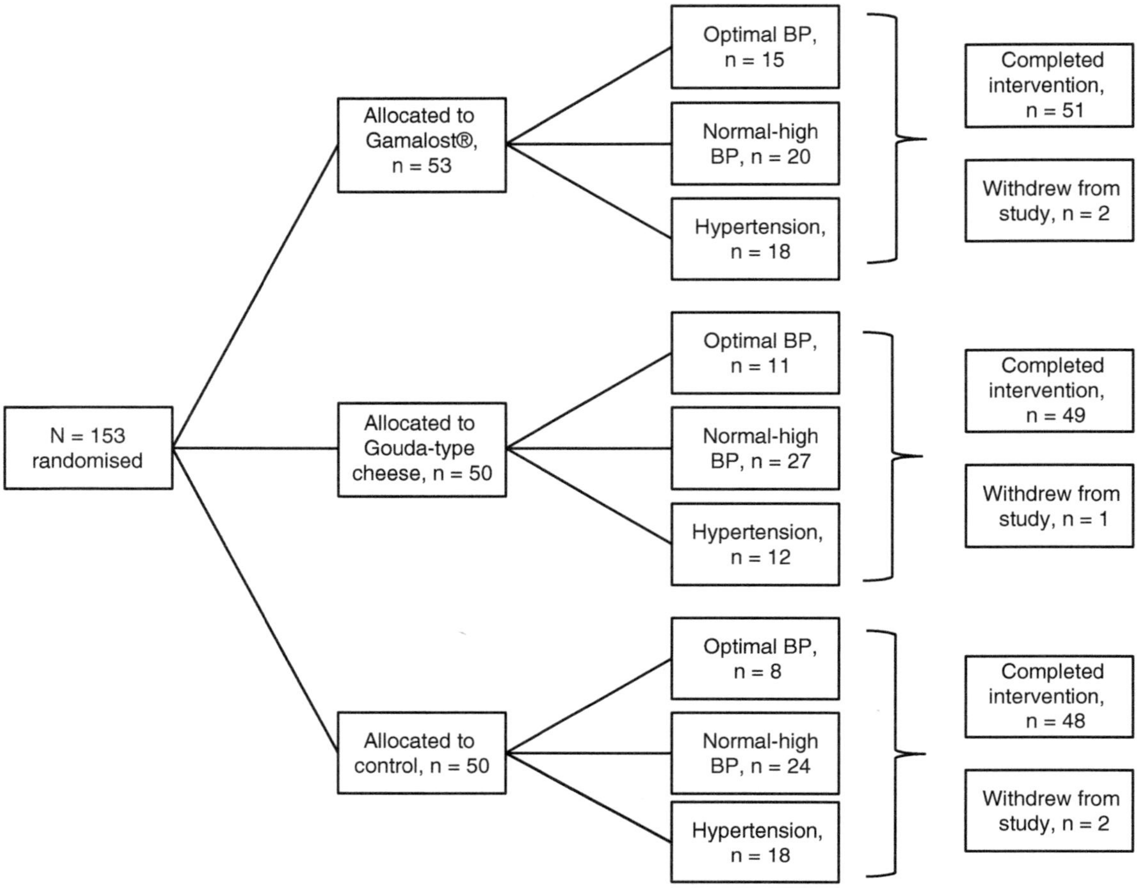

Fig. 1. Flow chart of a single-blinded, randomised, controlled trial of Gamalost® and Gouda-type cheeses and blood pressure in 153 Norwegian participants. BP, blood pressure.

same batch and were ripened for 3 months. The cheese needed for the duration of the trial was provided for all participants, and they were given more as needed. Furthermore, participants were instructed to freeze the Gamalost® cheese throughout the trial so that the rapid proteolysis occurring in the cheese would not change the activity of the ACE-inhibiting peptides, as freezing does not affect the ACE-inhibitory activity of the cheese. The nutritional properties and ACE-inhibitory activity of the two cheeses can be found in Table 1. A portion of the study population filled out charts of weighed daily cheese intake, used to evaluate compliance with the cheese intake.

Socio-demographic and dietary assessment

A questionnaire was developed for a cross-sectional trial on Gamalost® intake and BP in a Norwegian population (20), and it was based on the previously validated questionnaire from the Oslo Health Study (main questionnaire and second supplementary questionnaire 1 of the Oslo Health Study). Experience from this cross-sectional trial showed that the questionnaire was suitable, but a couple more questions on food intake were added. The questionnaire contained questions on age, education, health, leisure time physical activity, medication, and supplement use, as well as several questions on diet, including some focusing specifically on dairy product intake. A translated version of the questionnaire used at baseline can be found in Supplementary file 1. Total dairy product intake was calculated by summarising the frequency of intake of all cheese, all milk, and fermented milk products. A revised version of the questionnaire containing only questions on food intake was distributed at the midway measurements, whereas a third version, which included some of the questions on health and physical activity from the first questionnaire, was used at the end of the trial. The second and third questionnaires were used to assess whether any major changes to diet and physical activity pattern occurred during the intervention period. Participants were also asked to record any difficulties they had with compliance. The last questionnaire also included a question regarding discomforts the participants may have experienced during the intervention period.

BP measurements

BP was measured according to the American Heart Association recommendations (21). Participants rested

Table 1. Nutrient composition (per 100 g and daily intake) of intervention cheeses

	Gamalost®		Gouda-type cheese	
Nutrient	100 g	Daily intake, 50 g	100 g	Daily intake, 80 g
Energy[a], kcal	213	107	351	281
Protein[a], g	50	25	27	22
Fat[a], g	1	0.5	27	22
Carbohydrates[a], g	1	0.5	0	0
Calcium[a], mg	160	80	800	640
Sodium[a], mg	24	12	402	322
Magnesium[a], mg	13	7	33	26
Potassium[a], mg	98	49	77	62
IC_{50} ACE-inhibition[b]	0.34	0.34	0.59	0.59
ACE-inhibitory potential[c], mg	0.24	0.12	0.03	0.02

[a]From TINE SA, manufacturer of the two cheeses; [b]IC_{50} per unit weight of freeze-dried pH 4.6 soluble fraction (SF), expressed as mg pH 4.6 SF per ml. From Qureshi et al. (15); [c]ACE-inhibitory potential, expressed as mg captopril equivalents per cheese weight. From Qureshi et al. (15).

for approximately 10 min before the measurement was taken using a Microlife BP A200 sphygmomanometer (Microlife, Widnau, Switzerland). In a sitting position, three consecutive measurements were taken and the average of the second and third measurements was used for analysis (automatically calculated by the BP device). If needed, the device took four measurements to get a more accurate reading. All BP measurements were taken between 06:30 and 10:30, after an overnight fast. Participants were notified of their BP and whether the BP was within the normal range or not. Based on baseline BP, participants were grouped into categories according to the guidelines published by the European Society of Hypertension and the European Society of Cardiology (22). Consequently, participants were categorised as optimal if systolic BP was <120 mmHg and diastolic BP was <80 mmHg, normal-high if systolic BP was 120–139 mmHg and/or diastolic BP was 80–89 mmHg, and hypertensive if systolic BP was ≥ 140 mmHg and/or diastolic BP was $\geq$ 90 mmHg.

Anthropometric measurements

Height was measured to the nearest 0.1 cm using a portable stadiometer (Seca 217, Seca, Hamburg, Germany). Body weight was measured to the nearest 0.1 kg, without shoes or heavy clothing, using digital scales (TBF-300A Body Composition Analyzer, Tanita, Tokyo, Japan). Body mass index (BMI) was computed as weight (kg) divided by the square of height (m). Waist circumference was measured to the nearest 0.1 cm using a measuring tape (Seca 201 Circumference measuring tape, Seca), in accordance with World Health Organization recommendations, i.e. at the midpoint between the iliac crest and the lowest rib margin (23). All anthropometric measurements were also performed between 06:30 and 10:30.

Statistical analyses

Prior to statistical analysis, the dataset was recoded by an independent person to remove information on intervention groups, hence the primary researchers were blinded while performing the analyses. Statistical analyses were performed according to the intention-to-treat principle. One-way ANOVA with Bonferroni correction for multiple comparisons or the chi-square (χ^2) test were used as appropriate to assess differences between the intervention groups. Baseline characteristics are presented as mean (standard deviation) or percentages, where appropriate. The paired samples t-test was used to evaluate change in BP from start to end in each intervention group. Dunnett test was used to evaluate mean BP changes between each treatment group and the control group. A $p<0.05$ was considered statistically significant. All statistical analyses were performed using the SPSS 21.0 software package (IBM Corporation, Armonk, New York).

Results

Baseline characteristics

A total of 153 participants were included in the study from the beginning ($n=53$ in Gamalost® group, $n=50$ each in both Gouda-type cheese and control groups). At baseline, 22% had optimal BP, 46% had moderately high BP, and 31% were hypertensive. Some baseline characteristics of the total study sample and the three groups are presented in Table 2. There were no major differences between the groups in selected health variables, salt, alcohol, or dairy product intake. BP was not significantly different at baseline, even though the prevalence of hypertension was slightly lower in the Gouda-type cheese group compared to the control group. The participants consumed on average seven servings of cheese per week,

Table 2. Baseline characteristics (mean (standard deviation (SD))) or %, by intervention group

	Intervention group								
	All (n = 153)		Gamalost® (n = 53)		Gouda-type cheese (n = 50)		Control (n = 50)		
Characteristic	Mean	SD	Mean	SD	Mean	SD	Mean	SD	*p*
Gender, female (%)	52.3		50.9		60.0		46.0		0.4
Age (years)	43.1	16.4	41.2	17.0	42.7	15.8	45.5	16.4	0.4
Weight (kg)	77.2	14.8	75.6	13.7	76.0	13.6	79.9	16.8	0.3
Height (cm)	173.9	8.9	174.9	8.7	171.9	8.7	174.7	9.4	0.2
BMI (kg/m^2)	25.7	3.7	24.6	3.3	25.6	3.5	26.0	3.7	0.1
Waist circumference (cm)	83.1	11.8	80.9	11.3	82.8	10.9	85.8	12.9	0.1
Systolic BP (mmHg)	132.3	17.2	131.5	19.3	130.6	14.7	134.8	17.2	0.4
Diastolic BP (mmHg)	82.4	9.8	82.5	10.6	81.4	8.9	83.1	10.0	0.7
Hypertension[a] (%)	31.4		34.0		24.0		36.0		0.4
Education (years)	16.6	2.9	16.6	2.7	17.0	2.3	16.4	3.5	0.6
Smoking[b] (%)	3.3		3.8		2.0		4.1		0.9
Physical activity[c] (%)	38.4		39.6		36.7		38.8		0.9
Salt usage[d] (%)	72.5		71.7		72.0		74.0		0.9
Alcohol consumption[e] (%)	57.2		64.2		53.1		54.0		0.1
Total dairy[f]	18.4	11.9	19.7	12.9	17.5	10.1	18.0	12.7	0.6
Gouda-type cheese[f]	5.7	4.3	6.1	4.6	5.4	3.6	5.6	4.8	0.7
Gamalost®[f]	0.7	1.9	0.6	1.7	0.6	1.8	0.8	2.2	0.9

[a]Percentage who have either SBP > 140, or DBP > 90; [b]percentage daily smokers; [c]percentage who reported moderate to hard physical activity more than 4 h per week; [d]percentage who salt their food; [e]percentage who consume alcohol > 1/week; [f]servings per week.

whereas Gamalost® intake was predictably low with less than one serving per week.

BP changes

Paired samples *t*-test (Supplementary file 2) showed that both systolic and diastolic BP decreased significantly from baseline to midway, and from baseline to the end of the trial in the entire study population. All groups had significant decreases in systolic BP (Fig. 2a, Supplementary file 2), whereas, at the end of the trial, only the Gamalost® group had significantly decreased diastolic BP (Fig. 2b, Supplementary file 2). An intention-to-treat analysis of BP change, and comparing the intervention groups with the control group, showed no effect of the cheeses on midway or end BP (Supplementary file 3).

When stratifying by baseline BP category, the paired samples *t*-test (Supplementary file 4) showed that the participants with optimal BP at baseline did not have any reductions throughout the trial, as illustrated in Fig. 3. Figure 3a and b shows mean systolic and diastolic BP

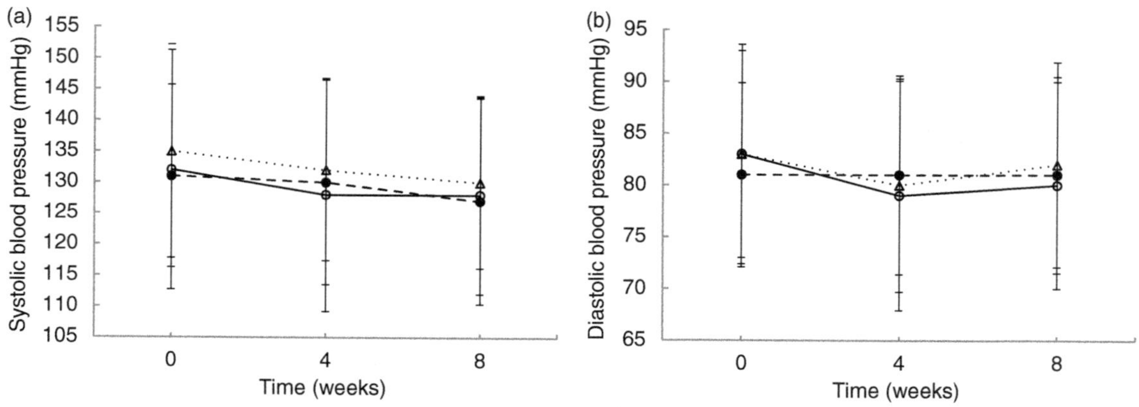

Fig. 2. Mean values (standard deviation) for systolic (a) and diastolic (b) blood pressure at baseline, midway, and end in the three groups. ○Gamalost®, ●Gouda-type cheese, ΔControl.

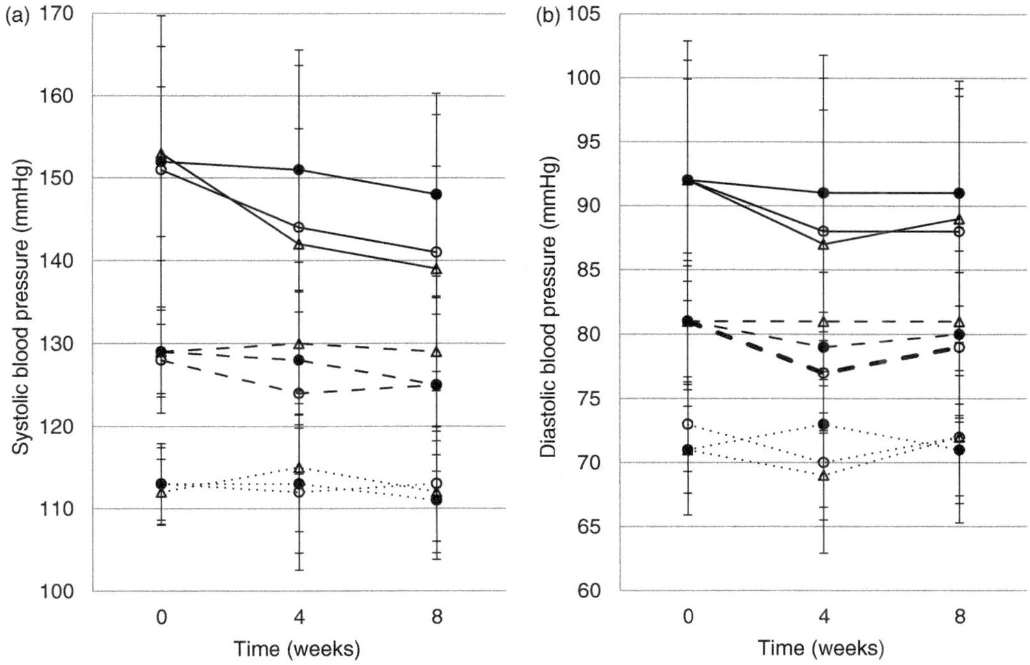

Fig. 3. Systolic (a) and diastolic (b) blood pressure (mean (SD)) at baseline, midway, and end, in the three intervention groups. Solid lines: participants with hypertension at baseline; dashed lines: participants with normal-high BP at baseline, and dotted lines: participants with optimal BP at baseline. ○Gamalost®, ●Gouda-type cheese, ΔControl.

changes through the trial, respectively, grouped by BP category at baseline. Systolic BP decreased significantly in the hypertensive subgroup in both the Gamalost® ($p = 0.001$) and control ($p < 0.001$) groups at both midway and end measurements. Systolic BP was also significantly lower at the end of the trial ($p = 0.049$) for participants with normal-high BP in the Gouda-type cheese group. At the end of the trial, diastolic BP was significantly decreased in the normal-high BP ($p = 0.038$) and hypertensive ($p = 0.004$) subgroups of the Gamalost® intervention group only.

Further analyses stratified by BP categories are presented in Table 3. Here, the intervention cheese groups are compared against the control group. Systolic BP shows a borderline significant effect of consuming Gamalost® compared to control also in the normal-high BP subgroup (−4.3 mmHg, 95% CI −9.8, 1.1, $p = 0.14$). Even though BP decreased overall in all groups, when comparing change in BP in those with hypertension at baseline, the Gouda-type cheese group had significantly higher midway and end systolic BP compared to the control group (midway: 10.5 mmHg, 95% CI 0.9, 20.2, $p = 0.03$, end: 10.1 mmHg, 95% CI 1.6, 18.6, $p = 0.02$). In the Gamalost® group, there seems to be a small borderline significant effect on diastolic BP compared to control at week 4, for participants with normal-high BP at baseline (−3.5 mmHg, 95% CI −7.3, 0.4, $p = 0.08$). At 8 weeks, the association remained but was less significant.

Other changes

At the end of the intervention, waist circumference decreased significantly in all three intervention groups ($p < 0.001$), whereas weight was only significantly reduced in the Gamalost® and control groups (data not shown). Dairy product and Gamalost® intake was significantly different between the groups at the end of the trial (ANOVA, data not shown, $p < 0.001$), with total dairy intake increasing in the two cheese groups and decreasing in the control group. Five participants failed to complete the trial, as illustrated in Fig. 1, due to adverse events unrelated to the study itself.

Discussion

This randomised, controlled trial showed systolic BP reductions in all intervention groups, and reductions in diastolic BP in the Gamalost® group after 8 weeks of intervention. However, compared to the control, there was no BP-lowering effect of Gamalost®, a cheese rich in ACE-inhibiting peptides, or of a standard Gouda-type cheese in 153 subjects recruited from a general healthy population. When participants were stratified by baseline BP, there was a non-significant effect of consuming Gamalost® compared to control at 4 weeks in participants with normal-high BP, but this was not present at 8 weeks.

In this trial, systolic BP was significantly reduced in hypertensive subjects in both the Gamalost® and control groups, but not the Gouda-type group. It is uncertain

Table 3. Stratified analysis based on blood pressure category at baseline, comparing control group with the two cheese diets

			4 weeks (midway)				8 weeks (end)			
		Baseline BP	Mean BP	BP change	Difference from control (95% CI)	*p*	Mean BP	BP change	Difference from control (95% CI)	*p*
Systolic BP										
Hypertensive	Control	152.7 (3.1)	141.8 (3.3)	−10.9 (2.2)			139.1 (2.9)	−13.7 (2.5)		
	Gamalost®	150.8 (4.4)	144.2 (4.6)	−6.7 (2.8)	4.3 (−4.3, 12.9)	0.43	141.3 (3.9)	−9.50 (2.5)	4.2 (−3.4, 11.8)	0.36
	Gouda-type	151.5 (2.6)	147.9 (3.5)	−0.4 (3.7)	10.5 (0.9, 20.2)	0.03	147.9 (3.5)	−3.6 (2.1)	10.1 (1.6, 18.6)	0.02
Normal-high	Control	129.2 (2.1)	129.7 (2.1)	0.3 (1.7)			128.7 (1.9)	−0.6 (1.7)		
	Gamalost®	128.4 (1.4)	124.4 (2.2)	−4.1 (1.7)	−4.3 (−9.8, 1.1)	0.14	125.4 (1.9)	−3.0 (1.7)	−2.4 (−8.1, 3.4)	0.55
	Gouda-type	128.6 (1.0)	127.9 (1.6)	−0.5 (1.5)	−0.8 (−6.0, 4.3)	0.91	124.9 (2.1)	−3.5 (1.7)	−2.9 (−8.3, 2.5)	0.37
Optimal	Control	111.5 (1.4)	114.9 (2.8)	3.4 (2.4)			111.8 (2.6)	0.3 (2.2)		
	Gamalost®	112.5 (1.3)	112.3 (2.5)	−0.1 (1.9)	−3.5 (−11.7, 4.7)	0.50	113.5 (2.0)	0.5 (1.6)	0.2 (−6.8, 6.4)	1.0
	Gouda-type	112.9 (1.3)	127.9 (1.6)	−0.4 (3.1)	−3.8 (−12.5, 5.0)	0.50	109.7 (2.3)	−3.5 (1.9)	−3.8 (−10.2, 2.7)	0.31
Diastolic BP										
Hypertensive	Control	91.9 (2.2)	141.8 (3.3)	−5.1 (2.0)			88.5 (2.3)	−3.4 (2.1)		
	Gamalost®	92.2 (2.6)	144.2 (4.6)	−4.1 (1.4)	1.0 (−4.5, 6.5)	0.89	87.6 (2.6)	−4.6 (1.4)	−1.2 (−6.8, 4.4)	0.85
	Gouda-type	92.0 (2.3)	147.9 (3.5)	−0.9 (2.1)	4.1 (−2.0, 10.3)	0.23	92.3 (2.5)	−0.8 (1.8)	2.6 (−3.6, 8.9)	0.54
Normal-high	Control	80.8 (1.0)	80.5 (1.6)	−0.1 (1.3)			80.6 (1.5)	0.1 (1.5)		
	Gamalost®	81.0 (1.2)	77.5 (1.1)	−3.6 (1.1)	−3.5 (−7.3, 0.4)	0.08	78.8 (1.3)	−2.2 (1.0)	−2.2 (−6.4, 2.1)	0.42
	Gouda-type	80.9 (0.8)	79.3 (1.1)	−1.4 (1.0)	−1.3 (−4.9, 2.4)	0.65	79.7 (1.3)	−0.9 (1.3)	−0.9 (−4.9, 3.1)	0.84
Optimal	Control	70.5 (1.2)	68.5 (1.2)	−2.0 (1.3)			71.8 (2.4)	1.3 (1.8)		
	Gamalost®	73.0 (1.0)	69.7 (1.9)	−3.7 (1.7)	−1.7 (−7.7, 4.3)	0.72	71.9 (1.4)	−1.5 (1.5)	−2.8 (−8.0, 2.4)	0.36
	Gouda-type	71.3 (1.5)	79.3 (1.1)	1.3 (2.0)	3.3 (−3.1, 9.7)	0.38	71.2 (1.1)	−0.8 (1.3)	−2.1 (−7.5, 3.4)	0.59

Values are mean (SE), 2-sided *p*-values for the difference from control (Dunnett test).

why BP was reduced in the control group, but it could be a result of the statistical phenomenon known as regression to the mean (24). Another reason for the reduction of systolic BP in the control group could be the seasonal variations in BP that are known to occur throughout the year (25). BP tends to be higher in the winter months and lower in the summer, which is consistent with the start of this study in April and ending in June. Even though there was no significant difference in baseline BP between the three groups, the Gouda-type cheese group had fewer subjects with hypertension compared to the Gamalost® and control groups. This could possibly explain why the hypertensive subgroup in the Gouda-type cheese group did not have the same reductions in BP as the other two groups. It was hypothesised that during the intervention, BP would decrease in the Gamalost® group compared to the control, due to the high intake of ACE-inhibiting bioactive peptides. A borderline significant reduction in diastolic BP in the Gamalost® group was seen in the subcategory of subjects with normal-high BP. The association was less significant at 8 weeks, which could be explained by regression to the mean or problems with compliance. This borderline significant change in diastolic BP is in accordance with a larger diet intervention trial on the effect of the Mediterranean diet on BP, which found a small significant effect on diastolic but not systolic BP (26). In the previous cross-sectional trial (20), the opposite occurred as systolic BP, but not diastolic BP, was significantly lower with higher intakes of Gamalost®. With the high prevalence of high BP and hypertension in the Norwegian and worldwide population, a small lowering of mean BP in the normal-high BP subgroup in the Gamalost® group compared to control at 4 weeks could be clinically meaningful if they were able to achieve a significant effect beyond 4 weeks. The normal-high BP category was the largest subgroup in all three intervention groups, leading to the assumption that results from these groups have the best statistical power. In the general population, this subgroup of people is also those who might benefit from lifestyle changes, for example, a diet including a cheese rich in ACE-inhibiting peptides, such as Gamalost®.

It has been estimated that a small reduction in diastolic BP of 2 mmHg could reduce the risk of coronary heart disease by 6% (27), indicating that only small reductions are needed for cheese and dairy products to have a clinically meaningful effect on BP. Previous randomised, controlled trials on the BP-lowering effect on milk-derived bioactive peptides showed mixed results. VPP and IPP, derived from casein, are usually considered the two lactotripeptides with the most promising antihypertensive potential (28). However, in a double-blinded placebo-controlled trial on subjects with elevated BP (SBP $\geq$ 140 mmHg) given concentrates of these two peptides, they did not exert any BP-lowering effect compared to the placebo group (28). A similar trial using a milk fermented with *Lactobacillus helveticus,* which gave a product naturally rich in VPP and IPP, found a significant BP-lowering effect on diastolic BP, which was not maintained after 4 weeks' intervention in the normal-high BP category, whereas both systolic and diastolic BP was decreased in the hypertensive category until 4 weeks (29). Many trials investigating the BP-lowering effect of foods have used extracts of foods or synthetic foods/drinks containing active ingredients that may occur naturally in foods. Trials that use actual foods as the intervention, such as the current trial, have mixed results in terms of BP reductions. A BP-lowering effect of foods consumed as part of a normal diet in a free living population has been observed for foods such as kiwifruit (male smokers) (30), flaxseed (peripheral artery disease patients) (31), and fermented milk (buttermilk) (moderately hypercholesterolemic subjects) (32), whereas no significant effects were found for other foods, such as walnuts (33).

Information obtained from participants in the cross-sectional trial (20), which included many people who regularly consumed Gamalost®, indicated that 50 grams of Gamalost® was a feasible daily intake of the cheese. It is possible that a true BP-lowering effect of Gamalost® would be observed if the serving was increased, but we judged that a bigger serving would be unlikely to be tolerated by regular and non-consumers. The study population in the current intervention trial was recruited from the general population and they had no underlying conditions and diseases. We were unable to recruit solely subjects with increased BP at baseline, as evidenced by the initial BP in the overall study population (132/82 mmHg). A significant correlation between initial BP and the change in BP has been found (34), with initial higher BP showing greater response to the BP-lowering agent, suggesting that, should further trials on the BP-lowering effect of Gamalost® be performed, subjects with optimal BP should be excluded. With the inclusion of normotensive participants in the trial, it is possible that this study is actually underpowered since we would not expect a reduction in BP in those with normal BP. Even though many cheeses have been found to be rich in ACE-inhibiting bioactive peptides, the results from the present trial suggest that the effect may not be transferrable to healthy human populations through the amount of cheese consumed in this trial. A meta-analysis of randomised, controlled trials on the effect of VPP and IPP on BP found that the response to treatment was generally greater in Japanese studies compared to European studies (35). The authors suggested that one cause was the typically higher habitual intake of dairy products in Europe, which may have an effect on the BP response to lactotripeptides treatment. The fact that participants in the control group in the current trial could consume dairy products could have confounded the results of this trial and contributed towards the null findings. Suggestions for future trials are to include a wash-out period before the baseline, during which participants do not consume dairy products, and to remove dairy products from the diet of the control group.

It is uncertain why waist circumference was reduced in all groups from baseline to the end of the trial. The questionnaire used in this trial was not detailed enough to detect changes in energy intake, but it did not seem that food intake changed significantly. The change in waist circumference could be caused by increased physical activity as the season changed from late winter/early spring to late spring/early summer. It is also possible that the reduction in waist circumference was due to the phenomenon known as the Hawthorne effect, in which participants in a trial will change their behaviour because they know they are being observed.

A limitation of this trial is the use of a sphygmomanometer for in-office BP measurements, as opposed to ambulatory 24-h BP measurements, which would produce values of higher accuracy. BP varies throughout the day and the current trial is therefore unable to distinguish whether the participants had an effect of the intervention on nocturnal BP. White-coat hypertension, reported to occur in about 15–35% of people (21, 36, 37), is a source of error that could be greatly reduced by ambulatory BP measurements (38). If the baseline BP measurements were falsely high, it is expected that BP will decrease slightly on subsequent visits, a result of getting used to the situation and regression to the mean. However, subjects were randomly allocated to groups and statistical analyses were adjusted according to the subject's baseline BP. At the baseline BP measurement, the participants were informed of their BP. They were not given any medical advice, but they were told if their BP was outside of the recommended range, they could make an appointment with their general practitioner. None of the participants reported starting any medical antihypertensive treatments during the trial. Furthermore, since the participants were of generally good health and had, on average, a BP within the normal range at baseline, the generalisability of these findings to populations with a higher BP may be somewhat limited. The participants were only provided with the intervention cheese, and though they were asked to maintain their habitual diet, we had only partial control of the diet during the trial.

The strengths of this study include the relatively long duration and design of the trial, specifically that it is a randomised, single-blinded controlled trial. The retention of participants in the trial was good, with only five subjects lost to follow-up, and the same number of subjects dropped out in the Gamalost® group and the control group.

In conclusion, when compared to the mean change in BP in the control group, there was no major effect of a cheese rich in ACE-inhibiting peptides or a standard Gouda-type cheese on BP in a general population. However, when stratified by BP category at baseline, there was a non-significant reduction in diastolic BP in the group that consumed the cheese rich in ACE-inhibiting peptides, compared to the control group of those participants with normal-high BP at 4 weeks of intervention. The current results suggest cheeses rich in ACE-inhibiting bioactive peptides may not have an effect on BP when consumed in moderate amounts, but further similar trials on other cheeses should be performed to evaluate these findings.

Authors' contributions

All authors contributed to formulating the research question, designing the study, carrying out the statistical analysis and critically revising the manuscript. Additionally, RN carried out the study and drafted the manuscript.

Acknowledgements

The authors are grateful to all participants in the trial. The staff in the dairy group at the Norwegian University of Life Sciences for all the practical help, and Eirin Huseby, who made the trial run smoothly for both the participants and the researchers, are all highly acknowledged.

Financial support for the current trial (grant number: 185041) was provided by the Norwegian Research Council (Oslo), the Norwegian Foundation for Research Levy on Agricultural Products (Oslo), the Norwegian Agricultural Agreement Research Fund, and TINE SA (Oslo, Norway). Cheeses for the trial were provided by TINE SA. The funders had no role in the design, analysis or writing of this article. A.H.P. was supported by the South-Eastern Norway Regional Health Authority.

Conflict of interest and funding

None of the authors have any conflicts of interest to declare.

References

1. Alwan A. Global status report on noncommunicable diseases 2010. World Health Organization; 2011. Available from: http://www.who.int/nmh/publications/ncd_report_full_en.pdf [cited 4 April 2015].
2. World Health Organization. The top 10 causes of death. 2014. Available from: http://www.who.int/mediacentre/factsheets/fs310/en/ [cited 22 August 2014].
3. MacMahon S, Peto R, Cutler J, Collins R, Sorlie P, Neaton J, et al. Blood pressure, stroke, and coronary heart disease. Part 1, Prolonged differences in blood pressure: prospective observational studies corrected for the regression dilution bias. Lancet 1990; 335(8692): 765–74.
4. Lim SS, Vos T, Flaxman AD, Danaei G, Shibuya K, Adair-Rohani H, et al. A comparative risk assessment of burden of disease and injury attributable to 67 risk factors and risk factor clusters in 21 regions, 1990–2010: a systematic analysis for the Global Burden of Disease Study 2010. Lancet 2012; 380: 2224–60. doi: http://dx.doi.org/10.1016/S0140-6736(12)61766-8
5. Appel LJ, Brands MW, Daniels SR, Karanja N, Elmer PJ, Sacks FM. Dietary approaches to prevent and treat hypertension:

a scientific statement from the American Heart Association. Hypertension 2006; 47(2): 296–308.
6. Sacks FM, Svetkey S, Vollmer WM, Appel LJ, Bray GA, Harsha D, et al. Effects on blood pressure of reduced dietary sodium and the Dietary Approaches to Stop Hypertension (DASH) diet. DASH-Sodium Collaborative Research Group. N Engl J Med 2001; 344(1): 3–10. doi: http://dx.doi.org/10.1056/NEJM200101043440101
7. He J, Wofford MR, Reynolds K, Chen J, Chen CS, Myers L, et al. Effect of dietary protein supplementation on blood pressure: a randomised, controlled trial. Circulation 2011; 124(5): 589–95.
8. Wang L, Manson JE, Buring JE, Lee IM, Sesso HD. Dietary intake of dairy products, calcium, and vitamin D and the risk of hypertension in middle-aged and older women. Hypertension 2008; 51(4): 1073–9. doi: http://dx.doi.org/10.1161/HYPERTENSIONAHA.107.107821
9. Houston M. The importance of potassium in managing hypertension. Curr Hypertens Rep 2011; 13: 309–17.
10. Korhonen H, Pihlanto A. Bioactive peptides: production and functionality. Int Dairy J 2006; 16: 945–60.
11. Silva SV, Malcata FX. Caseins as source of bioactive peptides. Int Dairy J 2005; 15: 1–15.
12. Pritchard SR, Phillips M, Kailasapathy K. Identification of bioactive peptides in commercial Cheddar cheese. Food Res Int 2010; 43: 1545–8.
13. Gomez-Ruiz JA, Ramos M, Recio I. Angiotensin-converting enzyme-inhibitory peptides in Manchego cheeses manufactured with different starter cultures. Int Dairy J 2002; 12: 697–706.
14. Lignitto L, Cavatorta V, Balzan S, Gabai G, Galaverna G, Novelli E, et al. Angiotensin-converting, enzyme inhibitory activity of water-soluble extracts of Asiago d'allevo cheese. Int Dairy J 2010; 20(1): 11–17.
15. Qureshi TM, Vegarud GE, Abrahamsen RK, Skeie S. Characterization of the Norwegian autochthonous cheese Gamalost and its angiotensin I-converting enzyme (ACE) inhibitory activity during ripening. Dairy Sci Technol 2012; 92(6): 613–25. doi: http://dx.doi.org/10.1007/s13594-012-0078-1
16. Pripp A. Effect of peptides derived from food proteins on blood pressure: a meta-analysis of randomised controlled trials. Food Nutr Res 2008; 52. doi: 10.3402/fnr.v52i0.1641
17. Pripp AH, Sorensen R, Stepamak L, Sorhaug T. Relationship between proteolysis and angiotensin-I-converting enzyme inhibition in different cheeses. LWT Food Sci Technol 2006; 39(6): 677–83. doi: http://dx.doi.org/10.1016/j.lwt.2005.03.018
18. Qureshi TM, Vegarud GE, Abrahamsen RK, Skeie S. Angiotensin 1-converting enzyme (ACE) inhibitory activity of the Norwegian autochthonous cheese Gamalost and Norvegia after in vitro human gastrointestinal digestion. J Dairy Sci 2013; 96(2): 838–53. doi: http://dx.doi.org/10.3168/jds.2012-5993
19. Sieber R, Butikofer U, Egger C, Portmann R, Walther B, Wechsler D. ACE-inhibitory activity and ACE-inhibiting peptides in different cheese varieties. Dairy Sci Technol 2010; 90(1): 47–73. doi: http://dx.doi.org/10.1051/dst/2009049
20. Nilsen R, Pripp AH, Høstmark AT, Haug A, Skeie S. Short communication: is consumption of a cheese rich in angiotensin-converting enzyme-inhibiting peptides, such as the Norwegian cheese Gamalost, associated with reduced blood pressure? J Dairy Sci 2014; 97(5): 2662–8. doi: http://dx.doi.org/10.3168/jds.2013-7479
21. Pickering TG, Hall JE, Appel LJ, Falkner BE, Graves J, Hill MN, et al. Recommendations for blood pressure measurement in humans and experimental animals. Hypertension 2005; 45(1): 142–61. doi: http://dx.doi.org/10.1161/01.HYP.0000150859.47929.8e
22. Mancia G, Fagard R, Narkiewicz K, Redon J, Zanchetti A, Bohm M, et al. 2013 ESH/ESC practice guidelines for the management of arterial hypertension. Blood Press 2014; 23(1): 3–16.
23. WHO (2011). Waist circumference and waist-hip ratio: report of a WHO expert consultation, Geneva, 8–11 December 2008. Geneva, Switzerland: WHO.
24. Barnett AG, van der Pols JC, Dobson AJ. Regression to the mean: what it is and how to deal with it. Int J Epidemiol 2005; 34: 215–20.
25. Modesti PA. Season, temperature and blood pressure: a complex interaction. Eur J Intern Med 2013; 24(7): 604–7.
26. Toledo E, Hu FB, Estruch R, Buil-Cosiales P, Corella D, Salas-Salvado J, et al. Effect of the Mediterranean diet on blood pressure in the PREDIMED trial: results from a randomised controlled trial. BMC Med 2013; 11: 207.
27. Cook NR, Cohen J, Hebert PR, Taylor JO, Hennekens CH. Implications of small reductions in diastolic blood pressure for primary prevention. Arch Intern Med 1995; 155(7): 701–9.
28. Engberink MF, Schouten EG, Kok FJ, van Mierlo LAJ, Brouwer IA, Geleijnse JM. Lactotripeptides show no effect on human blood pressure. Hypertension 2008; 51(2): 399–405. doi: http://dx.doi.org/10.1161/HYPERTENSIONAHA.107.098988
29. Aihara K, Kajimoto O, Hirata H, Takahashi R, Nakamura Y. Effect of powdered fermented milk with Lactobacillus helveticus on subjects with high-normal blood pressure or mild hypertension. J Am Coll Nutr 2005; 24(4): 257–65.
30. Karlsen A, Svendsen M, Seljeflot I, Laake P, Duttaroy AK, Drevon CA, et al. Kiwifruit decreases blood pressure and whole-blood platelet aggregation in male smokers. J Hum Hypertens 2013; 27(2): 126–30.
31. Rodriguez-Leyva D, Weighell W, Edel AL, LaVallee R, Dibrov E, Pinneker R, et al. Potent antihypertensive action of dietary flaxseed in hypertensive patients. Hypertension 2013; 62(6): 1081–9.
32. Conway V, Couture P, Gauthier S, Pouliot Y, Lamarche B. Effect of buttermilk consumption on blood pressure in moderately hypercholesterolemic men and women. Nutrition 2014; 30(1): 116–19.
33. Katz DL, Davidhi A, Ma Y, Kavak Y, Bifulco L, Njike VY. Effects of walnuts on endothelial function in overweight adults with visceral obesity: a randomised, controlled, crossover trial. J Am Coll Nutr 2012; 31(6): 415–23.
34. Sumner DJ, Meredith PA, Howie CA, Elliott HL. Initial blood pressure as predictor of the response to antihypertensive therapy. Br J Clin Pharmacol 1988; 26(6): 715–20.
35. Fekete AA, Givens DI, Lovegrove JA. Casein-derived lactotripeptides reduce systolic and diastolic blood pressure in a meta-analysis of randomised clinical trials. Nutrients 2015; 7: 659–81.
36. Franklin SS, Thijs L, Hansen TW, O'Brien E, Staessen JA. White-coat hypertension new insights from recent studies. Hypertension 2013; 62(6): 982–7.
37. Pickering TG, Coats A, Mallion JM, Mancia G, Verdecchia P. Blood pressure monitoring. Task force V: white-coat hypertension. Blood Press Monit 1999; 4(6): 333–41.
38. O'Brien E, Parati G, Stergiou G, Asmar R, Beilin L, Bilo G, et al. European Society of Hypertension position paper on ambulatory blood pressure monitoring. J Hypertens 2013; 31(9): 1731–68.

***Rita Nilsen**
Norwegian University of Life Science
P.O. Box 5003, 1432 Ås
Norway
Email: rita.nilsen@nmbu.no

17

Proprietary tomato extract improves metabolic response to high-fat meal in healthy normal weight subjects

Xavier Deplanque, Delphine Muscente-Paque and Eric Chappuis*

Naturalpha SAS, Parc Eurasanté, Loos, France

Abstract

Background: Low-density lipoprotein (LDL) oxidation is a risk factor for atherosclerosis. Lycopene and tomato-based products have been described as potent inhibitors of LDL oxidation.

Objectives: To evaluate the effect of a 2-week supplementation with a carotenoid-rich tomato extract (CRTE) standardized for a 1:1 ratio of lycopene and phytosterols, on post-prandial LDL oxidation after a high-fat meal.

Design: In a randomized, double-blind, parallel-groups, placebo-controlled study, 146 healthy normal weight individuals were randomly assigned to a daily dose of CRTE standardized for tomato phytonutrients or placebo during 2 weeks. Oxidized LDL (OxLDL), glucose, insulin, and triglyceride (TG) responses were measured for 8 h after ingestion of a high-fat meal before and at the end of intervention.

Results: Plasma lycopene, phytofluene, and phytoene were increased throughout the study period in the CRTE group compared to placebo. CRTE ingestion significantly improved changes in OxLDL response to high-fat meal compared to placebo after 2 weeks ($p < 0.0001$). Changes observed in glucose, insulin, and TG responses were not statistically significant after 2 weeks of supplementation, although together they may suggest a trend of favorable effect on metabolic outcomes after a high-fat meal.

Conclusions: Two-week supplementation with CRTE increased carotenoids levels in plasma and improved oxidized LDL response to a high-fat meal in healthy normal weight individuals.

Keywords: *cardiovascular*; *carotenoid-rich tomato extract*; *oxidative stress*; *tomato*; *oxidized LDL*

Aerobic metabolism generates reactive oxygen species (ROS) including superoxide anion, hydrogen peroxide, and hydroxyl radicals. Biological and physiological processes are regulated by ROS that act as signaling molecules, allowing environmental adaptations of mammalian cells; however, ROS also interact with different biological targets and are commonly associated with oxidative stress linked to the development of certain pathologies where lipids, proteins, and DNA damage might be involved (1). ROS have a causal role in atherosclerosis that consists of migration, accumulation, and proliferation of foam cells in intimal smooth muscle cell, leading to the development of fibrofatty plaque sclerosis and cardiovascular events. An understanding of the underlying mechanisms involved in atherogenesis has dramatically improved over recent years and has revealed that endothelial dysfunction, the first step in this process, is a consequence of decreased nitric oxide (NO) bioavailability and increased generation of ROS in the vascular wall. Circulating low-density lipoproteins (LDLs) are entrapped in the subendothelial space of the vascular endothelium and subjected to oxidative modification to form oxidized LDL (OxLDL) particles that are internalized by macrophages and accumulate in foam cells, leading to atherogenesis (2). Absorption of exogenous antioxidants such as ascorbate (vitamin C) and α-tocopherol (vitamin E) has been proposed as a strategy to inhibit atherogenesis through restoration of NO bioavailability and ability to limit LDL oxidation, but promising results from small trials have not been confirmed in large interventional trials (2). Other antioxidants such as lycopene, the strongest oxygen quencher amongst carotenoids, have a protective role toward cardiovascular diseases (3) and demonstrate an *in vitro* ability to protect lipoproteins from oxidation, but *in vivo* evidence is still conflicting (4, 5). Results of interventional trials suggest that lycopene alone is less effective than whole tomatoes or complex tomato extracts in improving cardiovascular risk factors linked to oxidative stress such as OxLDL (5, 6).

Carotenoid-rich tomato extract (CRTE) is a tomato extract displaying health benefits similar to that of whole tomato consumption. For example, evidence suggests that this complex improves blood pressure in never-treated grade I hypertensive subjects and in treated, but uncontrolled, hypertensive subjects (7, 8).

Administration of high-fat meals has been proposed as a challenge model for atherogenesis because it results in a postprandial (fed-state) response characterized by hypertriglyceridemia (9, 10), inducing an increase of plasma concentrations of OxLDL (11, 12), as well as other inflammatory and metabolic parameters (13–18).

Given the metabolic effects of tomato-based products, the aim of the present study was to investigate the effect of chronic administration of CRTE on postprandial OxLDL response after consumption of a high-fat meal challenge in healthy adults.

Methods

Participants

In total, 150 healthy males and females were recruited for this randomized, double-blind, parallel-groups, placebo-controlled study. Participants were required to be aged 18–70 years, with normal weight defined as body mass index (BMI) $\geq$18.5 and $<$25 kg/m^2, plasma LDL cholesterol (LDLc) $\geq$100 and $<$220 mg/dL, plasma fasting triglycerides (TGs) $<$340 mg/dL, and plasma fasting glycemia (FG) $<$126 mg/dL; absence of type 1 and type 2 diabetes and cardiovascular disease or stroke and significant gastrointestinal disease; and without history of cancer or bariatric surgery. Subjects taking drugs or supplements that altered blood lipid levels as well as smokers and subjects consuming more than one alcoholic drink daily were excluded.

This monocentric study took place at the Naturalpha Clinical Nutrition Center, Hôpital Saint Vincent de Paul, Lille, France, and was conducted in accordance with the Declaration of Helsinki and the (2008 revisions), International Conference on Harmonization Harmonized Tripartite Guideline for Good Clinical Practice and the laws and regulations of Israel and France. The study received approval from Ethics Committee and French Competent Authority (Agence Nationale de Sécurité du Médicament; permission no. ID-RCB 2013-A00346-39), and all participants signed a written informed consent form before enrollment. CONSORT guidelines 2010 were considered.

Intervention and study design

Subjects were selected during a screening visit (V1) up to 3 weeks before the baseline visit (V2), and eligible subjects were randomly assigned to take CRTE or placebo soft gel capsules. The treatment capsules were standardized for the levels of several phytonutrients such as lycopene and phytosterols in a 1:1 ratio (15 mg), as well as tocopherols and other tomato carotenoids, i.e. phytoene, phytofluene (4 mg), and β-carotene (0.5 mg). The capsules were taken once daily with the main meal (preferably lunch) for 2 weeks between V2 and the final visit (V3). During the intervention, participants received lifestyle and dietary recommendation aimed at controlling lycopene and tomato-based products intake.

At V2 and V3, blood was withdrawn to evaluate plasma lycopene, phytoene, and phytofluene baseline levels (at V2) and bioavailability and compliance (at V3). Then, subjects were served a high-fat breakfast (850 kcal; 50% of energy from fat; standardized in lycopene) that was ingested within 20 min. After ingesting the high-fat meals, blood was withdrawn during 8 h (except for insulin, 2 h) to evaluate efficacy (plasma OxLDL, glucose, TG, and insulin levels) of the intervention. Safety was evaluated by blood tests, a physical examination, vital signs, and reporting of adverse events (AEs). Compliance was assessed by collecting capsules at V3.

Randomization and blinding

Randomization was stratified according to gender. Random sequence was generated by an independent statistician and subjects were enrolled by a Clinical Nutrition Center investigator/staff. Study products (CRTE and placebo) were provided in a bottle containing the capsules, bearing a product number that was assigned to the subject's randomization number at V2. Neither the subject nor the investigator/staff knew the composition of the product.

Data collection

Physical examination, vital signs, AEs, and concomitant use of medication were recorded at each visit. Food recommendations were provided at each visit. Demographic data, medical history review, height and weight, and waist circumference were collected at V1. Safety parameters were collected at V1 and V3. Dietary instructions were provided to study participants at V1 and V2. Efficacy parameters were collected at V2 and V3, except for insulin (only at V3).

Blood collection for determination of plasma glucose and TGs was performed at 0, 30, 60, 90, 120, 240, 360, and 480 min after a high-fat meal. Blood collection for OxLDL was performed at 0, 180, 240, 360, and 480 min after high fat meal. Blood collection for insulin was performed at 0, 30, 60, 90, 120 and 180 min after high-fat meal.

Biochemical measurements

After collection, blood samples were immediately transferred into cooled test tubes (at approximately +4°C) preloaded with EDTA (K3) and vortexed to ensure that all blood came into contact with the test tube wall. Samples were centrifuged within 15 min of sampling in a cooled centrifuge (at approximately +4°C). The supernatant (plasma) was divided into two aliquots of approximately equal volume, and the aliquots were transferred to a deep-freezer and stored at −80°C.

OxLDL was measured using an oxidized LDL ELISA kit (catalog no. 10-1143-01, Mercodia, Uppsala, Sweden).

Quantitative determination of insulin was performed with an immunoassay method (catalog no. 33410, Beckman Coulter, Fullerton, CA), total TG with TG glycerol phosphate oxidase reagent (catalog no. 44580, Beckman Coulter), and plasma glucose with glucose reagent (catalog no. B24985, Beckman Coulter).

Lycopene, phytofluene, and phytoene in human plasma were determined with ultra-performance liquid chromatography with a C_{18} reverse phase column at multiple wavelengths by using photodiode array detector. For each sample, 500-μL plasma aliquots were spiked with 20 μL of an internal standard solution containing 20 μg/mL astaxanthin in reconstitution solution (100 μg/mL 2,6-di-*tert*-butyl-4-methylphenol [BHT] in isopropanol). Then, 500 μL of ethanol was added to the plasma by vortex for 5 sec followed by 4.0 mL of extraction solution (100 μg/mL BHT in hexane:dichloromethane, 80:20). The sample was then vortexed for 10 sec, sonicated for 5 min, and vortexed again for 5 sec. Samples were then centrifuged for 10 min at 4,000 rpm at room temperature, and 3.0 mL from the upper layer was transferred to evaporation tubes and dried in a SpeedVac trap under dark conditions for up to 50 min. A 500-μL aliquot of diethyl-ether was used to rinse down the dried sample from the walls of the evaporation tube to its base and subsequently dried in a SpeedVac trap under dark conditions for up to 20 min. The dried sample was then reconstituted in 200 μL of reconstitution solution, and 150 μL of the upper layer was transferred to autosampler vial with a glass insert.

Statistical analyses

The primary objective of the study was to evaluate the effect of the CRTE on the reduction of postprandial LDL oxidation in healthy weight men and women. Based on the previous work of Burton-Freeman (19), sample size was calculated to detect a decrease of −3.0 units in OxLDL between the CRTE and placebo groups, with 90% power and an α level of 0.05, assuming that the common standard deviation for OxLDL is 5.0 units.

Statistical analyses were performed by Medistat with SPSS SAS version 9.1 (SAS Institute, Cary, NC).

OxLDL changes from baseline as well as relative changes (%) on each time point were analyzed using the paired t-test or signed rank test for two means (paired observations), as appropriate, within study arms. Comparative analysis between active and placebo group at any time point was performed using the analysis of variance (ANOVA) model for repeated measurements or the mixed-effect model for repeated measures (MMRM), including the fixed effect time and product and adjusted for baseline measurement and for additional covariates (such as sex) as appropriate. Changes from baseline at every collected time point until 480 min within group in glucose, TGs, and insulin blood levels were analyzed using the paired t-test or signed rank test (as appropriate). Comparative analyses of the changes at all times between groups were analyzed using repeated measurements ANOVA or MMRM. Differences in OxLDL, blood glucose, and TGs at V2 and V3 for every time point after the high-fat meal were analyzed using the paired t-test. Area under the curve (AUC_{0-480}) was calculated over time for glucose, TGs, and insulin measurements. The changes from V2 to V3 in lycopene, phytofluene, and phytoene levels were analyzed using the paired t-test or signed rank test (as appropriate).

The intent-to-treat population included all randomized subjects who, as documented before the breaking of the study blind, (1) were dosed with the study product (either CRTE or placebo) and provided a baseline assessment and (2) provided at least part of the efficacy assessment (during the study day visit).

All tests were two tailed. A p value of 0.05 or less was considered statistically significant.

Results

Study flow, compliance, and adverse effects

One hundred and fifty subjects were enrolled in the study, and 146 completed the intervention between June and September 2013. One and three subjects withdrew from the CRTE and placebo groups, respectively.

Treatment compliance was similar in both study arms. An average of 6.2 ± 2.1 capsules was returned in the CRTE arm and an average of 6.6 ± 2.6 capsules was returned in the placebo arm.

CRTE was safe and well tolerated. No serious AEs occurred during the study. None of the subjects in the CRTE arm were discontinued from the study due to AEs, and none of the AEs led to an intervention or any significant additional concomitant therapy. No significant laboratory abnormalities or clinically significant changes in vital signs or physical findings were reported during the study.

Baseline characteristics of participants

Mean age of participants was 34.8 ± 11.7 and 34.9 ± 11.4 years in the CRTE and placebo groups, respectively. Females represented 55.3% of the CRTE group and 55.4% of the placebo group. Mean BMI was 22.4 ± 2.2 and 22.5 ± 2.2 kg/m^2 and mean waist circumference was 81.9 ± 7.6 and 81.9 ± 8.6 cm in CRTE and placebo groups, respectively.

Bioavailability

Serum levels of lycopene, phytofluene, and phytoene at V2 and V3 are displayed in Table 1. At V2, plasma lycopene, phytofluene, and phytoene levels were similar between groups. Between V2 and V3, plasma lycopene, phytofluene, and phytoene levels significantly increased in the CRTE group compared to the placebo group.

Table 1. Serum levels of lycopene, phytofluene, and phytoene during the study

	Placebo			CRTE			
	n	Mean ± SEM	*p** within treatment	*n*	Mean ± SEM	*p** within treatment	*p*** between treatments
Lycopene (ng/mL)							
V2	72	430.5 ± 12.8		75	404.6 ± 13.7		0.1634
V3	71	412.5 ± 14		75	501.4 ± 5.3		<0.0001
Change from V2 to V3		−16.8 ± 11	0.0922		96.8 ± 13.1	<0.0001	<0.0001
Phytofluene (ng/mL)							
V2	72	153.9 ± 9.1		75	148.6 ± 9.6		0.4663
V3	71	150.0 ± 9.4		75	284.1 ± 14.1		<0.0001
Change from V2 to V3		−5.1 ± 6.0	0.3190		135.5 ± 11.1	<0.0001	<0.0001
Phytoene (ng/mL)							
V2	72	56.5 ± 1.4		75	58.9 ± 2.4		0.8792
V3	71	57.8 ± 2.0		75	103.8 ± 4.7		<0.0001
Change from V2 to V3		1.2 ± 2.0	0.7741		45.0 ± 4.5	<0.0001	<0.0001

SEM, standard error of the mean; V, visit.
**p* by signed rank test indicates the statistical significance of the change within group.
***p* by Wilcoxon test indicates the statistical significance of difference in the changes between groups.

OxLDL levels after high-fat meal challenge

Changes in OxLDL levels after high-fat meal between V2 and V3 at different time points are illustrated in Fig. 1, and absolute values are reported in Table 2. At V2 and V3, no significant difference was noted between treatments at any time point after high-fat meal ingestion for absolute OxLDL values (Table 2). However, both treatments induced significant reductions in OxLDL levels for up to 6 h (360 min) after the high-fat meal. At the end of the intervention (V3), OxLDL levels were lower in the CRTE arm compared to their values at V2, whereas in the placebo arm OxLDL levels were higher than their levels at V2 (Fig. 1). Significant differences between study arms were observed at 0, 180, 360, and 480 min. Furthermore, changes in AUC_{0-480} of OxLDL from V2 to V3 were significantly different between CRTE and placebo arms ($p < 0.0001$).

TG, glucose, and insulin levels after high-fat meal challenge

Changes in TG and glucose serum levels after high-fat meal between V2 and V3 at different time points are shown in Fig. 2, and absolute values are reported in Table 2. Changes in TG response after the high-fat meal between V2 and V3 were not different between groups at any time point, and the change in TG AUC_{0-480} from V2 to V3 was close to significance ($p = 0.08$). At V3, lowering of TG response in the CRTE arm compared to the placebo was close to significance at 30 and 60 min after the high-fat meal ($p = 0.08$; Table 2). Changes in glycemic response were significantly improved at 30 and 60 min after a high-fat meal in the CRTE group compared to the placebo (Fig. 2b), whereas changes in glucose AUC_{0-480} from V2 to V3 were not different between groups ($p = 0.94$). Glycemic response at V3 (absolute values; Table 2) was significantly lower at 30, 60, 90, and 120 min after the high-fat meal in the CRTE arm compared to the placebo (Table 2).

Insulin levels measured at V3 (Fig. 3) were not lower in the CRTE group compared to the placebo, except at 120 min after the high-fat meal, as depicted in Fig. 3. Insulin AUC_{0-480} was not different between groups.

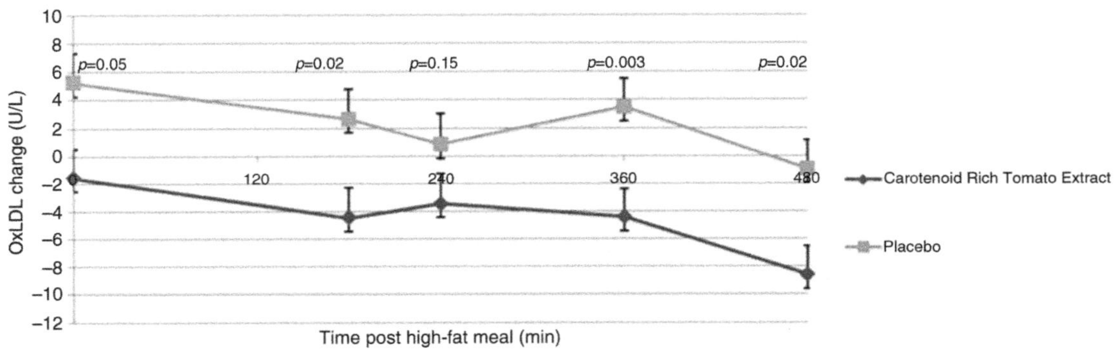

Fig. 1. Change of postprandial OxLDL levels from baseline at V2 to V3 by time points and treatment (mean ± SEM).

Table 2. Postprandial OxLDL, glucose, and TG serum levels during the study

		Placebo			CRTE			
	Time	*n*	Mean ± SEM	*p** within treatment	*n*	Mean ± SEM	*p** within treatment	*p** between treatments
OxLDL (U/L)								
V2	T0	71	62.30 ± 25.57		75	63.30 ± 27.75		0.821
	T180	71	53.66 ± 18.69	<0.001	75	54.88 ± 24.28	<0.001	0.7347
	T240	71	56.10 ± 22.11	<0.001	75	57.21 ± 27.44	<0.001	0.7898
	T360	71	55.31 ± 23.05	<0.001	75	58.61 ± 27.78	0.020	0.4376
	T480	71	59.20 ± 22.62	0.060	75	59.12 ± 27.27	0.015	0.9832
V3	T0	71	67.53 ± 25.63		75	61.73 ± 23.39		0.1547
	T180	71	64.95 ± 26.95	0.218	75	58.85 ± 27.32	0.030	0.1764
	T240	71	63.13 ± 25.77	0.706	75	59.76 ± 30.29	0.098	0.4713
	T360	71	65.79 ± 27.01	0.084	75	58.85 ± 25.06	0.015	0.1095
	T480	71	61.32 ± 29.47	0.634	75	54.69 ± 21.73	<0.001	0.1260
Glucose (g/L)								
V2	T0	71	0.91 ± 0.07		73	0.90 ± 0.07		0.6323
	T30	71	1.21 ± 0.20	<0.001	72	1.16 ± 0.19	<0.001	0.1210
	T60	71	1.02 ± 0.27	<0.001	73	0.93 ± 0.25	0.236	0.0455
	T90	71	0.85 ± 0.21	0.018	73	0.83 ± 0.24	0.005	0.5266
	T120	71	0.85 ± 0.17	0.007	73	0.82 ± 0.19	<0.001	0.3145
	T240	71	0.88 ± 0.14	0.109	75	0.83 ± 0.12	<0.001	0.0212
	T360	71	0.87 ± 0.06	<0.001	75	0.88 ± 0.09	0.044	0.6435
	T480	70	0.87 ± 0.05	<0.001	74	0.87 ± 0.06	<0.001	0.9076
V3	T0	71	0.91 ± 0.07		75	0.89 ± 0.07		0.1791
	T30	71	1.22 ± 0.17	<0.001	74	1.16 ± 0.18	<.001	0.0293
	T60	71	1.00 ± 0.24	0.001	75	0.91 ± 0.25	0.720	0.0237
	T90	70	0.85 ± 0.19	0.023	75	0.80 ± 0.17	<0.001	0.0595
	T120	71	0.87 ± 0.16	0.086	75	0.81 ± 0.16	<0.001	0.0172
	T240	71	0.86 ± 0.10	0.001	74	0.85 ± 0.12	<0.001	0.3805
	T360	71	0.88 ± 0.06	<0.001	73	0.89 ± 0.07	0.205	0.4851
	T480	71	0.89 ± 0.08	0.068	75	0.88 ± 0.06	0.101	0.8741
Triglycerides (g/L)								
V2	T0	71	0.86 ± 0.37		73	1.01 ± 1.49		0.4161
	T30	71	0.80 ± 0.34	0.004	72	0.97 ± 1.11	0.415	0.2142
	T60	71	1.01 ± 0.40	<0.001	73	1.16 ± 1.21	0.003	0.3133
	T90	71	1.17 ± 0.63	<0.001	73	1.26 ± 1.11	<0.001	0.5595
	T120	71	1.17 ± 0.44	<0.001	73	1.32 ± 1.05	<0.001	0.2625
	T240	71	1.16 ± 0.51	<0.001	75	1.28 ± 0.74	0.030	0.2274
	T360	71	1.02 ± 0.48	<0.001	75	1.05 ± 0.54	0.830	0.7469
	T480	71	0.78 ± 0.35	0.016	74	0.77 ± 0.41	0.142	0.8479
V3	T0	70	0.95 ± 0.40		75	0.87 ± 0.40		0.2381
	T30	71	0.95 ± 0.43	0.057	74	0.83 ± 0.39	0.263	0.0778
	T60	71	1.16 ± 0.48	<0.001	75	1.02 ± 0.43	0.920	0.0800
	T90	71	1.23 ± 0.53	<0.001	75	1.14 ± 0.49	0.388	0.2953
	T120	70	1.31 ± 0.58	<0.001	75	1.24 ± 0.49	0.146	0.4743
	T240	71	1.29 ± 0.63	<0.001	74	1.26 ± 0.62	0.121	0.7485
	T360	71	1.11 ± 0.45	<0.001	74	1.09 ± 0.52	0.688	0.8782
	T480	71	0.82 ± 0.36	0.287	75	0.76 ± 0.36	0.124	0.3250

STD, standard deviation; V, visit.

**p* value by t-test indicates the statistical significance of the change within or between group.

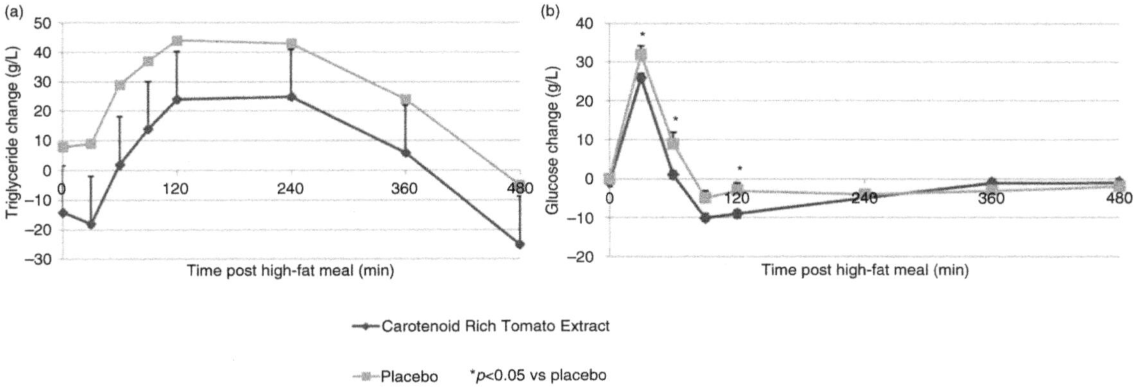

Fig. 2. Change of postprandial plasma triglycerides (a) and glucose (b) levels at V2 to V3 by time points and treatment (mean ± SEM).

Discussion

The effect of treatment with CRTE once daily for 2 weeks on postprandial OxLDL in healthy adult men and women with normal weight was evaluated in this single-center, randomized, double-blind, parallel-groups, placebo-controlled study. The power calculation, comparability of population features at baseline, low drop-out rate in the study, adequate compliance to intervention, and intention-to-treat statistical analysis support the validity of our trial results. The absence of follow-up on compliance to dietary and lifestyle recommendations is nevertheless a weakness of the study design.

Increased serum carotenoids at the end of intervention in the CRTE group witnessed the bioavailability of the product throughout the study period. This is in line with existing literature on tomato carotenoid bioavailability (20).

Concomitantly to this increase, the effects of 2-week supplementation with CRTE on OxLDL levels after a high-fat meal were evaluated. Reducing plasma OxLDL levels is considered a beneficial effect for atherosclerosis prevention and in the context of health claims for food products in the European Union (21). Interestingly, high inter-individual variability was observed in the OxLDL response to the high-fat meal, because only about one third of study population showed increased postprandial OxLDL levels. This explains why, on average, no significant increase in OxLDL levels was observed. The lack of deleterious effect of a high-fat meal on postprandial OxLDL levels was also reported in other studies. Reverri et al. (22) found no significant change in OxLDL concentration after consumption of a high-fat meal containing black beans or two control supplements. Another study (23) assessed the effect of a standardized high-fat meal on markers of inflammation and oxidative stress and found no significant changes in OxLDL concentrations in lean, obese non-diabetic, and type 2 diabetic men. A significant strength of this particular study included the evaluation of three well-defined patient populations and the use of a water control meal. In the current study, although a high-fat meal challenge did not exert the expected effect on metabolic response and flawed between-group comparisons in absolute OxLDL values at each visit, importantly the CRTE supplementation decreased changes in postprandial OxLDL levels for up to 8 h after ingestion of the high-fat meal, with a significant within treatment reduction in the CRTE, but not in the placebo group at 180, 360, and 480 min. Furthermore, when analyzing the change in OxLDL levels between V2 and V3 in the current study, the 2-week supplementation period resulted in a reduction of baseline levels (immediately before the meal) in the CRTE arm compared to placebo arm ($p \leq 0.05$). Although the elevation in baseline OxLDL values observed in the placebo group and not in the active treatment group at the V3 baseline is not fully understood, it can be hypothesized that this elevation was blocked in the active treatment group due to the anti-oxidative effect of the tested product (at this time point this group was already treated for 13 days). These results complete former observations from a pilot intervention trial (four healthy subjects) where a lycopene oleoresin administered before a high-fat meal challenge decreased LDL susceptibility

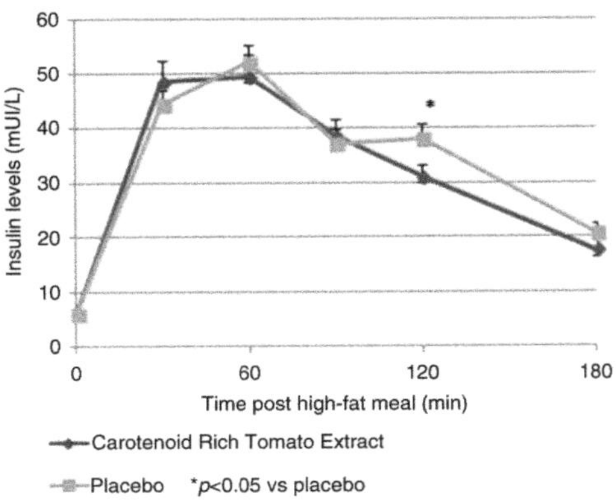

Fig. 3. Change of plasma insulin levels at V3 by time points and treatment (mean ± SEM).

to oxidation (24). Other plant-related substances and extracts have been reported to improve lipid peroxidation after either acute or chronic consumption, such as olive oil hydroxytyrosol (25, 26) or red wine polyphenols (27), but few have been investigated for their protective role after a high-fat meal challenge in healthy subjects. Additional studies should focus on acute and chronic effects of CRTE in normal life settings without metabolic challenge.

Changes observed in glucose, TG, and insulin values in the CRTE treatment arm (both in the change from baseline and AUC analysis) were not clinically meaningful by themselves, although together they may constitute an additive favorable effect of CRTE on metabolic outcomes after a high-fat meal. Longer exposure to treatment with CRTE may be required to see a more pronounced effect on the parameters assessed in the present study. The absence of insulin level measurements during the baseline visit did not allow us to draw a conclusion on the effect of the CRTE intervention on insulin response.

Additional information on the mechanisms of action of CRTE and its metabolic effects in response to a high-fat meal challenge could have been collected through analysis of inflammatory markers such as interleukin 8 (IL-8), a chemokine that has been recently described as an early marker of endothelial stress (15).

Results support safety and tolerance of CRTE in healthy normal weight subjects. No significant laboratory abnormalities or clinically significant changes in vital signs or physical finding were reported during the study.

Conclusions

Overall, the results of this study indicate that CRTE taken once daily for 2 weeks has a favorable effect on postprandial LDL oxidation, glucose, insulin, and TG levels for up to 8 h. CRTE was well tolerated throughout the study period, and additional trials are needed to prove the repeatability of these results in other sub-populations such as subjects at-risk of cardiovascular diseases.

Authors' contributions

XD and DMP were involved in the clinical study conductance, data analysis, and review of the manuscript. EC wrote the manuscript. All authors read and approved the final manuscript.

Acknowledgements

We thank Drs. Joseph Levy and Yoav Sharoni, Clinical Biochemistry and Pharmacology, Ben-Gurion University of the Negev, Beer-Sheva, Israel, for advice during the clinical trial and manuscript design and for critical reviews of this manuscript

Conflict of interest and funding

XD, DMP, and EC are employees of Naturalpha SAS, a private company that provides research and development services and that was mandated and financed by Lycored to conduct the human clinical trial presented in the present publication. XD, DMP, and EC declare that they have no competing interests.

CRTE tested in this study is commercialized by Lycored.

References

1. Schieber M, Chandel NS. ROS function in redox signaling and oxidative stress. Curr Biol 2014; 24(10): R453–62.
2. Lee R, Margaritis M, Channon KM, Antoniades C. Evaluating oxidative stress in human cardiovascular disease: methodological aspects and considerations. Curr Med Chem 2012; 19(16): 2504–20.
3. Mordente A, Guantario B, Meucci E, Silvestrini A, Lombardi E, Martorana GE, et al. Lycopene and cardiovascular diseases: an update. Curr Med Chem 2011; 18(8): 1146–63.
4. Chen J, Song Y, Zhang L. Effect of lycopene supplementation on oxidative stress: an exploratory systematic review and meta-analysis of randomized controlled trials. J Med Food 2013; 16(5): 361–74.
5. Burton-Freeman B, Sesso HD. Whole food versus supplement: comparing the clinical evidence of tomato intake and lycopene supplementation on cardiovascular risk factors. Adv Nutr 2014; 5(5): 457–85.
6. Sesso HD, Liu S, Gaziano JM, Buring JE. Dietary lycopene, tomato-based food products and cardiovascular disease in women. J Nutr 2003; 133(7): 2336–41.
7. Engelhard YN, Gazer B, Paran E. Natural antioxidants from tomato extract reduce blood pressure in patients with grade-1 hypertension: a double-blind, placebo-controlled pilot study. Am Heart J 2006; 151(1): 100.
8. Paran E, Engelhard YN, Hazan-Hallevy I, Sharoni Y, Levy J. P-565: effect of standardized tomato extract on blood pressure, endothelial function and plasma lycopene levels in treated hypertensive patients. Am J Hypertens 2005; 18(Suppl 4): 213A.
9. Bowen PE, Borthakur G. Postprandial lipid oxidation and cardiovascular disease risk. Curr Atheroscler Rep 2004; 6(6): 477–84.
10. Ursini F, Sevanian A. Postprandial oxidative stress. Biol Chem 2002; 383(3–4): 599–605.
11. Burton-Freeman B, Linares A, Hyson D, Kappagoda T. Strawberry modulates LDL oxidation and postprandial lipemia in response to high-fat meal in overweight hyperlipidemic men and women. J Am Coll Nutr 2010; 29(1): 46–54.
12. Graner M, Kahri J, Nakano T, Sarna SJ, Nieminen MS, Syvanne M, et al. Impact of postprandial lipaemia on low-density lipoprotein (LDL) size and oxidized LDL in patients with coronary artery disease. Eur J Clin Invest 2006; 36(11): 764–70.
13. Hyson D, Rutledge JC, Berglund L. Postprandial lipemia and cardiovascular disease. Curr Atheroscler Rep 2003; 5(6): 437–44.
14. Lundman P, Boquist S, Samnegard A, Bennermo M, Held C, Ericsson CG, et al. A high-fat meal is accompanied by increased plasma interleukin-6 concentrations. Nutr Metab Cardiovasc Dis 2007; 17(3): 195–202.
15. Esser D, Oosterink E, op 't Roodt J, Henry RM, Stehouwer CD, Muller M, et al. Vascular and inflammatory high fat meal responses in young healthy men; a discriminative role of IL-8 observed in a randomized trial. PLoS One. 2013; 8(2): e53474.
16. Ceriello A, Bortolotti N, Motz E, Pieri C, Marra M, Tonutti L, et al. Meal-induced oxidative stress and low-density lipoprotein

oxidation in diabetes: the possible role of hyperglycemia. Metabolism 1999; 48(12): 1503–8.
17. Ursini F, Zamburlini A, Cazzolato G, Maiorino M, Bon GB, Sevanian A. Postprandial plasma lipid hydroperoxides: a possible link between diet and atherosclerosis. Free Radic Biol Med 1998; 25(2): 250–2.
18. Tushuizen ME, Nieuwland R, Scheffer PG, Sturk A, Heine RJ, Diamant M. Two consecutive high-fat meals affect endothelial-dependent vasodilation, oxidative stress and cellular microparticles in healthy men. J Thromb Haemost 2006; 4(5): 1003–10.
19. Burton-Freeman B, Talbot J, Park E, Krishnankutty S, Edirisinghe I. Protective activity of processed tomato products on postprandial oxidation and inflammation: a clinical trial in healthy weight men and women. Mol Nutr Food Res 2012; 56(4): 622–31.
20. Engelmann NJ, Clinton SK, Erdman JW. Nutritional aspects of phytoene and phytofluene, carotenoid precursors to lycopene. Adv Nutr 2011; 2(1): 51–61.
21. European Food Safety Authority, EFSA Panel on Dietetic Products, Nutrition and Allergies (NDA). Guidance on the scientific requirements for health claims related to antioxidants, oxidative damage and cardiovascular health. EFSA J 2011; 9(12): 13.
22. Reverri EJ, Randolph JM, Steinberg FM, Kappagoda CT, Edirisinghe I, Burton-Freeman BM. Black beans, fiber, and antioxidant capacity pilot study: examination of whole foods vs. functional components on postprandial metabolic, oxidative stress, and inflammation in adults with metabolic syndrome. Nutrients 2015; 7(8): 6139–54.
23. Phillips LK, Peake JM, Zhang X, Hickman IJ, Briskey DR, Huang BE, et al. Postprandial total and HMW adiponectin following a high-fat meal in lean, obese and diabetic men. Eur J Clin Nutr 2013; 67(4): 377–84.
24. Fuhrman B, Volkova N, Rosenblat M, Aviram M. Lycopene synergistically inhibits LDL oxidation in combination with vitamin E, glabridin, rosmarinic acid, carnosic acid, or garlic. Antioxid Redox Signal 2000; 2(3 Fall): 491–506.
25. Marrugat J, Covas MI, Fito M, Schroder H, Miro-Casas E, Gimeno E, et al. Effects of differing phenolic content in dietary olive oils on lipids and LDL oxidation – a randomized controlled trial. Eur J Nutr 2004; 43(3): 140–7.
26. Weinbrenner T, Fito M, de la Torre R, Saez GT, Rijken P, Tormos C, et al. Olive oils high in phenolic compounds modulate oxidative/antioxidative status in men. J Nutr 2004; 134(9): 2314–21.
27. Gorelik S, Ligumsky M, Kohen R, Kanner J. A novel function of red wine polyphenols in humans: prevention of absorption of cytotoxic lipid peroxidation products. FASEB J 2008; 22(1): 41–6.

***Eric Chappuis**
Naturalpha
Parc Eurasanté
FR-59120 Loos
France
Email: eric.chappuisl@yahoo.fr

The association between adherence to the New Nordic Diet and diet quality

Helga Birgit Bjørnarå[1]*, Nina Cecilie Øverby[1], Tonje Holte Stea[1], Monica Klungland Torstveit[1], Elisabet Rudjord Hillesund[1], Lene Frost Andersen[2], Sveinung Berntsen[1] and Elling Bere[1]

[1]Department of Public Health, Sport and Nutrition, Faculty of Health and Sport Sciences, University of Agder, Kristiansand, Norway; [2]Department of Nutrition, University of Oslo, Oslo, Norway

Abstract

Background: Previous studies have reported a positive association between scoring on healthy Nordic diet scales and the intake of healthy foods and nutrients, and also with higher intake of meat, sweets, cakes, and energy in general. These studies have used the same food frequency questionnaire (FFQ) responses for constructing the diet score as for calculating intakes of foods and nutrients. Thus, it is not clear whether the coexistence of healthy and less healthy dietary aspects among adherers to Nordic diets would occur even though separate methods were applied for exploring these relations.
Objective: To assess the association between adherence to the New Nordic Diet (NND), derived from an FFQ, and diet quality, determined from two 24-h dietary recall interviews.
Design: In total, 65 parents of toddlers in Southern Norway answered the NND FFQ and two 24-h dietary recall interviews. NND adherence was determined from the FFQ and categorized into low, medium, and high adherence. The two 24-h recalls provided data for the intake of specific foods and nutrients, selected on the basis of the Norwegian food-based guidelines as an indicator of a healthy diet. The Kruskal–Wallis test was used for assessing differences in food and nutrient intake across NND groups.
Results: High NND adherence derived from FFQ was associated with a high intake of fruits ($p = 0.004$) and fiber ($p = 0.02$), and a low intake of meat ($p = 0.004$) and margarines ($p = 0.05$), derived from recalls. A larger proportion of high NND adherers (68%) complied with the national dietary recommendation targeting meat intake compared with low NND adherers (29%) ($p = 0.04$).
Conclusion: The present study showed that higher NND adherence measured with FFQ was associated with a higher intake of selected healthy foods and nutrients, measured with recalls. However, a higher intake of meat, sweets, and energy, as earlier reported, was not observed.

Keywords: *New Nordic Diet*; *diet score*; *Norwegian food-based guidelines*; *dietary intake*; *nutrient intake*

Responsible Editor: Per Ole Iversen, University of Oslo, Norway.

As a result of the demonstrated protective effects of the Mediterranean diet on disease (1–3) and mortality (2), the possible protective effects of other regional diets have gained attention. In the Nordic countries, dietary scores have been constructed in order to explore adherence to different aspects of the Nordic diets with expected health-promoting effects (4–6). Recently, observational studies have reported that compliance with Nordic diets is associated with lower mortality (4, 7) and a reduced risk of non-communicable diseases (5, 8–13). However, the evidence is not quite consistent, as other studies have failed to demonstrate associations between Nordic diets and breast cancer (14), colorectal cancer (15), or type 2 diabetes (16) and have reported equivocal associations with cardio-metabolic risk factors (17).

Three studies have examined dietary composition and nutrient intake related to three different Nordic diet scores, concluding that high scores were associated with an increased intake of healthy foods (5, 18) and essential nutrients (5, 6, 18). In a sample of Swedish women (18), higher scores on the Healthy Nordic Food Index (HNFI) were associated with a higher intake of the six food groups included in the score, that is, apples/pears, cabbage, root vegetables, whole grain bread, oatmeal, and fish/shellfish, in addition to fiber and higher micronutrient density. Likewise, participants in the Norwegian Mother and

Child Cohort Study (MoBa), who attained higher ratings in the New Nordic Diet (NND) score, reported a higher consumption of healthy foods like whole grains, fish, fruits, and vegetables, and thus increased fiber intake and overall higher nutrient density (5). In a representative sample of the Finnish population, increased compliance with the Baltic Sea Diet Score implied a higher intake of fiber, iron, vitamin D, and folate, and a decreased intake of saturated fatty acids (SFAs) and alcohol (6). Moreover, high diet scores were associated with being more physically active (6, 18) and more likely to exercise (5).

Nevertheless, not all reported associations between diet scores and food intake have been in a healthier direction. In Norway, 'high' NND adherers were reported eating slightly more meat, cakes, and desserts than 'low' NND adherers (5), while Swedish women with high scores on the HNFI also reported a higher intake of less healthy foods such as processed meat and sweets (18). Moreover, in the Finnish sample higher intake of sodium and lower intake of polyunsaturated fatty acids (PUFAs) was observed among adherers to the Baltic Sea Diet Score (6). In all three studies, a high score was positively associated with energy intake (5, 6, 18).

These three studies, examining the association between adhering to Nordic diets and food/nutrient intake, all used the same food frequency questionnaire (FFQ) for constructing the diet score as for calculating intakes of foods and nutrients. Therefore, based on the previously reported coexistence of healthy and less healthy dietary aspects among adherers to predefined healthy Nordic diets, the aim of the current study was to assess the association between adherence to the NND score, derived from an FFQ, and diet quality, determined from two 24-h dietary recall interviews.

Methods

Design and study sample

The present data originate from the project Healthy and Sustainable Lifestyle, which in 2014 collected data in collaboration with the Child Food Courage project (19). As part of these projects, a web-based questionnaire was constructed to explore lifestyle behaviors, self-perceived health and quality of life, as well as basic demographic and socioeconomic variables (e.g. sex, age, height, weight, ethnicity, and educational attainment) among parents of toddlers. For the current methodological study, a convenience sample, consisting of parents of toddlers born between 2008 and 2011, was recruited through kindergartens. The leader of each kindergarten was asked to distribute the study invitation to eligible parents who were able to speak and read Norwegian. For each child, either the mother or the father could participate. Parents were informed about the purpose and implications of the study through a web page and via e-mail distribution. In total, 1,191 parents from 19 kindergartens in the county of Vest-Agder, Southern Norway, were invited to participate. A total of 86 (7%) parents signed up. Parents provided consent electronically, followed by administration of the questionnaire survey by e-mail. Subsequently, two 24-h dietary recalls were conducted by telephone 2–4 weeks apart, level of physical activity was recorded objectively for seven consecutive days, and anthropometric measurements were undertaken (height and body mass). Data collection was conducted between March and August 2014. In total, 56 parents (65% of those who signed up) completed all measurements, that is, the electronic questionnaire, two dietary recalls, and the physical activity assessment, while 65 parents (76%) completed the questionnaire and two dietary recalls, and 75 parents (87%) completed the questionnaire only.

Measures

The New Nordic Diet score

The electronic questionnaire incorporated an FFQ assessing participants' habitual frequency of intake of selected foods, without specification of amounts consumed. The foods assessed included foods that are part of the concept of a NND, which has been suggested due to its inherent properties that potentially promote health, environmental sustainability, and food traditions (20), without compromising palatability (21). The NND consists of healthy foods native to the Nordic climate or foods that can be produced or cultivated in the Nordic climate, like certain fruits, berries, root vegetables, cabbages, whole grains, wild fish and game, potatoes, and rapeseed oil (20, 22). The NND score was previously developed to capture adherence to the NND in observational studies (5), and has recently shown acceptable test–retest reliability (23). The NND score comprises 10 subscales selected to summarize meal pattern and habitual intake of typical Nordic foods. Appendix 1 describes the components underlying the construction of the 10 subscales in the present study, including questionnaire items and frequency options. In the present study, the number of items forming the basis for each subscale ranged from 1 to 5, a total of 24 questions. Each subscale was dichotomized by the sex-specific median and assigned values of '0' or '1', with '1' indicating a more frequent consumption of main meals (subscale 1) or a more favorable intake of selected foods (subscale 2–10). Each subscale was assigned equal weightage, and adding the subscales yielded a score ranging from 0 to 10, with increasing scores indicating higher compliance with the NND. The total score was trichotomized grouping participants into 'low' (0–3 points), 'medium' (4–5 points), and 'high' (6–10 points) adherence to the NND (5), with cutoffs for groupings determined to obtain the most equally sized groups.

24-Hour dietary recall interviews
Two unannounced 24-h dietary recalls were collected by telephone, 2–4 weeks apart by two trained interviewers, after completion of the FFQ. Each interview lasted for approximately 20–30 min, aiming to obtain detailed information on all foods and beverages consumed by the participants in the period between waking up on the preceding day and waking up on the interview day. A booklet containing photographs of various portion sizes for common foods and standard sizes of glasses, cups, and plates (24) was available on the project's web page to ease the estimation of portion sizes from memory. Dietary intake was reported for one weekday and one weekend day by 21 participants (32%), of whom 18 participants (86%) reported for a Sunday, while 3 participants (14%) reported for a Saturday. The remaining 44 participants (68%) reported dietary intake for two weekdays, due to feasibility. Dietary information was converted into daily energy and nutrient intakes using the food calculation software KBS V 7.0, linked directly to the food composition database N3. The Norwegian food composition table from 2006 (25) forms the basis for this food composition database, which is also supplemented with additional food items from reliable sources. The 24-h recall functionality of the KBS program was developed specifically for the Norkost 3 study, which represents the latest national dietary survey conducted among a representative sample of Norwegian adults (24). Nutritional supplements were excluded from the calculations, as food intake per se was that of interest in this study, and what corresponds with the concept NND.

In order to assess diet quality across NND adherence, specific foods and nutrients assessed by the two 24-h dietary recalls were selected, based on the official Norwegian food-based guidelines (26) as an indicator of a healthy diet. Foods assessed were 'Vegetables (fresh and frozen)', 'Fruits and berries (fresh)', 'Fruit juice', 'Whole grain products', 'Refined grain products', 'Fish', 'Meat', 'Low fat dairy products', 'Fatty dairy products', 'Vegetable oils', 'Margarines', 'Butter', 'Chocolate, candies and sugar-sweetened beverages', and 'Water'. Selected nutrients were fiber, added sugar, and sodium. In addition, we assessed energy intake across NND groups. Also, the proportion from each NND adherence category meeting the following quantitative Norwegian food recommendations was calculated; 'Eat at least five portions of vegetables, fruits, and berries every day', 'Eat whole grains every day', 'Eat fish for dinner two to three times a week and preferably also as sandwich spread', 'Choose lean meat and lean meat products. Limit the amount of processed meat and red meat', 'Choose foods containing little salt, and limit the use of salt for cooking', and 'Avoid sugar rich foods and beverages for everyday use'. Calculations were performed in line with the methodology of the Norkost 3 study (24), entailing that for whole meal bread, 40% of the product weight was accounted for as whole grains, while for muesli/mixed cereals, 50% of the product weight was included. Further, cut-offs for compliance were set at 70 g whole grain/day for women and 90 g/day for men. Recommendations regarding fish intake and meat consumption were operationalized into daily intake, as recommended weekly amounts are 300–450 g of fish (ready to eat), and <500 g of red and processed meat (ready to eat), for both females and males. Consequently, due to the features of the food calculation software used (KBS V 7.0), 40% of the product weight of processed fish products was included (24), and for meat intake the recommended commodity weight (750 g/week) (27) represented the cut-off.

Moreover, the habitual frequency of consumption of selected foods (i.e. vegetables, fruits and berries, fruit juice, whole grain products, refined grain products, fish, meat, and sweet pastries, candies, and sugar-sweetened beverages) across NND adherence groups was assessed using FFQ data. Although amounts were not specified, frequencies would allow for an examination of tendencies across groups, using the same FFQ data for determining NND adherence as for assessing dietary intake, in line with the methodology applied in the earlier studies (5, 6, 18).

Physical activity and anthropometric measurements
To enable exploration of the physical activity level in the present sample, as one relevant sample characteristic, and also the relation between energy intake and energy expenditure, the monitor SenseWear Armband Mini (SWA; BodyMedia, Pittsburgh, Pennsylvania, USA) was used. SWA includes a 3-axis accelerometer, a heat-flux sensor, a skin temperature sensor, and a near-body ambient temperature sensor (28). Data from these sensors were combined with sex, age, body weight, and height to estimate physical activity intensity and energy expenditure using algorithms developed by the manufacturer. Participants were instructed to wear the monitor on the upper left arm (on the triceps, at mid humerus point) for seven consecutive days, only removing it for bathing, or any other water activity. Those with a nickel allergy were discouraged from participating ($n=5$), as wearing the monitor may cause skin rashes due to 8% nickel content. Data were downloaded using SenseWear Professional V.8.1 (BodyMedia, Pittsburgh, Pennsylvania, USA). A valid day was defined as at least 80% (19.2 h) wearing time, and a minimum of four valid days with at least one weekend day was required for participants to be included in the analyses (29, 30). Data were calculated and reported as mean values per day. Participants exceeding 21.5 min/day with moderate and vigorous physical activity, in bouts of at least 10 min duration, were classified as meeting the recommendations for physical activity (26, 31). The cut-off defining moderate to vigorous intensity was 3 metabolic equivalents (METs) (32). Anthropometric

measurements were obtained by trained staff, with subjects barefoot and dressed in light clothes. Height was measured using a portable stadiometer with the head in the Frankfort plane, two measurements were taken and added with a third if the first two differed by $>1\%$. The mean of the closest two measurements was calculated. Body mass was measured by a segmental multi-frequency bioelectrical impedance analysis (BIA), conducted with In Body 720 (Biospace Co., Ltd., Seoul, Korea). Body mass index (BMI) was computed, as this represents one significant and commonly included sample characteristic, and participants with a BMI ≥ 25 kg/m^2 were categorized as overweight/obese (33). In compliance with the measurement protocol, participants were instructed to abstain from exercise and food within 2 h of testing, and immediately prior to the measurement to avoid showering and sauna, and to empty their bladder. Pregnant women were excluded from the body composition measurements ($n=1$).

Statistical analysis

Statistical analyses were performed with the statistical software package IBM SPSS Statistics version 22.0 (IBM Corp., Somers, New York, USA). To explore differences in sample characteristics across NND adherence categories, Chi-square test for independence (χ^2) was used. Food consumption variables were skewed, thus the Kruskal–Wallis test was applied for assessing differences in food, nutrient and energy intakes, and energy expenditure, across NND categories. Results are presented as median and quartiles. Differences in compliance with the Norwegian quantitative food-based dietary guidelines according to NND adherence group was assessed with Chi-square. A two-sided p-value of <0.05 was considered statistically significant.

Results

A total of 65 participants were included in the final analyses. Mean age in the study sample was 35.2 years (SD$\pm$5.0 years), 55 participants (85%) were females, 58 participants (89%) were native Norwegians, and 37 participants (57%) reported four or more years of university or college education (Table 1). Furthermore, 13 participants (20%) were overweight or obese, while 46 participants (82%) met the national recommendations on physical activity (26). No significant differences were observed in sample characteristics across NND categories (Table 1). Participants were categorized according to the NND score into low ($n=17$), medium ($n=23$), or high ($n=25$) NND adherence, representing 26, 35, and 39% of the sample, respectively. Among the 21 participants (32%) reporting dietary intake for one weekday and one weekend day, distribution across NND adherence groups was: low ($n=5$), medium ($n=6$), and high ($n=10$), representing 24, 28, and 48%, respectively.

Table 1. Selected characteristics of the study sample in total ($n=65$), according to NND adherence

	Degree of NND adherence				
	Whole sample ($n=65$)	Low ($n=17$)	Medium ($n=23$)	High ($n=25$)	
	n (%)	n (%)	n (%)	n (%)	p*
Sex					
Female	55 (85)	14 (82)	20 (87)	21 (84)	0.92
Age (yrs)					
20–34	31 (48)	8 (47)	12 (52)	11 (44)	
≥35–47	34 (52)	9 (53)	11 (48)	14 (56)	0.85
Ethnicity					
Native Norwegian†	58 (89)	16 (94)	21 (91)	21 (84)	0.54
Educational attainment					
Higher education‡	37 (57)	13 (77)	9 (39)	15 (60)	0.06
Weight status					
Overweight/obese§	13 (20)	4 (24)	5 (22)	4 (16)	0.81
Physical activity level					
Physically active‖	46¶ (82)	11 (73)	16 (80)	19 (91)	0.40

NND, New Nordic Diet. *p-values calculated from Chi-square test for independence (χ^2). †Both parents born in Norway. ‡≥4 years of university or college education. §Body mass index ≥25 kg/m^2. ‖>21.5 min/day with moderate and vigorous physical activity, in bouts of at least 10 min duration, measured by the activity monitor SenseWear Armband Mini. ¶For physical activity level $n=56$; 15, 20, and 21 parents categorized into low, medium, and high NND, respectively.

Different consumption of selected foods (Table 2) across NND groups was detected for meat ($p=0.004$), fruits and berries ($p=0.004$), and margarines ($p=0.05$), entailing that those classified as 'low' NND adherers reported the highest consumption of meat and margarines, while 'high' NND adherers reported the largest intake of fruits and berries. For the other foods assessed, that is, fresh and frozen vegetables, fruit juice, whole grain products, refined grain products, fish, low-fat dairy products, fatty dairy products, vegetable oils, butter, chocolate, candies and sugar-sweetened beverages, and water, no significant differences were observed. The relative intake of dietary fiber (E%) differed significantly across NND groups; fiber contributed with 2.7 E%, 2.4 E%, and 2.1 E% ($p=0.02$), in 'high', 'medium', and 'low' NND adherers, respectively. For added sugar and sodium, no differences according to NND classifications were found. Likewise, energy intake and energy expenditure did not differ across NND groups (Table 2).

Regarding the frequency of habitual food intake (results not shown) measured with FFQ, significant differences across NND adherence groups were found for all foods except from fruit juice. 'High' NND reported to eat vegetables, fruits and berries, whole grain products,

Table 2. Daily energy expenditure, energy intake, and consumption of fiber, added sugar, sodium (Na), and selected foods, according to NND adherence

	Degree of NND adherence						
	Low ($n = 17$)		Medium ($n = 23$)		High ($n = 25$)		
	Median[†]	(Q1, Q3)	Median	(Q1, Q3)	Median	(Q1, Q3)	p*
Energy expenditure (kJ)[‡]	11,026	(10,041, 12,203)	10,621	(10,040, 11,870)	11,456	(10,074, 12,436)	0.65
Energy intake (kJ)	9,361	(7,762, 12,200)	8,308	(7,418, 10,992)	8,883	(7,225, 10,961)	0.46
Fiber (g)	24.5	(21.8, 27.7)	26.4	(22.0, 32.0)	30.2	(23.0, 40.3)	0.07
Fiber (E%)	2.1	(1.6, 2.6)	2.4	(2.1, 2.7)	2.7	(2.2, 3.1)	0.02
Added sugar (g)	38.1	(17.8, 60.4)	27.8	(10.7, 40.4)	21.1	(12.7, 36.2)	0.19
Added sugar (E%)	6.9	(3.4, 8.8)	4.7	(2.5, 7.5)	4.4	(2.7, 6.7)	0.17
Na (mg)	2738.0	(2214.5, 3795.0)	2786.0	(1828.0, 3860.0)	2789.0	(1984.5, 3778.5)	0.92
Vegetables (fresh and frozen)	139.9	(86.8, 218.6)	140.6	(76.0, 198.5)	164.4	(110.6, 243.5)	0.56
Fruits and berries (fresh)	102.5	(60.8, 207.8)	150.0	(120.5, 305.0)	267.5	(187.6, 348.8)	0.004
Fruit juice	93.8	(0.0, 312.5)	0.0	(0.0, 187.5)	0.0	(0.0, 122.5)	0.15
Whole grain products	57.7	(33.6, 110.0)	53.7	(30.1, 117.6)	67.2	(34.0, 136.0)	0.60
Refined grain products	130.2	(52.7, 169.7)	86.2	(51.3, 166.0)	74.9	(38.7, 162.7)	0.67
Fish‖	21.3	(0.0, 60.1)	5.0	(0.0, 85.3)	38.5	(0.0, 86.8)	0.53
Meat¶	167.4	(134.6, 233.8)	116.5	(54.2, 189.6)	102.0	(60.8, 128.8)	0.004
Low fat dairy products	110.0	(12.0, 283.15)	142.5	(62.5, 320.3)	125.0	(49.8, 406.3)	0.60
Fatty dairy products	146.0	(71.7, 187.3)	75.2	(40.0, 154.9)	88.0	(57.0, 155.4)	0.20
Vegetable oils	1.1	(0.0, 5.1)	0.0	(0.0, 3.0)	0.3	(0.0, 2.3)	0.63
Margarines	7.5	(0.7, 19.6)	5.5	(2.5, 11.6)	1.1	(0.0, 7.9)	0.05
Butter	5.6	(3.2, 12.1)	5.0	(1.6, 10.2)	6.8	(2.2, 16.7)	0.50
Chocolate, candies, and sugar-sweetened beverages	42.0	(6.3, 205.0)	24.5	(1.0, 163.1)	4.0	(0.0, 64.5)	0.15
Water	1000.0	(601.9, 1297.0)	1215.0	(812.5, 1893.8)	1120.0	(795.0, 1452.5)	0.33

NND, New Nordic Diet. *Kruskal–Wallis test was used to derive p-values. [†]Median and quartiles were calculated from two 24-h dietary recalls. [‡]For energy expenditure (measured by the activity monitor SenseWear Armband Mini) and energy intake (assessed by two 24-h dietary recalls). $n = 56$; 15, 20, and 21 parents categorized into low, medium, and high NND, respectively. ‖Includes lean fish, fatty fish, fish products, and selected fish toppings. ¶Includes poultry, pork, beef, game (all unprocessed), ground meat, and processed meat (salted meat, minced meat, sandwich meat, and liver paste).

and fish more frequently than 'low' NND, while 'low' NND recorded more frequent consumption of refined grain products, meat, and sweet pastries, candies, and sugar-sweetened beverages than 'high' NND.

Table 3 shows that a greater proportion of 'high' NND adherers complied with the guideline to 'Choose lean meat and lean meat products and limit the amount of processed meat and read meat', than 'low' NND adherers (68% versus 29%, $p = 0.04$). For the remaining five recommendations of interest, no significant differences between NND adherence groups were found.

Discussion

In the present study, the association between adherence to the NND, derived from an FFQ, and diet quality, determined from two 24-h dietary recall interviews, was assessed. In line with former findings, the trend was that 'high' NND adherers reported a more favorable diet in general (5, 6, 18), and a higher intake of fruits (5, 18) and dietary fiber (5, 6, 18). Contrasting previous findings (5, 18), neither higher intake of meat or sweets, nor higher energy intake or higher physical activity levels was observed among 'high' NND adherers (5, 6, 18).

The previously observed coexistence of healthy and less healthy dietary elements among adherers to predefined healthy Nordic diets could have different explanations. First, it may be real, that is, that those who achieve high scoring on the Nordic scales have higher intakes of a wide variety of foods, which may be characterized as both healthy and less healthy. High intake of healthy foods and beverages will most likely have positive health effects, in spite of unhealthy elements in the diet. This aspect may partly explain previous results, especially as higher scoring on the Nordic scales was associated with being more physically active, or more likely to exercise, as well. Dietary factors not included when constructing a specific diet score could confound true associations between the healthier aspects of the diet and relevant outcomes. An example is meat, which has been reported to associate positively with colorectal cancer (34), and also with

Table 3. Proportions meeting the quantitative recommendations incorporated in the official Norwegian food-based dietary guidelines, according to NND adherence

		Degree of NND adherence			
		Low ($n = 17$)	Medium ($n = 23$)	High ($n = 25$)	
Quantitative dietary recommendations	Behavior required for scoring	% adhering to recommendation	% adhering to recommendation	% adhering to recommendation	p*
3: 'Eat at least five portions of vegetables, fruits, and berries every day'[†]	>500 g/day	29	35	48	0.43
4: 'Eat whole grains every day'	>70 g/day (women) >90 g/day (men)	35	35	40	0.92
5: 'Eat fish for dinner two to three times a week and preferably also as toppings'[‡]	>43 g/day	29	39	48	0.48
6: 'Choose lean meat and lean meat products. Limit the amount of processed meat and read meat[§]'	<107 g/day	29	61	68	0.04
9: 'Choose foods containing little salt, and limit the use of salt for cooking'.	<6 g salt (NaCl) per day	24	39	36	0.56
10: 'Avoid sugar rich foods and beverages for everyday use'.	<10 E% sugar/day	88	87	96	0.51

NND, New Nordic Diet. *Proportions were calculated using chi-square. [†]For those with an average intake of at least 100 g of fruit juice, 100 g of juice were included. [‡]Includes lean fish, fatty fish, fish products, and selected fish toppings. [§]Includes lean, red meat (unprocessed), ground meat, and processed meat (salted meat, minced meat, sandwich meat, and liver paste).

compliance to the HNFI (18). These relations may partly explain the lack of an inverse association between greater scoring on the HNFI, and colorectal cancer (15). Second, the scales assessing adherence to the different Nordic diets might be biased as a result of *the consistency motif* (35), that is, participants falling into a pattern of similar responses when answering comparable questions, which is a tendency that could apply to FFQs. Those reporting to eat more of the healthy Nordic foods might also erroneously report eating more of certain less healthy foods. If so, it may be debatable whether the dietary scores actually capture what they intend to capture. Third, artificial covariance (35) could have biased the earlier reported associations, due to using the same questionnaire responses for deriving the dietary score and for calculating food and nutrient intakes. In turn, such false associations could result in invalid inferences regarding diet-health relations. Since measurement errors would be less correlated if applying separate methods for these two operations (36), it may be favorable to construct the diet score from an FFQ, while using dietary recalls for estimating intake of foods and nutrients.

The FFQ was unfortunately not tested for validity, and misreporting, especially the underreporting of foods generally considered unhealthy, is a common challenge when data are self-reported (36, 37). However, if randomly distributed, misreporting should still allow the ranking of participants into groups according to intake. Besides, although the underlying concept of interest was NND adherence at the group level, the limited sample size in this study ideally calls for more than two 24-h recall interviews to reduce the influence of day-to-day variations in food consumption. This uncertainty seems to be reflected through the lack of a consistent trend in the results, and especially foods eaten more seldom, like fish, are the most sensitive for day-to-day variations. Moreover, all groups reported considerably lower energy intake than the objectively measured energy expenditure. Possible explanations might be increased activity levels caused by awareness of being observed (38), low energy intake as a result of the misreporting or underreporting of food consumption, or poor repeatability (37), due to the wide variations in food intake from one day to another.

On the other hand, our findings concerning the frequency of habitual food consumption, determined from the FFQ, revealed the same trend as when using separate methods. Hence, although frequencies are not the same as amounts, different observations in the current study compared with the earlier studies on Nordic scales might be related to sample characteristics. A homogenous and selective sample in the present study, in addition to recently collected data, could possibly imply a sample following a healthier diet than parents of toddlers in general, and therefore reduced generalizability. And, since dietary patterns are likely to change over time, the Nordic scales may capture other dietary aspects today, than when exploring data collected 10–20 years ago. In other words, the present results might indicate that the NND score, and similar Nordic scores, capture healthy diets to a larger degree when applied in more contemporary samples.

The results of the current study should be interpreted in the context of several limitations. As mentioned above, the study sample was selective and homogenous, that is, the majority being females, native Norwegians, and highly educated, probably caused by a very low response rate (7%). Together with a small sample size, these characteristics restricted study power, eligible statistical analyses (e.g. sub-group analyses), and generalizability to the population in general. A notably larger amount of the present sample complied with the recommended physical activity level (26), and fewer were overweight or obese, compared with a representative sample of the Norwegian adult population (39), that is, 82% versus 32%, and 20% versus 48%, respectively. Participating parents might have been more health-conscious and more likely to adhere to a favorable lifestyle, including a healthier diet. Unlike the former studies exploring the HNFI (18), the NND (5), and the Baltic Sea Diet Score (6), differences across NND adherence categories were not detected concerning age, educational level, BMI, physical activity level, or energy intake, expressing the homogeneity of the sample. Yet, lack of differences could also be a result of the limited sample size.

Regarding dietary scores as a method for quantifying adherence to dietary patterns, subjectivity is introduced related to the selection and scoring of included components, cut-off points, and so on (40, 41). Importantly, although reflecting a larger part of the overall diet, diet scores do not cover all aspects of diet, meaning that other food items not incorporated into the scale could bias the associations under investigation. Also, as cut-offs for the NND score were determined by the median, dietary behavior required for scoring is sample specific, and caution must be exercised when generalizing the results. In light of the sample characteristics, it is plausible that the diet underlying 'low', 'medium', or 'high' NND adherence entailed higher diet quality in the present sample compared to a more representative sample. Still, this procedure for determining cut-offs is in line with the methods applied in previous studies exploring relations between predefined dietary patterns and various health parameters (4–6, 42).

In addition to the use of separate methods for determining NND adherence and calculating intakes of foods and nutrients, it may be a study strength that the questionnaire was recently developed, and thus provided contemporary data. Previous studies derived dietary scores from data collected between years 1991 and 1999 (18), 2002 and 2008 (5), and in 2007 (6), implying that dietary patterns might have changed. On the other hand, it could be a disadvantage if NND adherers in the current study were familiar with the proposed favorable characteristics of the foods included in the NND, and gave the anticipated most desirable answers to the questions. Moreover, repeated 24-h recall interviewing is considered one appropriate method for collecting representative dietary data at group level, entailing less participant burden than dietary records (36, 43).

Unequal methodological approaches, or a selective and more recent sample, might partly explain discrepancies in the present findings as compared with earlier studies (5, 6, 18), that is, the previously observed associations between adherence to healthy Nordic diets and the intake of less healthy foods not part of the diets under investigation (21, 22). Nevertheless, considering the limitations of the current study, these associations should be further explored in larger and more heterogeneous samples in order to draw conclusions. Also, when applied in epidemiological studies, potential confounding lifestyle and dietary factors not included in the dietary score should be accounted for, since residual confounding could distort explored associations. Increased knowledge concerning potential methodological bias, as discussed in the present study, would be of importance, due to the fact that such bias may result in false inferences regarding diet-disease relations.

Conclusions

The present study assessed the association between adherence to the NND measured with FFQ and diet quality measured with two 24-h dietary recall interviews, and showed that higher NND adherence was associated with a higher intake of selected healthy foods and nutrients. However, a higher intake of meat, sweets, and energy in general, as earlier reported in adherers to predefined healthy Nordic diets, was not observed, whether assessed by FFQ or 24-h dietary recall. Nonetheless, the methodological limitations in the current study imply replications in larger and more representative samples before inferences can be drawn regarding explanations for these partly differing results.

Authors' contributions

EB, MKT, NCØ, THS and HBB designed the present study; ERH, EB, and NCØ constructed the initial NND score; HBB, EB, MKT, NCØ, and LFA developed the HSL-questionnaire; HBB and EB prepared the dataset, SBS directed the physical activity assessments; HBB analyzed the data and wrote the paper; HBB and EB had primary responsibility for final content. All authors read and approved the final manuscript.

Disclosure

This study was conducted according to the guidelines laid down in the Declaration of Helsinki, and research clearance was obtained from The Norwegian Social Science Data Services. Written informed consent was obtained from all subjects.

Acknowledgements

The authors are grateful to participating parents for their indispensable contribution.

Conflict of interest and funding

The authors declare that they have no conflict of interest. This study was funded by the University of Agder.

References

1. Martinez-Gonzalez MA, Bes-Rastrollo M. Dietary patterns, Mediterranean diet, and cardiovascular disease. Curr Opin Lipidol 2014; 25: 20–6.
2. Sofi F, Cesari F, Abbate R, Gensini GF, Casini A. Adherence to Mediterranean diet and health status: meta-analysis. Br Med J 2008; 337a: 1344.
3. Gotsis E, Anagnostis P, Mariolis A, Vlachou A, Katsiki N, Karagiannis A. Health benefits of the Mediterranean diet: an update of research over the last 5 years. Angiology 2015; 66: 304–18.
4. Olsen A, Egeberg R, Halkjær J, Christensen J, Overvad K, Tjønneland A. Healthy aspects of the Nordic diet are related to lower total mortality. J Nutr 2011; 141: 639–44.
5. Hillesund ER, Bere E, Haugen M, Overby NC. Development of a New Nordic Diet score and its association with gestational weight gain and fetal growth – a study performed in the Norwegian Mother and Child Cohort Study (MoBa). Public Health Nutr 2014; 17: 1909–18.
6. Kanerva N, Kaartinen NE, Schwab U, Lahti-Koski M, Männistö S. The Baltic Sea Diet Score: a tool for assessing healthy eating in Nordic countries. Public Health Nutr 2014; 17: 1697–705.
7. Roswall N, Sandin S, Lof M, Skeie G, Olsen A, Adami HO, et al. Adherence to the healthy Nordic food index and total and cause-specific mortality among Swedish women. Eur J Epidemiol 2015; 30(6): 509–17. doi: http://dx.doi.org/10.1007/s10654-015-0021-x
8. Kyrø C, Skeie G, Loft S, Overvad K, Christensen J, Tjønneland A, et al. Adherence to a healthy Nordic food index is associated with a lower incidence of colorectal cancer in women: the Diet, Cancer and Health Cohort Study. Br J Nutr 2013; 109: 920–7.
9. Kanerva N, Kaartinen NE, Schwab U, Lahti-Koski M, Männistö S. Adherence to the Baltic Sea diet consumed in the Nordic countries is associated with lower abdominal obesity. Br J Nutr 2013; 109: 520–8.
10. Kanerva N, Kaartinen NE, Ovaskainen M-L, Konttinen H, Kontto J, Männistö S. A diet following Finnish nutrition recommendations does not contribute to the current epidemic of obesity. Public Health Nutr 2013; 16(5): 786–94.
11. Kanerva N, Loo BM, Eriksson JG, Leiviskä J, Kaartinen NE, Jula A, et al. Associations of the Baltic Sea diet with obesity-related markers of inflammation. Ann Med 2014; 46: 90–6.
12. Hillesund ER, Overby NC, Engel SM, Klungsoyr K, Harmon QE, Haugen M, et al. Associations of adherence to the New Nordic Diet with risk of preeclampsia and preterm delivery in the Norwegian Mother and Child Cohort Study (MoBa). Eur J Epidemiol 2014; 29: 753–65.
13. Lacoppidan SA, Kyrø C, Loft S, Helnæs A, Christensen J, Hansen CP, et al. Adherence to a healthy Nordic food index is associated with a lower risk of type-2 diabetes – the Danish Diet, Cancer and Health Cohort Study. Nutrients 2015; 7: 8633–44.
14. Li Y, Roswall N, Sandin S, Strom P, Adami HO, Weiderpass E. Adherence to a healthy Nordic food index and breast cancer risk: results from a Swedish Cohort Study. Cancer Causes Control 2015; 26(6): 893–902. doi: http://dx.doi.org/10.1007/s10552-015-0564-x
15. Roswall N, Li Y, Kyro C, Sandin S, Lof M, Adami HO, et al. No association between adherence to a healthy Nordic food index and colorectal cancer: results from a Swedish Cohort Study. Cancer Epidemiol Biomarkers Prev 2015; 24(4): 755–7. doi: http://dx.doi.org/10.1158/1055-9965.EPI-14-1314
16. Kanerva N, Rissanen H, Knekt P, Havulinna A, Eriksson J, Männistö S. The healthy Nordic diet and incidence of type 2 diabetes-10-years follow up. Diabetes Res Clin Pract 2014; 106: e34–7.
17. Kanerva N, Kaartinen NE, Rissanen H, Knekt P, Eriksson JG, Sääksjärvi K, et al. Associations of the Baltic Sea diet with cardiometabolic risk factors – a meta-analysis of three Finnish studies. Br J Nutr 2014; 112: 616–26.
18. Roswall N, Eriksson U, Sandin S, Löf M, Olsen A, Skeie G, et al. Adherence to the healthy Nordic food index, dietary composition, and lifestyle among Swedish women. Food Nutr Res 2015; 59: 26336, doi: http://dx.doi.org/10.3402/fnr.v59.26336
19. ISRCTN Registry. Available from: http://www.isrctn.com/search?q=%C3%98verby [cited 24 April 2015].
20. Bere E, Brug J. Towards health-promoting and environmentally friendly regional diets-a Nordic example. Public Health Nutr 2009; 12: 91–6.
21. Mithril C, Dragsted LO, Meyer C, Blauert E, Holt MK, Astrup A. Guidelines for the New Nordic Diet. Public Health Nutr 2012; 1: 1–7.
22. Mithril C, Dragsted LO, Meyer C, Tetens I, Biltoft-Jensen A, Astrup A. Dietary composition and nutrient content of the New Nordic Diet. Public Health Nutr 2013; 16: 777–85.
23. Bjørnarå HB, Hillesund ER, Torstveit MK, Stea TH, Øverby NC, Bere E. An assessment of the test-retest reliability of the New Nordic Diet score. Food Nutr Res 2015; 59: 28397, doi: http://dx.doi.org/10.3402/fnr.v59.28397
24. Melnæs BK, Lundberg-Hallén N, Helland-Kigen KM, Lund-Blix NA, Myhre JB, Johansen AMW, et al. 'Norkost 3', a national dietary survey conducted among Norwegian men and women aged 18–70 years, 2010–11. Oslo: The Norwegian Directorate of Health Affairs; 2012.
25. The Norwegian food composition table. 2006. Available from: http://www.matportalen.no/verktoy/the_norwegian_food_composition_table/old_tables [cited 17 April 2015].
26. Helsedirektoratet (2014). Anbefalinger om kosthold, ernæring og fysisk aktivitet. Oslo: Helsedirektoratet. Contract No: IS-2170.
27. The Norwegian Health Directorate: Nutrition Recommendations to Promote Public Health and Prevent Chronic Diseases (2011). Methodology and scientific knowledge base. Oslo: Norwegian Ministries. Contract No: IS-1881.
28. St-Onge M, Mignault D, Allison DB, Rabasa-Lhoret R. Evaluation of a portable device to measure daily energy expenditure in free-living adults. Am J Clin Nutr 2007; 85: 742–9.
29. Ward DS, Evenson KR, Vaughn A, Rodgers AB, Troiano RP. Accelerometer use in physical activity: best practices and research recommendations. Med Sci Sports Exerc 2005; 37(11 Suppl): 582–8.
30. Scheers T, Philippaerts R, Lefevre J. Variability in physical activity patterns as measured by the SenseWear Armband: how many days are needed? Eur J Appl Physiol 2012; 112: 1653–62.
31. World Health Organization. Global recommendations on physical activity for health. 2010. Available from: http://apps.who.int/iris/handle/10665/44399 [cited 13 November 2015].
32. Garber CE, Blissmer B, Deschenes MR, Franklin BA, Lamonte MJ, Lee IM, et al. American College of Sports Medicine Position Stand. Quantity and quality of exercise for developing and maintaining cardiorespiratory, musculoskeletal, and neuromotor fitness in apparently healthy adults: guidance for prescribing exercise. Med Sci Sports Exerc 2011; 43: 1334–59.

33. World Health Organization. Obesity and overweight. Fact sheet No. 311 [Updated January 2015]. 2011. Available from: http://www.who.int/mediacentre/factsheets/fs311/en/ [cited 18 November 2015].
34. World Cancer Research Fund | American Institute for Cancer Research (2007). Food, nutrition, physical activity, and the prevention of cancer: a global perspective. Washington, DC: American Institute for Cancer Research; 2007.
35. Podsakoff PM, MacKenzie SB, Lee J-Y, Podsakoff NP. Common method biases in behavioral research: a critical review of the literature and recommended remedies. J Appl Psychol 2003; 88: 879–903.
36. Willett W. Nutritional epidemiology. 3rd ed. New York: Oxford University Press; 2013.
37. Livingstone MBE, Black AE. Markers of the validity of reported energy intake. J Nutr 2003; 133: 895S–920S.
38. McCambridge J, Witton J, Elbourne DR. Systematic review of the Hawthorne effect: new concepts are needed to study research participation effects. J Clin Epidemiol 2014; 67: 267–77.
39. Helsedirektoratet (2015). Fysisk aktivitet og sedat tid blant voksne og eldre i Norge. Nasjonal kartlegging 2014–2015. Oslo: Helsedirektoratet.
40. Moeller SM, Reedy J, Millen AE, Dixon LB, Newby P, Tucker KL, et al. Dietary patterns: challenges and opportunities in dietary patterns research: an experimental biology workshop, April 1, 2006. J Am Diet Assoc 2007; 107: 1233–9.
41. Waijers PM, Feskens EJ, Ocké MC. A critical review of predefined diet quality scores. Br J Nutr 2007; 97: 219–31.
42. Bach A, Serra-Majem L, Carrasco JL, Roman B, Ngo J, Bertomeu I, et al. The use of indexes evaluating the adherence to the Mediterranean diet in epidemiological studies: a review. Public Health Nutr 2006; 9: 132–46.
43. Brussaard J, Löwik M, Steingrimsdottir L, Møller A, Kearney J, De Henauw S, et al. A European food consumption survey method – conclusions and recommendations. Eur J Clin Nutr 2002; 56(Suppl 2): S89–94.

***Helga Birgit Bjørnarå**
Department of Public Health
Sport and Nutrition, Faculty of Health and Sport Sciences
University of Agder
Post Box 422, NO-4604 Kristiansand
Norway
Email: helga.birgit.bjornara@uia.no

Appendix 1. The components underlying the construction of the 10 subscales within the NND score ($n = 75$)

Subscale	Related question(s)	Response alternatives and coding	Calculations (min-max)	Median = cut-off	Dietary behavior associated with scoring
Meal pattern	How often do you eat -Breakfast -Lunch -Dinner -Evening meal/supper	Never = 0 Less than once a week = 0.5 Once a week = 1 Twice a week = 2 Three times a week = 3 Four times a week = 4 Five times a week = 5 Six times a week = 6 Every day = 7	Sum of answers to the four questions (0–28)	Women: 25.0 Men: 25.0	Women: < 25.0 = 0 ≥ 25.0 = 1 Men: ≤ 25.0 = 0 > 25.0 = 1
Nordic fruits	How often do you eat typical Nordic fruits (apple, pear, plum)	Never = 0 Less than once a week = 0.5 Once a week = 1 Twice a week = 2 Three times a week = 3 Four times a week = 4 Five times a week = 5 Six times a week = 6 Every day = 7 Several times a day = 10	No calculation (0–10)	Women: 4.0 Men: 3.5	Women: ≤ 4.0 = 0 > 4.0 = 1 Men: ≤ 3.5 = 0 > 3.5 = 1
Root vegetables	How often do you eat root vegetables (e.g. carrot, rutabaga, onion)?	Never = 0 up to Several times a day = 10	No calculation (0–10)	Women: 5.0 Men: 4.5	Women: ≤ 5.0 = 0 > 5.0 = 1 Men: ≤ 4.5 = 0 > 4.5 = 1
Cabbages	How often do you eat cabbages (e.g. cauliflower, broccoli, Brussels sprouts, kale)?	Never = 0 up to Several times a day = 10	No calculation (0–10)	Women: 3.0 Men: 3.0	Women: ≤ 3.0 = 0 > 3.0 = 1 Men: < 3.0 = 0 ≥ 3.0 = 1
Potatoes vs. rice/pasta	How often do you eat -Potatoes -Rice -Pasta	Never = 0 up to Several times a day = 10	Frequency of eating potatoes relative to eating rice and pasta combined: potatoes/(0.1 + rice + pasta) (0–100)	Women: 0.49 Men: 0.39	Women: ≤ 0.49 = 0 > 0.49 = 1 Men: < 0.39 = 0 ≥ 0.39 = 1
Whole grain breads vs. white breads	How often do you eat -Refined breads/bread rolls -Whole grain breads -Whole grain hard breads	Never = 0 up to Several times a day = 10	Frequency of eating whole grain breads and whole grain hard breads combined relative to eating refined breads: (whole grain breads + whole grain hard breads)/(0.1 + refined breads) (0–200)	Women: 15.0 Men: 9.6	Women: ≤ 15.0 = 0 > 15.0 = 1 Men: ≤ 9.6 = 0 > 9.6 = 1

Appendix 1 (Continued)

Subscale	Related question(s)	Response alternatives and coding	Calculations (min-max)	Median = cut-off	Dietary behavior associated with scoring
Oatmeal	How often do you eat oatmeal?	Never = 0 up to Several times a day = 10	No calculation (0–10)	Women: 1.0 Men: 0.75	Women: < 1.0 = 0 ≥ 1.0 = 1 Men: ≤0.75 = 0 > 0.75 = 1
Foods from the wild countryside	How often do you eat -Game (e.g. moose, reindeer, deer) -Lean fish (e.g. cod, Pollock, haddock) -Fatty fish (e.g. mackerel, herring, halibut) -Other seafood (e.g. shrimps, crabs, mussels -Berries	Never = 0 up to Several times a day = 10	Sum of answers to the five questions (0–50)	Women: 4.5 Men: 4.5	Women: < 4.5 = 0 ≥4.5 = 1 Men: ≤4.5 = 0 >4.5 = 1
Milk vs. juice	How often do you drink -Milk -Fruit juice without added sugar	Never = 0 up to Several times a day = 10	Frequency of drinking milk relative to drinking fruit juice: milk/(0.1 + juice) (0–100)	Women: 1.29 Men: 2.5	Women: ≤ 1.29 = 0 > 1.29 = 1 Men: ≤2.5 = 0 >2.5 = 1
Water vs. sugar/ artificially sweetened beverages	How often do you drink -Water -Sugar-sweetened beverages -Artificially sweetened beverages	Never = 0 up to Several times a day = 10	Frequency of drinking water relative to drinking sugar-sweetened beverages and artificially sweetened beverages combined: water/(0.1 + sugar-sweetened beverages + artificially sweetened beverages) (0–100)	Women: 6.25 Men: 2.8	Women: ≤6.25 = 0 >6.25 = 1 Men: ≤2.8 = 0 >2.8 = 1

NND, New Nordic Diet.

19

Protective effects of *Trifolium alexandrinum* L. against lung injury induced by environmental toxin CCl_4 in experimental rats

Rahmat Ali Khan[1]*, Huda Mohammad Alkreathy[2], Abdus Saboorshah[1], Mushtaq Ahmed[1] and Samiullah Khan[3]

[1]Department of Biotechnology, Faculty of Biological Sciences, University of Science and Technology Bannu, Khyber Pakhtunkhwa, Pakistan; [2]Department of Pharmacology, King Abdulaziz University(KAU), Jeddah, Saudi Arabia; [3]Department of Microbiology, Faculty of Biological Sciences, Quaid-i-Azam University, Islamabad, Pakistan

Abstract

Background: In Pakistan numerous medicinal floras has used in the treatment of various human ailments. Among them *Trifolium alexandrinum* L. is traditionally used in the curing of disease. Presently we designed to ascertain the protective role of *Trifolium alexandrinum* methanolic extracts (TAME) against carbon tetrachloride (CCl_4)-induced lung injury and oxidative stress in rats.
Methods: Exposure to CCl_4 induces oxidative stress and causes tissue damage by the induction of CCl_4 free radicals. Twenty-four male albino rats were divided equally into four groups. Rats in group I had free access to drinking water and laboratory food. Group II was treated with 1 ml/kg body weight (b.w.) CCl_4 (30% in olive oil). Groups III and IV rats were fed (p.o.) 200 mg/kg b.w. TAME and 50 mg/kg b.w. silymarin after 24 h of CCl_4 treatment for 2 weeks.
Results: Administration of CCl_4 caused a significant ($p < 0.01$) decrease in the activities of antioxidant enzymes (catalase, peroxidase, glutathione peroxidase, glutathione-*S*-transferase), and glutathione contents were decreased; however, thiobarbituric acid-reactive substances were increased ($p < 0.01$). The alterations caused by CCl_4 were significantly ($p < 0.01$) reversed toward control levels by supplementation of TAME and silymarin.
Conclusion: These results suggest that in rats TAME and silymarin could protect the lungs against CCl_4-induced oxidative damage.

Keywords: *lungs*; *CCl_4*; *lipid peroxidation*; Trifolium alexandrinum

The epithelium cells of the lungs are frequently exposed to the highest concentration of oxygen and gaseous exchanges that make them susceptible to pulmonary toxicity (1). Pulmonary toxicity is caused by the generation of ROS (highly reactive oxygen species) that alter the structure of protein, nucleic acid, and other macro molecules (2). During aerobic metabolism, in normal situations, the toxic metabolites of oxygen are formed in low quantity in lung cells (3, 4). This normal production of ROS performs an essential role in a number of physiological activities but, in excess, the generation of ROS embraces several ailments (5). Pulmonary diseases like asthma, hyperoxia, and sarcoidosis are believed to be linked with oxidative stress. Chronic pulmonary disease (CPD) is the foremost cause of death, both in the industrialized and developing countries. It is associated with a progressive decrease in lung function that ultimately results in emphysema and chronic bronchitis (6). Different environmental factors like sunlight, UV light exposure, smoking, and chemicals are the main causes of the generation of ROS (7). Carbon tetrachloride (CCl_4) is a synthetic industrial chemical that induces hepatic and renal toxicity in workers as well as in experimental animals (8) via ingestion, skin absorption or intraperitoneal intoxication, or by the inhalation of CCL_4 lipid peroxidation, which increases while the antioxidant defense enzymes and total tissue proteins decreases (9). CCl_4 is metabolized into trichloromethyl radical ($^{\bullet}CCl_3$) that combines with oxygen and forms a more reactive peroxy trichloromethyl radical ($^{\bullet}OOCCl_3$). These free radicals produce alkoxy ($R^{\bullet}$) and peroxy radicals ($ROO^{\bullet}$) that form lipid peroxides, and cause enzymatic inactivity and tissue injury (10). CCl_4 also decreases tissue proteins and the antioxidant enzymes like SOD, peroxidase (POD), and catalase (CAT) (11, 12). Oxidative stress initiates and continues a range of lung, liver, and kidney damages. Therefore, it is of the utmost importance to evaluate agents with powerful antioxidant potential against the attack of CCl_4 (13). The majority of foodstuff and natural products have been reported to be excellent means of chemo-protection. *Curcuma longa* has been reported to have therapeutic activity due to its antioxidant potential (14, 15). Similarly, the methanolic extract of *Ephorbia prostrata* is a potential phototoxic and antioxidant that markedly inhibits free radicals due to the presence of flavonoids and polyphenolic compounds (16). The phytochemical assessment of *Trifolium alexandrinum* has revealed the presence of steroids, terpenoinds, flavonoids, and isoflavonoids (17). Hence it was selected for the present study for the evaluation of the capability of *T. alexandrinum* to reduce the toxicity induced by CCl_4 in the lungs of albino rats.

Materials and methods

Chemicals

Methanol, glutathione reduced (GSH), glutathione oxidized (GSSG), glutathione peroxidase (GSH-Px), glutathione-*S*-transferase (GST), bovine serum albumin (BSA), 5,5-dithio-bis-(2-nitrobenzoic acid) (DTNB), 1-chloro-2,4-dinitrobenzene (CDNB), reduced nicotinamide adenine dinucleotide phosphate (NADPH), CCl_4, thiobarbituric acid (TBA), trichloroacetic acid (TCA), Folin–Ciocalteu reagent, sodium hydroxide, disodium hydrogen phosphate, sodium dihydrogen phosphate, and DMSO of Sigma Aldrich Chemicals Co. were utilized in this experiment.

Plant preparation and extraction

During the maturity period, *T. alexandrinum* (L.) plants (leaves, stem, and flowers) grown in the north region of Bannu District, Pakistan, were collected. Then it was taxonomically identified by Prof. Abdur Rahman, serving in the Department of Botany, the Post Graduate College of Bannu. The plant extract was chopped and dried under shade for a period of one month. Then, after drying, the chopped plant was grinded into 1-mm fine powder with the help of a mechanical grinder. The powdered material (700 g) was soaked in 2.5 liter (80%) methanol for a period of 1 week at room temperature and then filtered. The filtrate was collected and concentrated with the help of a rotary evaporator at 38°C, under reduced pressure, and the crude extract was stored at 4°C for further assessment.

Animals and treatment

The study protocol was approved by the ethical committee of University of Science and Technology of Bannu, for laboratory and experimental animal feed and care. The present experiment was designed with 24 adult albino rats. The rats, weighing 200–210 g, were divided equally into four groups; kept under normal laboratory conditions on 12 h light/darkness, at room temperature; and fed standard feed and water. Group I was the control and remained untreated, while group II was treated with 1 ml/kg body weight (b.w.; 30% in olive oil i.p.) CCl_4. Group III received 50 mg/kg b.w. silymarin, and group IV was treated with 200 mg/kg b.w. *T. alexandrinum* methanolic extracts (TAME) after 24 h of CCl_4 treatment. At the end of the experiment, after 24 h of the last dose, the rats were weighed and sacrificed. Lungs were removed, washed with saline, then dried with filter paper, and weighed. Lung tissues were stored at −70°C for further enzymatic analysis.

Assessment of protein, CAT, and POD

Homogenized lung tissue (200 mg) was placed in four volumes of 0.1 mM NaH_2PO_4 buffer (pH 7.4) and centrifuged at 6,000 × g for 30 min. The supernatant was collected and used for the analysis of antioxidant enzymes and protein. Protein was determined in the lung homogenate by the method of Lowry et al. (18), using BSA as standard. The activities of CAT and POD were carried out by the protocol of Chance and Maehly (19). In brief, the CAT activity was examined using hydrogen peroxide (H_2O_2). Change in absorbance was noted at 240 nm. The activity of POD was determined at 470 nm by the use of guaiacol as a substrate. One unit of enzymes (CAT and POD) was defined as an absorbance change of 0.01 as units/min.

GST assay

GST activity was determined by the method of Habig et al. (20), using CDNB as a substrate. GST was measured at 340 nm using a molar extinction coefficient of $9.6 \times 10^3\ M^{-1}\ cm^{-1}$.

GSH-Px assay

An assay of GSH-Px was determined by the method of Mohandas et al. (21). NADPH was used as a substrate and the absorbance measured at 340 nm. The molar coefficient was $6.22 \times 10^3\ M^{-1}\ cm^{-1}$.

Glutathione reductase activity

Activity of glutathione reductase in the lungs homogenate of rats was determined by the protocol of Carlberg

Table 1. Effect of TAME on the protein and lung marker enzymes of rats

Treatment	Protein (μg/mg tissue)	CAT (U/min)	POD (U/min)
Control	$280.7 \pm 9.6^{++}$	$1.7 \pm 0.4^{++}$	$3.1 \pm 0.5^{++}$
CCl_4	$187.4 \pm 13.2^{**}$	$0.9 \pm 0.2^{**}$	$1.7 \pm 0.3^{**}$
CCl_4 + silymarin	$277.8 \pm 10.6^{++}$	$1.5 \pm 0.3^{++}$	$3.0 \pm 0.6^{++}$
CCl_4 + TAME	$230.5 \pm 12.3^{++}$	$1.1 \pm 0.1^{++}$	$2.7 \pm 0.5^{++}$

Mean ± SEM ($n = 6$).

**Indicate significance from the control group at $p < 0.01$ probability level.

++Indicate significance from the CCl_4 group at $p < 0.01$ probability level.

Table 2. Effect of TAME on GSH-Px and GST in rat lungs

Treatment	GST (nmol/min/mg protein)	GSH (mol/g tissue)	GSH-Px (mol/g tissue)
Control	$34.9 \pm 3.2^{++}$		$110.8 \pm 5.3^{++}$
CCl_4	$23.3 \pm 2.5^{**}$	$13.93 \pm 1.4^{++}$	$99.7 \pm 4.8^{**}$
CCl_4+silymarin	$34.5 \pm 2.7^{++}$	$8.14 \pm 0.9^{**}$	$112.2 \pm 6.3^{++}$
CCl_4+TAME	$28.7 \pm 3.1^{++}$	$13.78 \pm 1.3^{++}$	$108.1 \pm 5.7^{++}$

Mean ± SEM ($n = 6$).
**Indicate significance from the control group at $p < 0.01$ probability level.
++Indicate significance from the CCl_4 group at $p < 0.01$ probability level.

and Mannervik (22), with some modifications. The change in absorbance was measured at 340 nm. NADPH was used as a substrate. An extinction coefficient of $6.22 \times 10^3\ M^{-1}\ cm^{-1}$ was used for calculations.

Estimation of TBARS

Thiobarbituric acid–reactive substances (TBARS) in lungs homogenate were estimated by the TBA method described by Wright et al. (23). Change in absorbance was noted at 535 nm. An extinction coefficient of $1.56 \times 10^5\ M^{-1}\ cm^{-1}$ was used for TBARS calculation.

Results

Results of this study have shown that CCl_4 toxicity significantly ($p < 0.01$) reduced the antioxidant enzyme level of the lung compared to the control group (Table 1). The co-treatment of 50 mg/kg b.w. silymarin and TAME at doses of 200 mg/kg b.w. significantly ($p < 0.01$) restored the activities of CAT and POD in the lungs of rats. TAME at the dose of 200 mg/kg b.w. restored completely the CAT and POD activities closely toward control level.

The activities of GST and GSH-Px in the lungs of rats were significantly ($p < 0.01$) decreased by intoxication of CCl_4 that were partially reversed by the supplementation of 200 mg/kg b.w. TAME. The results shown by silymarin group also effectively ($p < 0.01$) reduced the impact of CCl_4 on these considerations as shown in Table 2.

The contents of GSH in the lungs were significantly ($p < 0.01$) decreased while the TBARS contents increased in the CCl_4 intoxicated group as shown in Table 2 and Fig. 1, respectively. The altered level of GSH and TBARS by CCl_4 was reduced by the oral addition of methanolic extract of *T. alexandrinum* (L.). Silymarin also reduced the CCl_4-induced perturbations in the above markers.

The protective role of *T. alexandrinum* (L.) against CCl_4 intoxication in rat on lungs weight and relative lungs weight and body weight are shown in Table 3. CCl_4 significantly increased ($p < 0.01$) lung weight, relative lung weight, and body weight as compared to control group treatment of 200 mg/kg b.w. *T. alexandrinum* (L.) concentrations ameliorated the CCl_4 toxicity and reduced ($p < 0.01$) the lung weight, relative lung weight, significantly like that of standard silymarin.

Discussion

In this experiment, the recovery potential of the TAME was taken under consideration against CCl_4 toxicity in the lungs of rats. The main observations in these experiments were the capability of TAME to recover the inflammatory-oxidant activity of CCl_4. It is reported that CCl_4 induced toxicity due to its conversion to CCl_3, which is a highly reactive free radical. These CCl_3 free radicals damage DNA and lipids, and contribute to the loss in protein and enzyme activity (24). Results shown in Table 3 have revealed that CCl_4 intoxication in the rats significantly lowers the percent increase in body weight. The absolute weights of the rat lungs and the relative lung weights increased as compared to those of the control rats in the CCl_4 group. Minimal increase in the body weights may be due to the degeneration of body tissue while the increase in the lung weights may be the effect of the inflammatory response of the rat's lungs, as was evidenced in another study (25). Supplementations of TAME and silymarin possibly change the response and restore the changes in body and lung weights to those closer to the weights of the control group. CCl_4 intoxication significantly reduces the activities of CAT, and POD in lungs, which might be due to a depletion of GSH contents (26). The low level of GST and GSH-Px correlates to oxidative stress and the depletion of GSH in the lungs resulting from the treatment of CCl_4 administered to the rats. Normally, GSH is converted into GSSG, which is then reduced by glutathione reductase

Table 3. Effect of TAME on the body and lung weight of rats

Treatment	Initial body wt (g)	Final body wt (g)	% increase body wt	Absolute lungs wt	Relative lungs wt
Control	$190.3 \pm 5.7^{++}$	$198.2 \pm 5.2^{++}$	$4.2 \pm 0.7^{++}$	$1.5 \pm 0.5^{++}$	$0.75 \pm 0.05^{++}$
CCl_4	$185.2 \pm 6.2^{**}$	$192.3 \pm 9.0^{**}$	$3.8 \pm 0.5^{**}$	$1.9 \pm 0.2^{**}$	$0.98 \pm 0.07^{**}$
CCl_4+silymarin	$185.7 \pm 6.1^{++}$	$195.8 \pm 7.8^{++}$	$5.4 \pm 0.9^{++}$	$1.5 \pm 0.4^{++}$	$0.76 \pm 0.04^{++}$
CCl_4+TAME	$185.4 \pm 7.3^{++}$	$194.6 \pm 5.7^{++}$	$4.8 \pm 0.5^{++}$	$1.5 \pm 0.3^{++}$	$0.77 \pm 0.09^{++}$

Mean ± SEM ($n = 6$).
** Indicate significance from the control group at $p < 0.01$ probability level.
++Indicate significance from the CCl_4 group at $p < 0.01$ probability level.

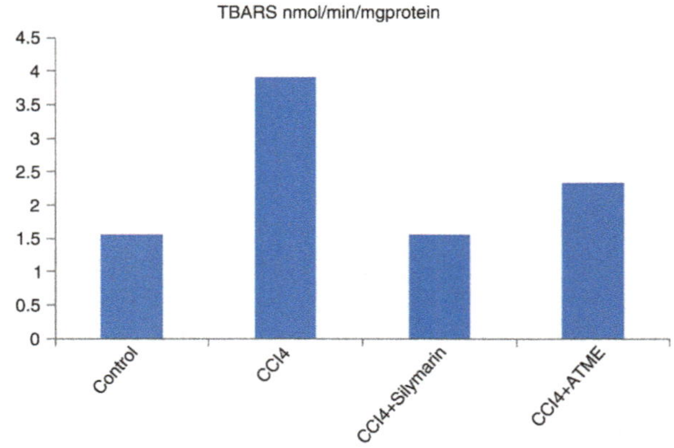

Fig. 1. Effects of TAME on TBARS in rat lungs.

to GSH. TBARS is a highly reactive aldehyde formed as a result of the peroxidation of polyunsaturated fatty acids. TBARS formation is considered a sign of tissue damages (27). The high level of TBARS accumulation in the lungs, as a result of CCl_4 treatment, indicates the extensive oxidative damage to lung tissues. The TAME extract contains polyphenols and flavonoids which have antioxidant and anti-inflammatory roles and reduce the risk of oxidative ailments. The reduction in the level of lipid peroxidation and the improved activity of antioxidant enzymes proved that TAME and silymarin are capable of protecting against various pathological conditions, including oxidative stress (28).

Conclusion

In rats, TAME significantly protects the lungs against oxidative damages, which might be due to the presence of bioactive constituents in the extract.

Conflicts of interest and funding

The authors have not received any funding or benefits from industry or elsewhere to conduct this study.

References

1. Jackson RM. Molecular, pharmacologic, and clinical aspects of oxygen-induced lung injury. Clin Chest Med 1990; 11: 73–86.
2. Fisher AB, Forman HJ, Glass M. Mechanisms of pulmonary oxygen toxicity. Lung 1984; 162: 255–9.
3. Clark JM, Lambertsen CJ. Pulmonary oxygen toxicity: a review. Pharmacol Rev 1971; 23: 37–133.
4. Crystal RG. Oxidants and respiratory tract epithelial injury: pathogenesis and strategies for therapeutic intervention. Am J Med 1991; 91: 39S–44S.
5. Conner EM, Grisham MB. Inflammation, free radicals, and antioxidants. Nutrition 1996; 12: 274–7.
6. Mannino DM, Homa DM, Akinbami LJ, Ford ES, Redd SC. Chronic obstructive pulmonary disease surveillance – United States, 1971–2000. MMWR Surveill Summ 2002; 51: 1–16.
7. Cerutti PA. Oxidant stress and carcinogenesis. Eur J Clin Invest 1991; 21: 1–5.
8. Abraham P, Wilfred G, Cathrine SP. Oxidative damage to lipids and proteins of the lungs, testis and kidney of rats during CCl_4 intoxication. Clin Acta 1999; 289: 177–9.
9. Daniels WM, Reiter RJ, Melchiorri D, Sewerynek E, Pablos MI, Ortiz GG. Melatonin counter acts lipid peroxidation induced by carbon tetrachloride but does not restore glucose-6-phosphatase activity. J Pineal Res 1995; 19: 1–6.
10. Weber LW, Boll M, Stampfl A. Hepatotoxicity and mechanism of action of haloalkanes: carbon tetrachloride as a toxicological model. Crit Rev Toxicol 2003; 33: 105–36.
11. Dogukan A, Akpolat N, Celiker H, Ilhan N, Bahcecioglu IH, Gunal AI. Protective effect of interferon-alpha on carbon tetrachloride-induced nephrotoxicity. J Nephrol 2003; 16: 81–4.
12. Adewole SO, Salako AA, Doherty OW, Naicker T. Effect of melatonin on carbon tetrachloride-induced kidney injury in Wistar rats. Afr J Biomed Res 2007; 10: 153–64.
13. Pradeep K, Mohan CV, Gobianand K, Karthikeyan S. Silymarin modulates the oxidant-antioxidant imbalance during diethylnitrosamine induced oxidative stress in rats. Eur J Pharmacol 2007; 560(2–3): 110–16.
14. Danciu C, Vlaia L, Fetea F, Hancianu M, Coricovac DE, Ciurlea SA, et al. Evaluation of phenolic profile, antioxidant and anticancer potential of two main representants of Zingiberaceae family against B164A5 murine melanoma cells. Biol Res. 2015; 48(1): 1.
15. Antunes LMG, Darin JDC, Bianchi MLP. Effects of the antioxidants curcumin or selenium on cisplatin-induced nephrotoxicity and lipid peroxidation in rats. Pharm Res 2001; 43(2): 145–50.
16. Khar A, Ali AM, Pardhasaradhi BV. Induction of stress response renders human tumor cell lines resistant to curcumin-mediated apoptosis: role of reactive oxygen intermediates. Cell Stress Chap 2001; 6(4): 368–76.
17. Khan AV, Ahmed QU, Shukla I, Khan AA. Antibacterial activity of leaves extracts of *Trifolium alexandrinum* Linn. against pathogenic bacteria causing tropical diseases. Asian Pac J Trop Biomed 2012; 3: 189–94.
18. Lowry OH, Rosenberg NJ, Farr AL, Randall RJ. Protein measurement with Folin Phenol reagent. J Biol Chem 1951; 193: 265–75.
19. Chance B, Maehly AC. Assay of catalase and peroxidases. Methods Enzymol 1955; 11: 764–75.
20. Habig WH, Pabst MJ, Jakoby WB. Glutathione-*S*-transferases: the first enzymatic step in mercapturic acid formation. J Biol Chem 1974; 249: 7130–9.
21. Mohandas J, Marshal JJ, Duggin GG, Horvath JS, Tiller DJ. Differential distribution of glutathione and glutathione-related enzymes in rabbit kidney. Possible implications in analgesic nephropathy. Biochem Pharmacol 1984; 33: 1801–7.
22. Carlberg I, Mannervik EB. Glutathione level in rat brain. J Biol Chem 1975; 250: 4475–80.
23. Wright JR, Colby HD, Miles PR. Cytosolic factors that affect microsomal lipid peroxidation in lung and liver. Arch Biochem Biophys 1981; 206: 296–304.
24. Venkatesan N, Punithavathi V, Chandrakasan G. Curcumin protects bleomycin-induced lung injury in rats. Life Sci 1997; 61(6): 51–8.
25. Khan RA, Khan MR, Sahreen S. Protective effect of *Sonchus asper* extracts against experimentally-induced lung injuries in rats: a novel study. Exp Toxicol Pathol 2012; 64: 725–31. doi: http://dx.doi.org/10.1016/j.etp.2011.01.007
26. Singh N, Kamath V, Narasimhamurthy K, Rajini PS. Protective effects of potato peel extract against carbon tetrachloride-

induced liver injury in rats. Environ Toxicol Pharmacol 2008; 26: 242–6.
27. Ohkawa H, Ohishi N, Yogi K. Assay for lipid peroxidation in animal tissues by thiobarbituric acid reaction. Anal Biochem 1979; 95: 351–8.
28. Vardavas CI, Majchrzak D, Wagner K-H, Elmadfa I, Kafatos A. The antioxidant and phylloquinone content of wildly grown greens in Crete. Food Chem 2006; 99: 813–21.

*Rahmat Ali Khan
Department of Biotechnology
Faculty of Biological Sciences
University of Science and Technology Bannu
Khyber Pakhtunkhwa, Pakistan
Email: Rahmatgul_81@yahoo.com

Quality of life in parents of preterm infants in a randomized nutritional intervention trial

Trond Nordheim[1,2]*, Tone Rustøen[3,4], Per O. Iversen[5,6] and Britt Nakstad[1,2]

[1]Department of Pediatric and Adolescent Medicine, Akershus University Hospital, Nordbyhagen, Norway; [2]Institute for Clinical Medicine, Campus Ahus, University of Oslo, Nordbyhagen, Norway; [3]Department of Research and Development, Division of Emergencies and Critical Care, Oslo University Hospital, Oslo, Norway; [4]Department of Nursing Science, Institute of Health and Society, University of Oslo, Oslo, Norway; [5]Department of Nutrition, Institute of Basic Medical Sciences, Faculty of Medicine, University of Oslo, Oslo, Norway; [6]Department of Haematology, Oslo University Hospital, Oslo, Norway

Abstract

Background: Being a parent of a very-low birth weight (VLBW, birth weight <1,500 g) infant is challenging because of the numerous complications these infants may encounter, many of which are caused by inadequate nutrition. Whether the burden to the parents increases when their VLBW infant participates in a randomized intervention trial (RCT) and is thus exposed to additional risk is unknown.
Objective: To examine parental qualify of life (QoL) and well-being after participation of their VLBW infants in a nutrition RCT.
Design: QoL and symptoms associated with well-being of parents of VLBW infants participating in a nutrition RCT ($n = 31$) and of a reference group (parents of nonparticipating VBLW infants, $n = 31$) were examined. Assessments were performed when their infants were in the neonatal intensive care unit (NICU) (time point T1) and concurrently at 3.5 years of age (time point T2). The parents completed the following questionnaires: Quality of Life Scale, Hospital Anxiety and Depression Scale, Lee Fatigue Scale (LFS), and General Sleeping Disturbance Scale (GSDS).
Results: At T1, the QoL was better among RCT parents ($p = 0.02$). At T2, the RCT parents reported less sleep disturbance symptoms (GSDS) ($p = 0.03$) and more energy (LFS) ($p = 0.03$).
Conclusion: The RCT participation of VLBW infants may have improved parental QoL. While in the neonatal unit, symptoms of anxiety and depression were common among all parents. The high incidence of anxiety and depression in parents must be considered in the care of parents in the NICU. Long-term effects of participation seem to be less sleep problems and more energy.

Keywords: *anxiety*; *depression*; *parents*; *premature*; *quality of life*; *very low birth weight*

For most parents, the sudden arrival of a premature infant is unexpected, overwhelming, and frightening. Being a parent of a critically sick newborn has been described as being in another world, alien from what they knew and had experienced earlier (1). Various studies have described the preterm children's health-related quality of life (QoL) (2–5), but less is known about parental QoL over time (6).

Researchers perform randomized studies to improve treatment and outcome of premature infants. The effect that participation may have on parents is unknown. Parents are invited to enroll their sick child in a study that has no guarantee of benefit to the infant. In an interview study, parents reported that they were grateful for the opportunity to participate, pleased that they could help other infants in the future, and believed that the participation could give access to better medical care and technology for their own infant (7). To our knowledge, no study has evaluated symptoms and QoL among parents of very-low birth weight infants (VLBW, birth weight <1,500 g) enrolled in a clinical randomized intervention trial (RCT). If the parents experience low QoL, symptoms of anxiety, depression, worse physical condition, and/or sleep disturbance, this could affect their children negatively. A Finnish study found an association between poor parental well-being and subsequent behavioral and emotional problems in their VLBW children (8), and a meta-analysis on parental depression stated that both parental and maternal depression affected child development (9).

Fifteen million preterm births worldwide yearly is a global health challenge (10). To address the putative importance of an adequate nutritional intake among VLBW infants, we have performed an intervention RCT – the PreNu study – to enhance their nutrient supply of protein and energy (11, 12). The PreNu study was originally powered to halve the proportion of infants discharged as growth restricted. A preplanned safety analysis revealed increased occurrence of late-onset septicemia in the intervention group (11). Further inclusion of infants was therefore stopped, a decision supported by the Regional Committee for Medical and Health Research Ethics.

In the present study, we explored the parent's QoL and selected symptoms – anxiety, depression, sleep disturbance, and fatigue – during their infant's hospital stay and at age 3.5 years. We compared parents in the PreNu study with parents whose VLBW infants never participated in a clinical research trial.

Subjects and methods

Parent cohort

Parents of VLBW infants were enrolled in the PreNu study at Akershus and Oslo University hospitals in Norway. Fifty of 57 eligible infants were recruited from August to December 2010 (12). Inclusion criteria were birth weight <1,500 g and born in the study hospitals. Exclusion criteria were congenital malformations, chromosomal abnormalities, critical illness with short life expectancy, and clinical syndromes known to affect growth and development.

In total, 26 eligible PreNu couples represented by 30 single parents at time point 1 (T1) and 31 single parents at time point 2 (T2) were enrolled in our study. For the purposes of the current study, the PreNu intervention and the PreNu control groups are analyzed together as one group denoted as the PreNu group. All infants received the same attention and follow-up by the researchers. Parents of children in foster care and parents who did not master the Norwegian language were not invited. Some were twins (four pairs) and triplets (one set).

A reference cohort of 25 eligible couples represented by 31 single parents whose VLBW infants never participated in a clinical study was randomly recruited with identical inclusion criteria. They were recruited at the study hospitals during the 3 months before and 3 months after the PreNu inclusion period by a neonatologist not involved in the PreNu study.

Time points of data collection

Data for the hospitalized period was collected retrospectively 3 years after birth (T1). The follow-up study of parental well-being was conceived in 2014, that is, 3.5 years after the inclusion period of the PreNu study (T2). We analyzed measures of self-report in the PreNu parent group and compared these measures with those of the reference group, both for their in the neonatal intensive care unit (NICU) period and at age 3.5 years. The T1 measures came with a clear instruction to answer as they would have done at the time their infant was in the NICU, and the items of the measures were phrased in 'past tense'. In the follow-up (T2), parents were invited to complete a new set of questionnaire.

Data collection

In addition to demographic parental characteristics, these questionnaires were used to collect data about quality of life (QoL) and symptoms in parents.

Quality of Life Scale-Norwegian version (QoLS-N) was used to measure QoL (13, 14). The QoLS-N consists of 18 items to which respondents rate their satisfaction with various aspects of life on a 9-point scale from 1 to 9. A higher score indicates better QoL. This scale is found to have solid psychometric properties, validity and reliability are well established, and the scale is commonly used in the Norwegian population. As a measure of internal consistency and reliability, we used Cronbach's alpha; in the present study, this value was 0.91 for the total QoLS-N scale.

Hospital Anxiety and Depression Scale (HADS) was used to measure anxiety and depression (15). HADS consists of 14 items: 7 measure anxiety and 7 measure depression on a scale from 0 (not at all) to 3 (very much). A cut-off of 8 points is identified for both anxiety and depression (16): mild (8–10), moderate (11–14), and severe (15–21) (15). HADS has been widely used and shows satisfactory psychometric properties for somatic, psychiatric, and primary care patients and in the general population, including Norwegian samples (17). The Cronbach's alpha was 0.80 for anxiety and 0.84 for depression in the present study.

General Sleep Disturbance Scale (GSDS) uses 21 items that measure different aspects in relation to sleep: quality, awakening, and rhythm. Each question ranges from 0 (never) to 7 (every day) on a numeric rating scale. Each of the individual scores can be added to a total score from 0 (no disturbance) to 147 (extremely disturbed) (18). The cut-off point for sleep disturbance versus normal sleep is established at 43 points. Validity and reliability are well established in many patient populations and in healthy individuals, including Norwegian patients with pulmonary disease (19). The Cronbach's alpha was 0.73 in the present study.

Lee Fatigue Scale (LFS) was used to measure fatigue (20). LFS consists of 18 items and two subscales: fatigue and energy. Severity score is documented on both scales from 0 to 10, where higher scores indicate more fatigue. LFS is used in a diversity of populations and also in healthy individuals (20). Validity and internal consistency are well established, and the instrument has been applied to many Norwegian samples and shows satisfactory psychometric properties (21). In the present study, Cronbach's alpha was 0.94 for LFS fatigue and 0.85 for LFS energy.

Self-Administered Comorbidity Questionnaire (SCQ) (22) was used to measure comorbidity. SCQ explores presence of disease, treatment, and whether the disease limits level of activity. The questionnaire is used in different patients groups, including Norwegians (23).

Stressful Likert Scale was used to classify and grade how stressful PreNu parents found the PreNu study participation, on a scale ranging from 1 (not stressful at all) to 5 (very stressful).

Statistical analyses
The software program IBM SPSS 22 (IBM Corp., Armonk, NY) was used to analyze all data. Normality of the data was tested visually by Q-Q plots. Mean scores and standard deviations were calculated for measure-indices. Missing items were handled according to the recommended method for each individual questionnaire. We used *t*-tests to evaluate differences in mean scores between groups for normally distributed data. The significance level was set at 0.05.

Approvals
The PreNu study and this follow-up study were both approved by the Regional Committee for Medical and Health Research Ethics. The PreNu study was registered in Clinical Trials with identifier NCT 01103219.

Results

Characteristics of the two-parent cohorts and their children
Thirty-one PreNu parents and 31 reference parents, both fathers and mothers, gave their informed consent to participate. There were 51 families at T1 and 35 accepted to participate in the follow-up (T2); response rates at T2 were 69 and 68%, respectively for the groups. Parents in the PreNu group were significantly older than the parents in the reference group (T1, $p = 0.04$; T2, $p < 0.01$) (Table 1). At T2, but not at T1, the PreNu group had more additional children than the reference group ($p = 0.02$) (Table 1).

QoL and symptom burden at T1
At T1, there was a significant difference in QoL between parents in the PreNu group compared with the reference group, with better QoL scores for the PreNu parents (Table 2). No significant differences were found between the two groups for anxiety or depression, or in fatigue, energy, or sleep disturbances. However, compared with the general population, parents in these premature cohorts had scores above the clinical cut-offs (≥ 8) for both anxiety (50.8; 43.3 and 58.1% of the PreNu and reference parents, respectively) and depression (48.4%; no difference between PreNu and reference parents) at T1 (Table 3).

Changes in symptom scores from T1 to T2
There was a significant improvement in anxiety, depression, sleep disturbance, fatigue, and energy for both groups of parents pooled between T1 and T2 (Table 4).

QoL and symptom burden at T2
There was no significant difference between the PreNu and the reference group at T2 regarding QoL, anxiety, depression, or fatigue, but the PreNu group reported significantly more energy and less sleep disturbance at T2 (Table 2).

Table 1. Demographics and clinical characteristics of participants at time points 1 and 2

	Time point 1			Time point 2		
	PreNu ($n = 30$) (%)	Reference ($n = 31$) (%)	p	PreNu ($n = 31$) (%)	Reference ($n = 28$) (%)	p
Male sex	43.3	51.5	0.52	45.2	50.0	0.72
Lives with other parent	96.7	100	0.31	93.5	96.4	0.66
Have additional children	56.7	32.3	0.06	61.3	37.0	0.07
	Mean (SD)	Mean (SD)	p	Mean (SD)	Mean (SD)	p
No. of children/family	1.67 (0.7)	1.45 (0.6)	0.21	1.71 (0.7)	1.35 (0.5)	0.02
Age (years)	34.9 (5.6)	31.7 (5.9)	<0.01	34.8 (5.5)	29.8 (5.4)	<0.01
Comorbidity (SCQ score)	1.53 (2.7)	1.74 (2.5)	0.26	0.55 (1.1)	0.61 (1.4)	0.90
Infant characteristics:						
GA (weeks)	28.4 (2.7)	29.7 (2.9)	0.08	28.8 (3.0)	29.5 (3.2)	0.40
Birth weight (g)	1,045 (248)	1,169 (259)	0.06	1,044 (244)	1,128 (270)	0.22

SCQ, Self-Administered Comorbidity Questionnaire; GA, gestational age.

Table 2. Differences in scores between parents in the PreNu group compared to the reference group at time points 1 and 2

	Score at time point 1				Score at time point 2			
	PreNu (n = 30)	Reference (n = 31)			PreNu (n = 31)	Reference (n = 28)		
	Mean (SD)	Mean (SD)	p	95% CI	Mean (SD)	Mean (SD)	p	95% CI
QoLS	85.3 (12.6)	76.9 (2.6)	0.02	1.5 to 15.3	88.8 (11.6)	83.1 (12.8)	0.08	−0.7 to 12.1
HADS depression	6.3 (4.1)	7.8 (5.3)	0.23	−3.9 to 1.0	2.4 (2.6)	2.8 (3.2)	0.61	−2.0 to 1.2
HADS anxiety	7.9 (3.5)	8.9 (4.4)	0.34	−3.0 to 1.0	3.3 (2.6)	5.1 (4.6)	0.07	−3.7 to 0.1
HADS (total)	14.2 (6.7)	16.7 (9.0)	0.23	−6.5 to 1.6	5.7 (5.1)	7.9 (7.2)	0.62	−5.5 to 1.0
GSDS	35.8 (12.0)	40.2 (19.9)	0.30	−12.9 to 4.0	27.1 (8.0)	32.2 (8.8)	0.03	−9.7 to −0.4
LFS fatigue	3.3 (1.8)	3.9 (1.8)	0.20	−1.7 to 0.4	2.4 (1.8)	2.7 (2.1)	0.61	−1.3 to 0.8
LFS energy	4.3 (1.6)	3.6 (2.4)	0.14	−0.2 to 1.5	6.2 (1.4)	5.3 (1.8)	0.03	0.1 to 1.8

CI, confidence interval of the difference between the two groups; QoLS, Quality of Life Scale; HADS, Hospital and Anxiety Depression Scale; GSDS, General Sleep Disturbance Scale; LFS, Lee Fatigue Scale.

At T2, only 13.6% of all parents scored above cut-off (≥ 8) for anxiety and 5.1% for depression (Table 3).

Stress related to participation in PreNu study

Twenty-six percent of the PreNu parents found their infant's participation in the PreNu study to be mildly or a little stressful. None rated participation to be clearly or very stressful. Those who reported participation to be stressful experienced significantly more anxiety and sleep disturbance at T1, but not at T2 (Table 5).

Discussion

Parents of VLBW infants enrolled in the nutrition RCT PreNu trial reported significantly better QoL compared to reference parents during participation in the trial while hospitalized in the NICU. The reference group reported QoL scores similar to those of unemployed men and women (mean, 74.6; SD, 16.8) and individuals with various health problems (mean, 79.6; SD, 13.8) in the general Norwegian population (14). At T1, the parent PreNu group had higher QoL scores than comparable age groups in the general population (mean score for 30–39 years, 83.1; SD, 12.5) (14). At T2, the QoL in both parent groups had improved, with mean scores similar to those in the general population (14).

The difference in QoL between the PreNu parents and the reference group may be explained by a closer follow-up, more time spent in conversations, and interest shown by the research group members. The effect of the amount of follow-up on positive outcome is in accordance with other studies (24). Extensive contact with relevant health professionals during a hospital stay is shown to be beneficial for adults and can reduce symptoms of anxiety and depression (25).

Table 3. Differences between parents in the PreNu group compared to the reference group on level of anxiety and depression at time points 1 and 2

		Time point 1			Time point 2		
		PreNu (n = 30)	Reference (n = 31)	Total	PreNu (n = 31)	Reference (n = 28)	Total
		% (n)	% (n)	% (n)	% (n)	% (n)	% (n)
HADS anxiety	Normal	56.7 (17)	41.9 (13)	49.2 (30)	93.5 (29)	78.6 (22)	86.4 (51)
	Mild	20 (6)	19.4 (6)	19.7 (12)	6.5 (2)	10.7 (3)	8.5 (5)
	Moderate	20 (6)	29 (9)	24.6 (15)	0	3.6 (1)	1.7 (1)
	Severe	3.3 (1)	9.7 (3)	6.6 (4)	0	7.1 (2)	3.4 (2)
HADS depression	Normal	60 (18)	51.6 (16)	55.7 (34)	96.8 (30)	92.9 (26)	94.9 (56)
	Mild	26.7 (8)	19.4 (6)	23 (14)	0	0	0
	Moderate	10 (3)	16.1 (5)	13.1 (8)	3.2 (1)	7.1 (2)	5.1 (3)
	Severe	3.3 (1)	12.9 (4)	8.2 (5)	0	0	0

HADS, Hospital and Anxiety Depression Scale.

Table 4. Differences on anxiety, depression, sleep disturbances, and fatigue at time points 1 and 2

	Time point 1				Time point 2				Difference between the two time points				
	Mean	*n*	Range	SD	Mean	*N*	Range	SD	Mean	SD	*N*	*P*	95% CI
HADS anxiety	8.4	61	0 to 17	4.0	4.2	59	0 to 20	3.8	4.1	3.7	45	<0.01	3.0 to 5.2
HADS depression	7.0	61	0 to 18	4.8	2.6	59	0 to 13	3.0	4.5	4.1	45	<0.01	3.2 to 5.7
HADS total	15.5	61	1 to 35	8.0	6.7	59	0 to 32	6.3	8.6	6.2	45	<0.01	6.7 to 10.4
GSDS	38.0	61	0 to 76	16.5	29.4	53	13 to 56	8.7	7.9	14.5	42	<0.01	3.4 to 12.4
QoLS	81	61	40 to 109	14.0	86.2	58	59 to 112	12.4	−3.6	12.3	45	0.05	−7.3 to 0.6
LFS fatigue	3.6	61	0 to 8.2	2.0	2.5	59	0 to 7.9	1.9	1.1	1.8	45	<0.01	−0.5 to 1.6
LFS energy	4.0	61	0.2 to 8.0	1.7	5.8	59	1.6 to 9.6	1.7	2.2	2.2	45	<0.01	−2.5 to 5.6

Data are from both study groups pooled. CI, confidence interval of the difference between the time points; HADS, Hospital and Anxiety Depression Scale; GSDS, General Sleep Disturbance Scale; QoLS, Quality of Life Scale; LFS, Lee Fatigue Scale.

One fourth of the PreNu parents thought participating in the trial was stressful, even though they scored better on QoL than those whose infant never participated in a RCT. This 'stressed' group had more symptoms of anxiety and sleep disturbance compared to the 'non-stressed' group. Being a VLBW infant parent is stressful, and it is difficult for the parent to evaluate the possible additive stress effect due to participation in an RCT. Cartwright et al. (7) found that parental stress is caused by having a sick infant in the NICU rather than by participating in the RCT. We found symptoms of anxiety in both in the PreNu and the reference group, which may impact on the reported stress (26).

QoL may affect a parent's ability to accept his or her infant and be sensitive to that infant's needs. Adverse life conditions and symptom burden in parents and caregivers may result in suboptimal nurture of their infant (8). It is important to explore whether participation in an intervention study can negatively impact on the burden of stress, and whether this impact is within the ethical standards for clinical research. We found no significant difference between the PreNu parents and reference group parents regarding anxiety and depression. This observation is important because severe maternal depression has been associated with poor child developmental outcome, including in VLBW infants (9). Not surprisingly, symptoms of anxiety and depression were very common in both parent groups while the infant was hospitalized. This finding can be attributed to the experience of becoming parents to a sick prematurely born infant. Clinical staff need to be aware of this and should offer support to parents in this vulnerable situation.

Table 5. Levels of anxiety, depression, and sleep disturbance related to level of stress among the PreNu parents

	Stressful (*n* = 8)	Not stressful (*n* = 22)		
	Mean (SD)	Mean (SD)	*p*	95% CI
HADS anxiety	11 (3.3)	6.8 (2.8)	<0.01	1.7 to 6.7
HADS depression	8.1 (2.6)	5.6 (4.4)	0.15	−0.9 to 5.9
HADS total	19.1 (5.2)	12.4 (6.3)	0.01	−1.6 to 11.8
GSDS	43.8 (11.9)	22.9 (10.8)	0.03	1.5 to 20.3

CI, confidence interval of the difference between those who thought participation in the randomized intervention trial was stressful and those who did not think it was stressful; HADS, Hospital and Depression Scale; GSDS, General Sleep Disturbance Scale.

The PreNu parents reported less sleeping disturbance and were more energetic than the reference group 3.5 years after the birth of their child (T2). One speculation could be that a higher QoL and satisfaction with life at the time the infants were hospitalized could be protective for sleeping problems. Sleep is important to health and recovery from illness, and postpartum psychological reactions and quality of sleep are related problems (27).

Parents in the PreNu group were slightly older than those in the reference group. Advancing age may be associated with lower QoL (14); however, in the present study, parents in the PreNu group were older and had higher QoL. Adjusting for age had no effect on the QoL. At T2, the parents in the PreNu group had significantly more children than the reference parents. In spite of having more children, the PreNu group had less sleep disturbance and more energy than the reference group.

Several considerations may explain the positive effect of attending an RCT. A Danish study of the effect of supportive communication on parental stress in a NICU found no effect on parental stress, but it raised concern about the need to support parents also in periods where the infant's clinical condition was stable and around discharge from the NICU (28). In our study, PreNu parents were closely followed from birth until 52 weeks age, several weeks after discharge. In addition comes the plausible benefit of providing the infant with a putative better nutrition regime.

The main motivating factor for consenting to their child's participation in an RCT is a belief in a direct benefit for the child (29). Parents may have felt more secure that their infant received the best possible treatment and thus relaxed more, despite the fact that the spoken and written invitation to PreNu was neutral, emphasizing that we did not know whether the intervention was good or bad for the infant. In an interview study focusing on parents' perceptions of their infants' participation in an RCT (7), parents thought their infants were given the best possible care because of their participation. Furthermore, the parents appreciated being given the choice of consent, thus putting them in a situation where they have the perception of being in control. At the core of the concept of sense of coherence (SOC) are the individual's experiences of comprehensibility, meaningfulness, and manageability of one's life (8). SOC is shown to be related to the psychosocial effects of health problems. Consenting may make the parents feel that they do something good for their infants and that they are actively exercising parental authority. Participation in an RCT could make the parents feel that their stay in the NICU is more purposeful.

The small number of respondents and the retrospective design at T1 are the main limitations in our study. The number of parents in the present study was determined by the number of participating children in the PreNu study. Because this study was planned after the PreNu recruitment period, we could only assess the parent situation at T1 retrospectively, and the quantitative information of the parent's well-being in this period was therefore retrospective. Both groups of parents had infants hospitalized in the same hospitals with the same routines and staff. To avoid bias, we invited and enrolled parents from the immediate period before and after the PreNu trial was run in these neonatal units. The two study groups were comparable regarding sex, comorbidity, the birth weight, and gestational age, and we did control for age of parent and number of children. The PreNu parents may be a selected group simply because of their sustained participation in the trial. In general, pediatric trials obtain a high participation rate (30), and this trial is no exception. Seventy percent of all eligible parents were recruited, implying that the PreNu parents are a representative group of VLBW parents.

Retrospective assessment may not be accurate, making it difficult to generalize and compare with prospective studies with the same measures. Self-report is by nature subjective and often makes the subject view his or her situation retrospectively. We believe that the experience of becoming a parent of a VLBW infant is remembered very vividly because of the emotional salience. A strength of this study is that our outcome measures had excellent internal consistency for both the retrospectively assessed T1 and the concurrently assessed T2 (with the exception of sleep disturbance).

It was not possible to control every psychosocial variable related to well-being, and correcting p values for multiple testing may have decreased the likelihood of false positives. However, because of the small size of our groups, it is unlikely that any clear and relevant difference would have been proven statistically significant on correction for multiple testing. Nevertheless, we believe that our extensive battery of measurement tools, the logical consistence of the findings, and relationships between the measures add credence to our results.

Conclusions

Parents of an infant born VLBW who participated in the PreNu intervention RCT experienced better QoL when the infant was hospitalized, compared to a reference group. Symptoms of anxiety and depression affected half of the parents, but this number improved and was normalized when their infant was 3.5 years of age. The high incidence of anxiety and depression in parents must be considered in the care of parents in the NICU. Long-term effects of participation seem to be less sleep problems and more energy. In recruiting newborn VLBW infants for an RCT trial, researchers can most likely be confident that participation in itself is not a burden for the parents and thus does not constitute an unacceptable risk for the infant. Parents in an RCT trial may feel more secure because of extra follow-up, but this hypothesis warrants more research.

Contributor statement

The first author contributed to all aspects of the study including conceptualization of the protocol, data collection, analysis, and drafting the manuscript. The other authors contributed to conceptualization of the protocol, supervision, analysis, and critical review of the manuscript. All authors approved the final manuscript.

Acknowledgements

We thank the parents who participated in this study.

Conflict of interest and funding

We declare that we have no conflicts of interest.

Financial support was obtained from the Health Region South Eastern Trust of Norway and Akershus University Hospital.

References

1. Hall EO. Being in an alien world: Danish parents' lived experiences when a newborn or small child is critically ill. Scand J Caring Sci 2005; 19: 179–85.
2. Baumgardt M, Bucher HU, Mieth RA, Fauchere JC. Health-related quality of life of former very preterm infants in adulthood. Acta Paediatr 2012; 101: E59–63.
3. Scheinberg AM. Screening for children born extremely preterm and at extremely lowbirthweight – a role for health-related quality of life measures? Dev Med Child Neurol 2011; 53: 878–80.
4. Vieira ME, Linhares MB. Developmental outcomes and quality of life in children born preterm at preschool- and school-age. J Pediatr (Rio J) 2011; 87: 281–91.
5. Vederhus BJ, Markestad T, Eide GE, Graue M, Halvorsen T. Health related quality of life after extremely preterm birth: a matched controlled cohort study. Health Qual Life Outcomes 2010; 8: 53.
6. Doering LV, Moser DK, Dracup K. Correlates of anxiety, hostility, depression, and psychosocial adjustment in parents of NICU infants. Neonatal Netw 2000; 19: 15–23.
7. Cartwright K, Mahoney L, Ayers S, Rabe H. Parents'perceptions of their infants' participation in randomized controlled trials. J Obstet Gynecol Neonatal Nurs 2011; 40: 555–65.
8. Huhtala M, Korja R, Lehtonen L, Haataja L, Lapinleimu H, Rautava P, et al. Parental psychological well-being and behavioral outcome of very low birth weight infants at 3 years. Pediatrics 2012; 129: E937–44.
9. Goodman JH. Paternal postpartum depression, its relationship to maternal postpartum depression, and implications for family health. J Adv Nurs 2004; 45: 26–35.
10. Blencowe H, Cousens S, Oestergaard MZ, Chou D, Moller AB, Narwal R, et al. National, regional, and worldwide estimates of preterm birth rates in the year 2010 with time trends since 1990 for selected countries: a systematic analysis and implications. Lancet 2012; 379: 2162–72.
11. Moltu SJ, Strommen K, Blakstad EW, Almaas AN, Westerberg AC, Braekke K, et al. Enhanced feeding in very-low-birth-weight infants may cause electrolyte disturbances and septicemia – a randomized, controlled trial. Clin Nutr 2013; 32: 207–12.
12. Blakstad EW, Strømmen K, Moltu SJ, Wattam-Bell J, Nordheim T, Almaas AN, et al. Improved visual perception in very low birth weight infants on enhanced nutrient supply. Neonatology 2015; 108: 30–7.
13. Burckhardt CS, Anderson KL. The Quality of Life Scale (QOLS): reliability, validity, and utilization. Health Qual Life Outcomes 2003; 1: 60.
14. Wahl AK, Rustoen T, Hanestad BR, Lerdal A, Moum T. Quality of life in the general Norwegian population, measured by the Quality of Life Scale (QOLS-N). Qual Life Res 2004; 13: 1001–9.
15. Zigmond AS, Snaith RP. The hospital anxiety and depression scale. Acta Psych Scand 1983; 67: 361–70.
16. Bjelland I, Dahl AA, Haug TT, Neckelmann D. The validity of the hospital anxiety and depression scale – an updated literature review. J Psychosom Res 2002; 52: 69–77.
17. Nortvedt MW, Riise T, Sanne B. Are men more depressed than women in Norway? Validity of the hospital anxiety and depression scale. J Psychosom Res 2006; 60: 195–8.
18. Lee KA. Self-reported sleep disturbances in employed women. Sleep 1992; 15: 493–8.
19. Borge CR, Wahl AK, Moum T. Association of breathlessness with multiple symptoms in chronic obstructive pulmonary disease. J Adv Nurs 2010; 66: 2688–700.
20. Lee KA, Hicks G, Nino-Murcia G. Validity and reliability of a scale to assess fatigue. Psych Res 1991; 36: 291–8.
21. Rustoen T, Wahl AK, Hanestad BR, Lerdal A, Paul S, Miaskowski C. Prevalence and characteristics of chronic pain in the general Norwegian population. Eur J Pain 2004; 8: 555–65.
22. Sangha O, Stucki G, Liang MH, Fossel AH, Katz JN. The Self-Administered Comorbidity Questionnaire: a new method to assess comorbidity for clinical and health services research. Arthr Rheum 2003; 49: 156–63.
23. Schjolberg TK, Dodd M, Henriksen N, Rustoen T. Factors affecting hope in a s ample of fatigued breast cancer outpatients. Palliat Support Care 2011; 9: 63–72.
24. McCarney R, Warner J, Iliffe S, van Haselen R, Griffin M, Fisher P. The Hawthorne Effect: a randomised, controlled trial. BMC Med Res Methodol 2007; 7: 8.
25. Cano Giménez E, Sánchez-Luna M. Providing parents with individualised support in a neonatal intensive care unit reduced stress, anxiety and depression. Acta Paediatr 2015; 104: E476.
26. Shields-Poe D, Pinelli J. Variables associated with parental stress in neonatal intensive care units. Neonatal Netw 1997; 16: 29–37.
27. Lawson A, Murphy KE, Sloan E, Uleryk E, Dalfen A. The relationship between sleep and postpartum mental disorders: a systematic review. J Affect Disord 2015; 176: 65–77.
28. Weis J, Zoffmann V, Greisen G, Egerod I. The effect of person-centred communication on parental stress in a NICU: a randomized clinical trial. Acta Paediatr 2013; 102: 1130–6.
29. Vanhelst J, Hardy L, Bert D, Duhem S, Coopman S, Libersa C, et al. Effect of child health status on parents' allowing children to participate in pediatric research. BMC Med Ethics 2013; 14: 9.
30. Campbell H, Surry SAM, Royle EM. A review of randomised controlled trials published in Archives of Disease in Childhood from 1982–96. Arch Dis Child 1998; 79: 192–7.

***Trond Nordheim**
Department of Pediatric and Adolescent Medicine
Akershus University Hospital
P.O. Box 1000, NO-1478 Lørenskog
Norway
Email: trond.nordheim@medisin.uio.no

PERMISSIONS

All chapters in this book were first published in FNR, by Taylor & Francis Online; hereby published with permission under the Creative Commons Attribution License or equivalent. Every chapter published in this book has been scrutinized by our experts. Their significance has been extensively debated. The topics covered herein carry significant findings which will fuel the growth of the discipline. They may even be implemented as practical applications or may be referred to as a beginning point for another development.

The contributors of this book come from diverse backgrounds, making this book a truly international effort. This book will bring forth new frontiers with its revolutionizing research information and detailed analysis of the nascent developments around the world.

We would like to thank all the contributing authors for lending their expertise to make the book truly unique. They have played a crucial role in the development of this book. Without their invaluable contributions this book wouldn't have been possible. They have made vital efforts to compile up to date information on the varied aspects of this subject to make this book a valuable addition to the collection of many professionals and students.

This book was conceptualized with the vision of imparting up-to-date information and advanced data in this field. To ensure the same, a matchless editorial board was set up. Every individual on the board went through rigorous rounds of assessment to prove their worth. After which they invested a large part of their time researching and compiling the most relevant data for our readers.

The editorial board has been involved in producing this book since its inception. They have spent rigorous hours researching and exploring the diverse topics which have resulted in the successful publishing of this book. They have passed on their knowledge of decades through this book. To expedite this challenging task, the publisher supported the team at every step. A small team of assistant editors was also appointed to further simplify the editing procedure and attain best results for the readers.

Apart from the editorial board, the designing team has also invested a significant amount of their time in understanding the subject and creating the most relevant covers. They scrutinized every image to scout for the most suitable representation of the subject and create an appropriate cover for the book.

The publishing team has been an ardent support to the editorial, designing and production team. Their endless efforts to recruit the best for this project, has resulted in the accomplishment of this book. They are a veteran in the field of academics and their pool of knowledge is as vast as their experience in printing. Their expertise and guidance has proved useful at every step. Their uncompromising quality standards have made this book an exceptional effort. Their encouragement from time to time has been an inspiration for everyone.

The publisher and the editorial board hope that this book will prove to be a valuable piece of knowledge for researchers, students, practitioners and scholars across the globe.

LIST OF CONTRIBUTORS

Amjad Iqbal
Department of Food Safety and Food Quality, University of Gent, Gent, Belgium
Department of Agriculture, Abdul Wali Khan University Mardan, Mardan, Pakistan

Farooq Shah
Department of Agriculture, Abdul Wali Khan University Mardan, Mardan, Pakistan

Muhammad Hamayun and Anwar Hussain
Department of Botany, Abdul Wali Khan University Mardan, Mardan, Pakistan

Muhammad Waqas, Sang-Mo Kang and In-Jung Lee
School of Applied Biosciences, College of Agriculture and Life Science, Kyungpook National University, Daegu, South Korea

Ayaz Ahmad
Department of Biotechnology, Abdul Wali Khan University Mardan, Mardan, Pakistan

Tanja Kongerslev Thorning, Anne Raben, Tine Tholstrup and Arne Astrup
Department of Nutrition, Exercise and Sports, Faculty of Science, University of Copenhagen, Copenhagen, Denmark

Sabita S. Soedamah-Muthu
Division of Human Nutrition, Wageningen University, Wageningen, The Netherlands

Ian Givens
Centre for Food, Nutrition and Health, University of Reading, Reading, UK

Ru Zhang, Jun Jiao, Wei Zhang, Zheng Zhang, Li-Qiang Qin and Shu-Fen Han
Jiangsu Key Laboratory of Preventive and Translational Medicine for Geriatric Disease, Department of Nutrition and Food Hygiene, School of Public Health, Soochow University, Suzhou, China

Weiguo Zhang
DSM Nutritional Products Human Nutrition and Health, Beijing, China

Haitao Pan, Qingyun Yang, Guidong Huang, Chen Ding, Peiqiu Cao, Lanlan Huang, Jiao Guo and Zhengquan Su
Key Research Center of Liver Regulation for Hyperlipidemia SATCM/Class III Laboratory of Metabolism SATCM, Guangdong TCM Key Laboratory for Metabolic Diseases, Guangdong Pharmaceutical University, Guangzhou, China

Tiancun Xiao
Inorganic Chemistry Laboratory, Oxford University, Oxford, United Kingdom
Guangzhou Boxabio Ltd, D-106 Guangzhou International Business Incubator, Guangzhou Science City, Guangzhou, China

Wen-Dee Chiang
Department of Food Science, College of Agriculture, Tunghai University, Taichung, Taiwan

Chih Yang Huang
Graduate Institute of Basic Medical Science, China Medical University, Taichung, Taiwan
School of Chinese Medicine, China Medical University, Taichung, Taiwan
Department of Health and Nutrition Biotechnology, Asia University, Taichung, Taiwan

Catherine Reena Paul
Graduate Institute of Basic Medical Science, China Medical University, Taichung, Taiwan
Department of Hospitality Management, College of Agriculture, Tunghai University, Taichung, Taiwan

Zong-Yan Lee and Wan-Teng Lin
Department of Hospitality Management, College of Agriculture, Tunghai University, Taichung, Taiwan

Karin Jonsson, Malin Barman and Ann-Sofie Sandberg
Division of Food and Nutrition Science, Department of Biology and Biological Engineering, Chalmers University of Technology, Gothenburg, Sweden

My Green
Department of Internal Medicine and Clinical Nutrition, University of Gothenburg, Gothenburg, Sweden

Agneta Sjöberg
Department of Food and Nutrition, and Sport Science, University of Gothenburg, Gothenburg, Sweden

Hilde K. Brekke
Department of Nutrition, Institute of Basic Medical Sciences, University of Oslo, Oslo, Norway

Agnes E. Wold
Clinical Bacteriology Section, Department of Infectious Diseases, University of Gothenburg, Gothenburg, Sweden

Grace K. M. Muhoozi
Department of Nutrition, Institute of Basic Medical Sciences, University of Oslo, Oslo, Norway
Department of Human Nutrition and Home Economics, Kyambogo University, Kampala, Uganda

Prudence Atukunda
Department of Nutrition, Institute of Basic Medical Sciences, University of Oslo, Oslo, Norway

Robert Mwadime
School of Food Technology, Nutrition and Bioengineering, Makerere University, Kampala, Uganda

Per Ole Iversen
Department of Nutrition, Institute of Basic Medical Sciences, University of Oslo, Oslo, Norway
Department of Hematology, Oslo University Hospital, Oslo, Norway

Ane C. Westerberg
Institute of Health Sciences, Kristiania University College, Oslo, Norway

Helena Filipsson Nyström
Institute of Medicine, Sahlgrenska Academy, University of Gothenburg, Gothenburg, Sweden
Department of Endocrinology, Sahlgrenska University Hospital, Gothenburg, Sweden

Anne Lise Brantsæter
Norwegian Institute of Public Health, Oslo, Norway

Iris Erlund
National Institute for Health andWelfare, Helsinki, Finland

Ingibjörg Gunnarsdottir
Unit for Nutrition Research, University of Iceland and Landspitali National University Hospital, Reykjavik, Iceland

Lena Hulthén
Department of Clinical Nutrition, Sahlgrenska Academy, University of Gothenburg, Gothenburg, Sweden

Peter Laurberg
Department of Endocrinology, Aalborg University Hospital, Aalborg, Denmark
Department of Clinical Medicine, Aalborg University, Aalborg, Denmark

Irene Mattisson
National Food Agency, Uppsala, Sweden

Lone Banke Rasmussen
Department of Endocrinology, Bispebjerg University Hospital, Copenhagen, Denmark

Suvi Virtanen
National Institute for Health andWelfare, Helsinki, Finland
School of Health Sciences, University of Tampere, Finland

Helle Margrete Meltzer
Norwegian Institute of Public Health, Oslo, Norway

Mduduzi Paul Mokoena, Taurai Mutanda and Ademola O. Olaniran
Discipline of Microbiology, School of Life Sciences, College of Agriculture, Engineering and Science, University of KwaZulu-Natal (Westville Campus), Durban, South Africa

Ting Li
Shaanxi Engineering Laboratory for Food Green Processing and Safety Control, College of Food Engineering and Nutritional Science, Shaanxi Normal University, Xi'an, China
Centre for Cancer and Inflammation Research, School of Chinese Medicine, Hong Kong Baptist University, Hong Kong, China

Xinshan Lu, Yanfei Sun and Xingbin Yang
Shaanxi Engineering Laboratory for Food Green Processing and Safety Control, College of Food Engineering and Nutritional Science, Shaanxi Normal University, Xi'an, China

Rubén Díaz-Rúa, Andreu Palou and Paula Oliver
Laboratory of Molecular Biology, Nutrition and Biotechnology, Universitat de les Illes Balears and CIBER de Fisiopatologı´a de la Obesidad y Nutricio´n (CIBERobn), Palma de Mallorca, Spain

Filiz Yangılar
Department of Nutrition and Dietetics, Faculty of Health Sciences, Erzincan University, Erzincan, Turkey

Hanna Sepp and Karin Höijer
Food and Meal Science, School of Education and Environment, Kristianstad University, Kristianstad, Sweden

Julie Carillon
Nutrition & Metabolism, UMR 204 NutriPass, University of Montpellier, Montpellier, France
Bionov Research, Montpellier, France

Bernard Jover
EA7288, University of Montpellier, Montpellier, France
PhyMedExp, INSERM U1046, UMR CNRS 9214, University of Montpellier, Montpellier, France

Jean-Paul Cristol, Sylvain Richard and Anne Virsolvy
PhyMedExp, INSERM U1046, UMR CNRS 9214, University of Montpellier, Montpellier, France

Jean-Max Rouanet
Nutrition & Metabolism, UMR 204 NutriPass, University of Montpellier, Montpellier, France

Francisco Navarro and Zaida Montero
Department of Environmental Biology and Public Health, Cell Biology, Faculty of Experimental Sciences, University of Huelva, Huelva, Spain
Algal Biotechnology Group, CIDERTA and Faculty of Sciences, University of Huelva and Marine International Campus of Excellence (CEIMAR), Huelva, Spain

Eduardo Forján, María Vázquez, Elisabeth Bermejo, María José Domínguez, Inés Garbayo and Carlos Vílchez
Algal Biotechnology Group, CIDERTA and Faculty of Sciences, University of Huelva and Marine International Campus of Excellence (CEIMAR), Huelva, Spain

Miguel Ángel Castaño
University Hospital Complex of Huelva Juan Ramón Jiménez, Huelva, Spain

Alberto Toimil
Department of Environmental Biology and Public Health, Cell Biology, Faculty of Experimental Sciences, University of Huelva, Huelva, Spain

Enrique Chagüaceda
CIDERTA Investigation Center, University of Huelva, Huelva, Spain

Miguel Ángel García-Sevillano
Department of Chemistry Materials Science, Faculty of Experimental Sciences, University of Huelva, Huelva, Spain

Marisa Sánchez
Riotinto Hospital, Huelva, Spain

Rosario Pásaro and José María Vega
Department of Physiology, Faculty of Biology, University of Seville, Seville, Spain
Department of Plant Biochemistry and Molecular Biology, Faculty of Chemistry, University of Seville, Seville

Rita Nilsen and Siv Skeie
Department of Chemistry, Biotechnology and Food Science, Norwegian University of Life Sciences, Ås, Norway

Are H. Pripp
Oslo Centre of Biostatistics and Epidemiology, Research Support Services, Oslo University Hospital, Oslo, Norway

Arne T. Høstmark
Institute of Health and Society, University of Oslo, Oslo, Norway

Anna Haug
Department of Animal and Aquacultural Sciences, Norwegian University of Life Sciences, Ås, Norway

Xavier Deplanque, Delphine Muscente-Paque and Eric Chappuis
Naturalpha SAS, Parc Eurasanté, Loos, France

Helga Birgit Bjørnarå, Nina Cecilie Øverby, Tonje Holte Stea, Monica Klungland Torstveit, Elling Bere, Elisabet Rudjord Hillesund and Sveinung Berntsen
Department of Public Health, Sport and Nutrition, Faculty of Health and Sport Sciences, University of Agder, Kristiansand, Norway

Lene Frost Andersen
Department of Nutrition, University of Oslo, Oslo, Norway

Rahmat Ali Khan, Abdus Saboorshah and Mushtaq Ahmed
Department of Biotechnology, Faculty of Biological Sciences, University of Science and Technology Bannu, Khyber Pakhtunkhwa, Pakistan

Huda Mohammad Alkreathy
Department of Pharmacology, King Abdulaziz University (KAU), Jeddah, Saudi Arabia

Samiullah Khan
Department of Microbiology, Faculty of Biological Sciences, Quaid-i-Azam University, Islamabad, Pakistan

Trond Nordheim and Britt Nakstad
Department of Pediatric and Adolescent Medicine, Akershus University Hospital, Nordbyhagen, Norway Institute for Clinical Medicine, Campus Ahus, University of Oslo, Nordbyhagen, Norway

Tone Rustøen
Department of Research and Development, Division of Emergencies and Critical Care, Oslo University Hospital, Oslo, Norway
Department of Nursing Science, Institute of Health and Society, University of Oslo, Oslo, Norway

Per O. Iversen
Department of Nutrition, Institute of Basic Medical Sciences, Faculty of Medicine, University of Oslo, Oslo, Norway
Department of Haematology, Oslo University Hospital, Oslo, Norway

Index